Early Diagnosis and Treatment of Cancer

Series Editor: Stephen C. Yang, MD

Breast Cancer
Edited by Lisa Jacobs and Christina A. Finlayson

Colorectal Cancer
Edited by Susan L. Gearhart and Nita Ahuja

Head and Neck Cancer
Edited by Wayne M. Koch

Ovarian Cancer
Edited by Robert E. Bristow and
Deborah K. Armstrong

Prostate Cancer
Edited by Li-Ming Su

EARLY DIAGNOSIS AND TREATMENT OF CANCER

Series Editor: Stephen C. Yang, MD

Colorectal Cancer

Edited by

Susan L. Gearhart, MD
Assistant Professor of Colorectal Surgery and Oncology
Department of Surgery
The Johns Hopkins University
Baltimore, Maryland

Nita Ahuja, MD
Assistant Professor of Surgery and Oncology
Department of Surgery
The Johns Hopkins University
Baltimore, Maryland

SAUNDERS

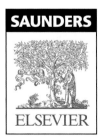

ELSEVIER

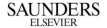

1600 John F. Kennedy Boulevard
Suite 1800
Philadelphia, PA 19103-2899

EARLY DIAGNOSIS AND TREATMENT OF CANCER: ISBN-13: 978-1-4160-4686–8
COLORECTAL CANCER
Copyright © 2011 by Saunders, an imprint of Elsevier Inc.

Notices

Knowledge and best practice in this field are constantly changing. As new research and experience
broaden our understanding, changes in research methods, professional practices, or medical
treatment may become necessary.

Practitioners and researchers must always rely on their own experience and knowledge in
evaluating and using any information, methods, compounds, or experiments described herein.
In using such information or methods they should be mindful of their own safety and the safety
of others, including parties for whom they have a professional responsibility.

With respect to any drug or pharmaceutical products identified, readers are advised to check
the most current information provided (i) on procedures featured or (ii) by the manufacturer of
each product to be administered, to verify the recommended dose or formula, the method and
duration of administration, and contraindications. It is the responsibility of practitioners, relying on
their own experience and knowledge of their patients, to make diagnoses, to determine dosages
and the best treatment for each individual patient, and to take all appropriate safety precautions.

To the fullest extent of the law, neither the Publisher nor the authors, contributors, or editors,
assume any liability for any injury and/or damage to persons or property as a matter of products
liability, negligence or otherwise, or from any use or operation of any methods, products,
instructions, or ideas contained in the material herein.

Library of Congress Cataloging-in-Publication Data

Early diagnosis and treatment of cancer: colorectal cancer / edited by Susan L. Gearhart, Nita Ahuja.
    p. ; cm.—(Early diagnosis and treatment of cancer series)
    Includes bibliographical references and index.
    ISBN 978-1-4160-4686-8
    1. Colon (Anatomy)—Cancer. 2. Rectum—Cancer. I. Gearhart, Susan L. II. Ahuja, Nita.
III. Series: Early diagnosis and treatment of cancer series.
    [DNLM: 1. Colorectal Neoplasms—diagnosis. 2. Colorectal Neoplasms—therapy. 3. Early
Diagnosis. WI 529 C719035 2010]
    RC280.C6C6627 2011
    616.99′4347—dc22
                                                                    2010012920

Acquisitions Editor: Dolores Meloni
Design Direction: Steven Stave

Print in the United States of America

Last digit is the print number: 9 8 7 6 5 4 3 2 1

Working together to grow
libraries in developing countries

www.elsevier.com | www.bookaid.org | www.sabre.org

ELSEVIER   BOOK AID International   Sabre Foundation

This book is dedicated to all the patients with colorectal cancer that we have had the privilege to treat. Your courage in facing this disease inspires us to continue to seek a cure for colorectal cancer both as surgeons and as scientists.

Series Preface

Seen on a graph, the survival rate for many cancers resembles a precipice. Discovered at an early stage, most cancers are quickly treatable, and the prognosis is excellent. In late stages, however, the typical treatment protocol becomes longer, more intense, and more harrowing for the patient, and the survival rate declines steeply. No wonder, then, that one of the most important means in fighting cancer is to prevent or screen for earlier stage tumors.

Within each oncologic specialty, there is a strong push to identify new, more useful tools for early diagnosis and treatment, with an emphasis on methods amenable to an office-based or clinical setting. These efforts have brought impressive results. Advances in imaging technology, as well as the development of sophisticated molecular and biochemical tools, have led to effective, minimally invasive approaches to cancer in its early stages.

This series, *Early Diagnosis and Treatment of Cancer*, gathers state-of-the-art research and recommendations into compact, easy-to-use volumes. For each particular type of cancer, the books cover the full range of diagnostic and treatment procedures, including pathologic, radiologic, chemotherapeutic, and surgical methods, focusing on questions like these:

- What do practitioners need to know about the epidemiology of the disease and its risk factors?
- How do patients and their families wade through and interpret the myriad of testing?
- What is the safest, quickest, least invasive way to reach an accurate diagnosis?
- How can the stage of the disease be determined?
- What are the best initial treatments for early-stage disease, and how should the practitioner and the patient choose among them?

- What lifestyle factors might affect the outcome of treatment?

Each volume in the series is edited by an authority within the subfield, and the contributors have been chosen for their practical skills as well as their research credentials. Key Points at the beginning of each chapter help the reader grasp the main ideas at once. Frequent illustrations make the techniques vivid and easy to visualize. Boxes and tables summarize recommended strategies, protocols, indications and contraindications, important statistics, and other essential information. Overall, the attempt is to make expert advice as accessible as possible to a wide variety of health care professionals.

For the first time since the inception of the National Cancer Institute's annual status reports, the 2008 "Annual Report to the Nation on the Status of Cancer," published in the December 3 issue of the *Journal of the National Cancer Institute*, noted a statistically significant decline in "both incidence and death rates from all cancers combined." This mark of progress encourages all of us to press forward with our efforts. I hope that the volumes in *Early Diagnosis and Treatment of Cancer* will make health care professionals and patients more familiar with the latest developments in the field, as well as more confident in applying them, so that early detection and swift, effective treatment become a reality for all of our patients.

Stephen C. Yang, MD
The Arthur B. and Patricia B. Modell
Professor of Thoracic Surgery
Chief of Thoracic Surgery
The Johns Hopkins Medical Institutions

Preface

In the United States, colorectal cancer ranks as the third most common cancer in both incidence and death for both men and women. In 2009, an estimated 146,970 new patients were diagnosed with colorectal cancer, and 49,920 colorectal cancer-related deaths occurred. Worldwide, colorectal cancer has an estimated incidence of 1.02 million cases, making it the third most common cancer. The highest incidences of colorectal cancer have been reported in North America, Australia/New Zealand, and Western Europe, with the lowest incidence in parts of Africa and Asia.

Recent advances have made the future of colorectal cancer patients more promising. Colorectal cancer is considered to be a disease that goes in a stepwise progression from normal colon to adenoma and then to invasive cancer. Knowledge of this stepwise progression presents an opportunity to intervene and identify pre-invasive lesions using endoscopic techniques and population-wide screening. The introduction of widespread screening in the United States occurred in the 1970s and 1980s, when researchers demonstrated the feasibility of testing for occult blood in stool and initiated randomized clinical trials. In 1985, the diagnosis of colon cancer in President Ronald Reagan led to increased public awareness of this disease. Finally, the introduction of Medicare reimbursement for all individuals in 2001 led not only to improvements in adherence to screening guidelines but also to increased likelihood of diagnosing the cancer at an early stage.

This volume on *Early Diagnosis and Treatment of Cancer: Colorectal Cancer* is meant as an introduction to the current understanding of the epidemiology, risk factors, and treatment options for colorectal cancer. Like the rest of this series, this book is designed to provide up-to-date information regarding safe and effective methods to reach a diagnosis, obtain accurate clinical staging of the disease, and choose the best method of treatment.

Included in this volume are discussions of hereditary colon cancer syndromes, indications for genetic screening, and potential chemoprevention methods. Since the stage of diagnosis is the most significant predictor of outcome, the book includes several chapters on screening techniques for early diagnosis of colorectal cancer. The book is also designed to guide the reader in formulating a logical, step-by-step treatment or patient care plan. Each chapter regarding treatment is comprehensive and timely, and key points emphasize the important aspects of each individual step in the process.

We thank the contributors—all leaders in their respective fields—for their dedication and tireless efforts in putting together this volume. We hope that the book will serve as an important resource guide for health care providers who strive to improve the lives of patients with both early and advanced stages of colorectal cancer. Finally, this volume is dedicated to all our patients with colorectal cancer who continue to inspire us to seek a cure.

Susan L. Gearhart, MD
Nita Ahuja, MD

Contents

Contributors

Nita Ahuja, MD
Assistant Professor of Surgery and Oncology, Department of Surgery, The Johns Hopkins University, Baltimore, Maryland

Vanita Ahuja, MD, MPH
Associate Program Director, York Hospital–Wellspan Health, York, Pennsylvania

Debashish Bose, MD, PhD
Fellow, Department of Surgical Oncology, The University of Texas MD Anderson Cancer Center, Houston, Texas

David Chang, MPH, PhD
Johns Hopkins University School of Medicine, Baltimore, Maryland

Kathryn M. Chu, MD, MPH
Clinical Assistant Professor, Johns Hopkins University School of Medicine, Baltimore, Maryland

Stephanie R. Downing, MD
General Surgery, Department of Surgery, Howard University Hospital, Howard University College of Medicine, Washington, DC; Research Associate, Department of Surgery, Johns Hopkins University School of Medicine, Baltimore, Maryland

Khaled El-Shami, MD, PhD
Assistant Professor of Oncology and Medicine, Lombardi Comprehensive Cancer Center at Georgetown University; Attending Oncologist, Georgetown University Hospital, Washington, DC

Susan L. Gearhart, MD
Assistant Professor of Colorectal Surgery and Oncology, Department of Surgery, The Johns Hopkins University, Baltimore, Maryland

Francis M. Giardiello, MD
John G. Rangos Sr. Professor of Medicine, Johns Hopkins University School of Medicine, Baltimore, Maryland

Samuel A. Giday, MD
Robert E. Meyerhoff Professor, Director, Endoscopic Ultrasound Unit, Division of Gastroenterology and Hepatology, Johns Hopkins University School of Medicine, Johns Hopkins Hospital, Baltimore, Maryland

Joseph M. Herman, MD, MSc
Assistant Professor of Radiation Oncology, The Johns Hopkins University School of Medicine, Baltimore, Maryland

Karen M. Horton, MD
Professor of Radiology, The Russell H. Morgan Department of Radiology and Radiological Science, Johns Hopkins Medical Institutions, Baltimore, Maryland

Matthew T. Hueman, MD, FACS
Assistant Professor of Surgery, Uniformed Services University; Surgical Oncologist and Associate Program Director, General Surgery, Department of Surgery, Walter Reed Army Medical Center, Washington, DC

Ajay Jain, MD
Assistant Professor of Surgery, University of Maryland Medical Center, Baltimore, Maryland

Michel I. Kafrouni, MD
Gastroenterology, Johns Hopkins Hospital, Baltimore, Maryland; Private Practice, Gastroenterology Consultants, P.A., Houston, Texas

John H. Kwon, MD
Assistant Professor, University of Chicago, Chicago, Illinois

Wells Messersmith, MD
Assistant Professor, Director, GI Cancers Program, University of Colorado Denver, Denver, Colorado

Melissa A. Munsell, MD
Associate Physician, Southern California Permanente Medical Group, Anaheim, California

Jamila Mwidau, MD
Johns Hopkins University School of Medicine, Baltimore, Maryland

Sujatha Nallapareddy, MD
Developmental Therapeutics and GI Malignancies, University of Colorado Denver, Denver, Colorado

Emmanouil P. Pappou, MD
Department of Surgery, The Johns Hopkins University School of Medicine, Baltimore, Maryland

Timothy M. Pawlik, MD, MPH
Associate Professor of Surgery and Oncology, Johns Hopkins University, Johns Hopkins Hospital, Baltimore, Maryland

Cheryl J. Pendergrass, MS, CGC
Genetic Counselor, The Johns Hopkins University School of Medicine, Baltimore Maryland

Nicole A. Phillips, BS
University of Chicago, Chicago, Illinois

Richard Schulick, MD
Professor of Surgery and Oncology, Chief, Cameron Division of Surgical Oncology, Johns Hopkins University, Baltimore, Maryland

Eun Ji Shin, MD
Assistant Professor of Medicine, Johns Hopkins University School of Medicine, Baltimore, Maryland

Jason K. Sicklick, MD
Chief Administrative Fellow, Department of Surgery, Memorial Sloan-Kettering Cancer Center, New York, New York

Jerry Stonemetz, MD
Clinical Associate, Johns Hopkins Medical Institutions, Baltimore, Maryland

Eden R. Stotsky, BSN, RN
Nurse Clinician, Johns Hopkins Hospital, Baltimore, Maryland

Susan Tsai, MD
Surgical Oncology Fellow, Johns Hopkins Medical Institutions, Baltimore, Maryland

Elizabeth C. Wick, MD
Assistant Professor of Colorectal Surgery, Johns Hopkins University; Attending Surgeon, Johns Hopkins Hospital, Baltimore, Maryland

Michelle N. Zikusoka, MD
Department of Medicine, Johns Hopkins University, Baltimore, Maryland

Epidemiology and Risk Factors of Colorectal Cancer

Kathryn M. Chu

KEY POINTS

- Colorectal cancer (CRC) is the third most common cancer and the third most common cause of cancer death in the United States.
- Over the past 20 years, the incidence of CRC has declined.
- Developed countries have a higher incidence of CRC than do developing countries.
- Adenocarcinoma is the most common type of CRC.
- Persons over 50 years of age have the greatest risk for CRC.
- A higher incidence of CRC is found among blacks than among other races.
- Men have a slightly higher risk of developing CRC than do women.
- Known risk factors for CRC include family history, obesity, poor diet, alcohol and cigarette use, and lack of exercise.

Epidemiology

Types of Colon and Rectal Cancer

Several types of primary cancer are located in the colon and rectum.[1] These include adenocarcinoma, carcinoid tumor, gastrointestinal stromal tumor, lymphoma, and squamous cell cancer of the anus. The majority (95%) of cancers of the colon and rectum are adenocarcinomas or tumors arising from intestinal glands. The epidemiology of this type of tumor is discussed in this chapter. Metastases to the colon and rectum are rare but can occur with melanoma and breast cancer. Carcinoid tumors arise more commonly in the small bowel and appendix, although on occasion these tumors can be identified in the rectum (Fig. 1-1A). Carcinoid tumors develop from gastrointestinal neuroendocrine cells. Gastrointestinal stromal tumors develop from interstitial cells of Cajal and can be found anywhere in the gastrointestinal tract (Fig. 1-1B). Lymphoma may originate in the colon and rectum but is more commonly found in the lymphatic system. Squamous cell cancer of the anus is associated with human papilloma virus infection (Fig. 1-1C).

Incidence of Adenocarcinoma of the Colon and Rectum

Colorectal cancer (CRC) is found throughout the world, but the incidence of this disease varies widely (Fig. 1-2). Developed countries have a higher incidence of CRC than do developing countries, with the highest incidences occurring in Australia, North America, and Northern and Western Europe. The United States has one of the highest rates of CRC in the world. The incidence is almost 10-fold lower in parts of Africa and Asia.[2,3]

CRC is the third most common cancer in the United States for men and women[4,5] (Fig. 1-3). Approximately 147,000 people (76,000 men and 71,000 women) will be diagnosed in 2010 (Fig. 1-4). The incidence of CRC has been decreasing over the last 20 years. In 2004, the reported incidence of CRC was 48.2 per 100,000, whereas in 1985 the reported incidence was 66.3 per 100,000. This decline is believed to be related to an increase in screening for CRC (detection and removal of colorectal polyps),[4,5] although changes in lifestyle may also play a role.

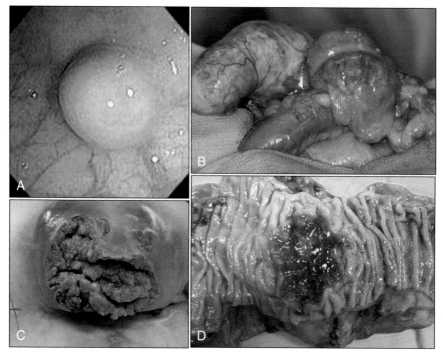

Figure 1-1. **A,** Carcinoid tumor of the rectum. **B,** Gastrointestinal stromal tumor of the colon. **C,** Squamous cell cancer of the anus. **D,** Adenocarcinoma of the colon.

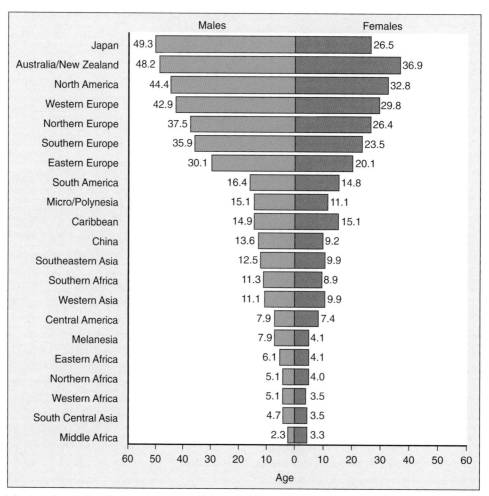

Figure 1-2. Age-standardized incidence rates per 100,000 for colorectal cancer by gender. (From Parkin DM, Bray F, Ferlay J, Pisani P: Global cancer statistics, 2002. CA Cancer J Clin 55:74–108, 2005.)

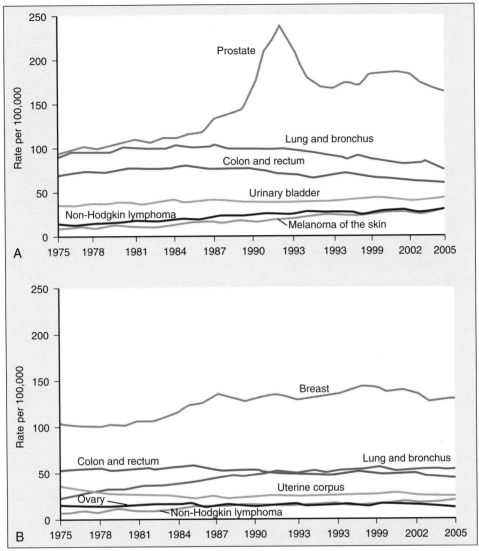

Figure 1-3. A, Age-adjusted cancer incidence rates for various cancers in men in the United States, 1975–2004. **B,** Age-adjusted cancer incidence rates for various cancers in women in the United States, 1975–2004. Data are age adjusted to the 2000 United States standard population and adjusted for delays in reporting. (From Cancer Statistics, 2008. American Cancer Society Statistics on Cancer 2008.)

Stage at Time of Diagnosis

There are several historical colorectal staging systems, including the Dukes and Astler-Coller systems. The most widely used staging system is the TNM system of the American Joint Committee on Cancer (AJCC).[6] In this system, the four stages are based on the depth of invasion of the primary tumor (T), lymph node status (N), and distant metastasis (M) (Table 1-1 and Box 1-1). Approximately 39% of colon and rectum cancer cases are diagnosed while the cancer is still confined to the primary site (localized stage or stage I/IIa), 36% are diagnosed after the cancer has spread to regional lymph nodes (stage III) or directly beyond the primary site (stage IIb), 19% are diagnosed after the cancer metastasized (distant stage or stage IV), and for 5% the staging information is unknown.[5] The most common site of metastasis for stage IV CRC is the liver.

In recent years, a greater proportion of CRC has been diagnosed at earlier stages.[7] This shift reflects the trend toward increased and improved screening. Gross and associates demonstrated that when Medicare began to reimburse for screening colonoscopy in 1998, a significantly higher percentage of cancers were diagnosed at an early stage (stage I).[8]

Estimated New Cases*		Estimated Deaths	
Male	**Female**	**Male**	**Female**
Prostate 192,280 (25%)	Breast 192,370 (27%)	Lung and bronchus 88,900 (30%)	Lung and bronchus 70,490 (26%)
Lung and bronchus 116,090 (15%)	Lung and bronchus 103,350 (14%)	Prostate 27,360 (9%)	Breast 40,170 (15%)
Colon and rectum 75,590 (10%)	Colon and rectum 71,380 (10%)	Colon and rectum 25,240 (9%)	Colon and rectum 24,680 (9%)
Urinary bladder 52,810 (7%)	Uterine corpus 42,160 (6%)	Pancreas 18,030 (6%)	Pancreas 17,210 (6%)
Melanoma of the skin 39,080 (5%)	Non-Hodgkin lymphoma 29,990 (4%)	Leukemia 12,590 (4%)	Ovary 14,600 (5%)
Non-Hodgkin lymphoma 35,990 (5%)	Melanoma of the skin 29,640 (4%)	Liver and intrahepatic bile duct 12,090 (4%)	Non-Hodgkin lymphoma 9,670 (4%)
Kidney and renal pelvis 35,430 (5%)	Thyroid 27,200 (4%)	Esophagus 11,490 (4%)	Leukemia 9,280 (3%)
Leukemia 25,630 (3%)	Kidney and renal pelvis 22,330 (3%)	Urinary bladder 10,180 (3%)	Uterine corpus 7,780 (3%)
Oral cavity and pharynx 25,240 (3%)	Ovary 21,550 (3%)	Non-Hodgkin lymphoma 9,830 (3%)	Liver and intrahepatic bile duct 6,070 (2%)
Pancreas 21,050 (3%)	Pancreas 21,420 (3%)	Kidney and renal pelvis 8,160 (3%)	Brain and other nervous system 5,590 (2%)
All sites 766,130 (100%)	All sites 713,220 (100%)	All sites 292,540 (100%)	All sites 269,800 (100%)

*Excludes basal and squamous cell skin cancers and in situ carcinoma except urinary bladder.

Figure 1-4. Leading sites of new cancer cases and deaths in the United States by gender, 2009 estimates. (From Cancer Facts and Figures 2009. © 2009, American Cancer Society, Inc. Surveillance Research.)

Table 1-1. American Joint Committee on Cancer Staging of Colorectal Cancer

Stage	T	N	M
Stage I	T1–2	N0	M0
Stage IIA	T3	N0	M0
Stage IIB	T4a	N0	M0
Stage IIC	T4b	N0	M0
Stage IIIA	T1–2	N1	M0
	T1	N2a	M0
Stage IIIB	T3–4	N1	M0
	T2–3	N2a	M0
	T1–2	N2b	M0
Stage IIIC	T4a	N2a	M0
	T3–4a	N2b	M0
	T4b	N1–2	M0
Stage IVA	Any T	Any N	M1a
Stage IVB	Any T	Any N	M1b

Adapted from Greene FL: AJCC Cancer Staging Manual, 7th ed. New York: Springer, 2010, p 199.

Location of Primary Tumor

Approximately 30% of CRC is located in the right colon, 10% in the transverse colon, 15% in the left (descending) colon, 25% in the sigmoid colon, and 20% in the rectum (Fig. 1-5). In the

Box 1-1. American Joint Committee on Cancer TNM Classification of Colorectal Cancer

Primary Tumor (T)

T0   No evidence of primary tumor
T1   Tumor invades submucosa
T2   Tumor invades muscularis propria
T3   Tumor invades through muscularis propria into pericolorectal tissue
T4a   Tumor penetrates the surface of the visceral peritoneum
T4b   Tumor directly invades or is adherent to other organs or structures

Regional Lymph Nodes (N)

N0   No invasion of regional lymph nodes
N1a   Invasion into one regional lymph node
N1b   Invasion into two to three regional lymph nodes
N1c   Tumor deposits without invasion into regional lymph nodes
N2a   Invasion into four to six regional lymph nodes
N2b   Invasion into seven or more regional lymph nodes

Distant Metastasis (M)

M0   No distant metastasis present
M1a   Single distant metastasis
M1b   Multiple distant metastasis

Adapted from Greene FL: AJCC Cancer Staging Manual, 7th ed. New York: Springer, 2010, pp 197–198.

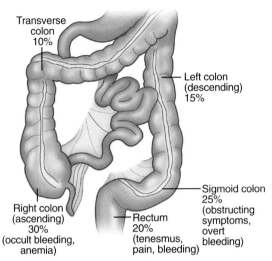

Figure 1-5. Distribution of colon and rectal cancer.
(From Hopkins Colon Cancer website. Used with permission from author, Michael Choti, MD. http://hopkinsgi.nts.jhu.edu/pages/latin/templates/index.cfm?pg=disease1&organ=6&disease=36&lang_id=1. Digestive Diseases Library—Colon Cancer. Sporadic Colon Cancer. Accessed June 24, 2007.)

past 20 years, epidemiologic studies have shown that the ratio of proximal to distal cancers has been increasing.[9-12] This is due to a slight increase in proximal cancers and a decrease in cancers of the descending colon and rectum. Older persons are more at risk for proximal lesions (Fig. 1-6), and the aging and growing population has contributed to this increase. The decrease in distal cancers is likely due to improved screening of the sigmoid and rectum.

Risk Factors

Although much has yet to be learned about why some individuals develop colon cancer and others do not, certain factors are known to increase a person's chance of developing the disease. These factors are both genetic and environmental.

Genetic Factors

Personal or Family History of Colorectal Cancer

A family history of CRC increases the likelihood that an individual will develop CRC. A prospec-

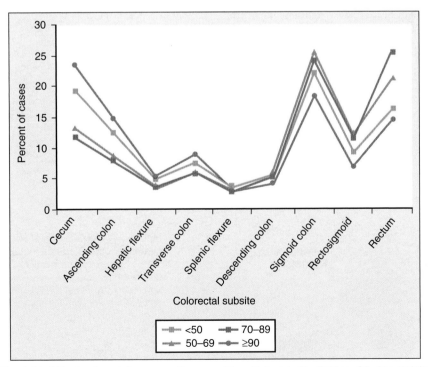

Figure 1-6. The right shift of colorectal cancer with age. (From Saltzstein SL, Behling, CA: Age and time as factors in the left-to-right shift of the subsite of colorectal adenocarcinoma: A study of 213,383 cases from the California Cancer Registry. J Clin Gastroenterol 41(2):173–177.)

tive study of 119,116 individuals examined the relative risk of developing CRC for those with a first-degree relative with a history of CRC compared with those with unaffected relatives. The age-adjusted relative risk of CRC was 1.7. The relative risk among individuals with two or more affected first-degree relatives was 2.7. For those younger than 45 years who had one or more affected first-degree relatives, the relative risk was 5.4.[13] Most patients with CRC who also have a family history of CRC do not have a genetically inherited syndrome. Overall, genetically inherited syndromes that cause CRC such as hereditary nonpolyposis colon cancer (HNPCC) and familial adenomatous polyposis (FAP) are rare (5% to 10%) (Fig. 1-7). These syndromes are discussed in Chapter 3, Hereditary Cancer Syndromes. A personal history of CRC increases a person's risk of developing another CRC.[14]

Personal History of Inflammatory Bowel Disease

A personal history of inflammatory bowel disease (ulcerative colitis or Crohn's disease) increases a person's risk of CRC. Individuals with primary sclerosing cholangitis, severe longstanding disease, and young age at diagnosis have the highest risk.[15-17] In a meta-analysis of 19 studies, the cumulative risk of CRC for those with ulcerative colitis was 2% at 10 years, 8% at 20 years, and 18% at 30 years.[18] The extent of disease is also associated with an increased risk of CRC. In a population-based cohort study of 3117 persons in Sweden with ulcerative colitis, the odds of developing CRC for isolated procti-

tis was 1.7 compared with 2.8 for left-sided colitis and 14.8 for pancolitis. Moreover, for those with pancolitis of more than 35 years' duration, the risk of CRC was 30%. For those with pancolitis for more than 35 years, which was diagnosed before the age of 15 years, the risk was 40%.[19]

Age

Age is a significant risk factor for CRC, with more than 90% of cases developing after age 50. The median age at diagnosis is 73 years for colon cancer and 67 years for rectal cancer.[5] Although the overall incidence of CRC is decreasing in the United States, some evidence suggests that its incidence among younger people is increasing. Moreover, younger individuals often present with more advanced disease and poorly differentiated tumors than do older adults.[20]

Gender

Men have a slightly higher risk of developing colon cancer compared with women (odds ratio = 1.4).[21] This risk is more pronounced in rectal cancer (odds ratio = 1.7).[22] From 2001 to 2005, the incidence of CRC was 59.2 per 100,000 for men compared with 43.8 per 100,000 for women.[5]

Race

Significant racial disparities exist in CRC (Fig. 1-8). There is a higher incidence in blacks compared with whites (62.1 versus 51.2 per

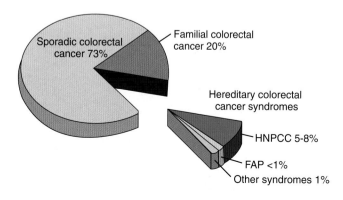

Figure 1-7. Contribution of familial and hereditary causes to colorectal cancer cases. FAP, familial adenomatous polyposis; HNPCC, hereditary nonpolyposis colon cancer. (From http://www1.geneticsolutions.com/?id=4338:22210. Lynch and de la Chapelle, 2003. © Clinical Tools, Inc.)

Sporadic colorectal cancer 73%

Familial colorectal cancer 20%

Hereditary colorectal cancer syndromes

HNPCC 5-8%

FAP <1%

Other syndromes 1%

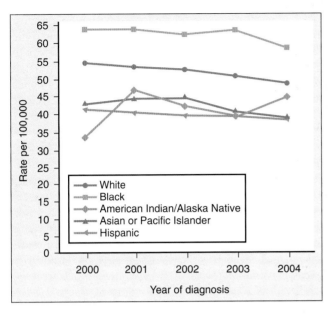

Figure 1-8. Age-adjusted incidence rates by race for colon and rectal cancer in the United States, 2000–2004. (Data from the Surveillance, Epidemiology, and End Results Program, http://www.seer.cancer.gov. Accessed May 1, 2007.)

100,000),[5] whereas Asian and Pacific Islanders have the lowest incidence of all ethnic groups.[5] Blacks are more likely to be diagnosed at an earlier age and with a more advanced stage of disease.[23] The reasons for these racial disparities are still being investigated. Certain racial and ethnic minorities may have lower rates of screening and poorer access to care.

Environmental Factors

Environmental factors are known to affect incidence rates. When individuals from one community move to another, they take on the risk of their new environment, often within one generation. For example, a study of Japanese immigrants to Hawaii revealed that the risk of CRC within this population was similar to that of Hawaiians rather than to that of residents of Japan.[24] Environmental factors that have been implicated in the incidence of CRC include diet, lack of exercise, obesity, smoking, alcohol consumption, and type 2 diabetes.

Diet

Consumption of animal fat is associated with CRC. In the U.S. Nurses Health Study, 88,751 women were prospectively followed up for 512,488 person-years. Women who consumed beef, pork, or lamb more than once per month were 2.5 times more likely to develop CRC compared with women who consumed meat less than once per month. No increased risk was found with consumption of vegetable fat.[25] The protective effect of fiber on CRC is controversial.[26] Recent meta-analyses have demonstrated that those in the highest quartile of fiber consumption had a decreased risk of CRC compared with those who were in the lowest quartile of fiber consumption. However, when controlling for other dietary factors, high fiber failed to demonstrate any protective effect.[27,28]

Exercise

Physical activity is inversely correlated with CRC. In a prospective study of 45,906 Swedish men, even moderate physical activity was associated with a 32% decreased risk of CRC.[29] This relation is stronger in men than in women.[30]

Smoking, Alcohol, Obesity, and Diabetes

CRC has been linked to long-term smoking and alcohol consumption of more than two drinks per day.[4] Obesity is associated with an increased risk of CRC. A study from Framingham, Massachusetts, demonstrated that individuals with a body mass index (BMI) of more than 30 have a 1.5 to 2.4 times increased risk of CRC.[31] Furthermore, centripetal obesity is significantly associated with CRC.[32]

Those with type 2 non–insulin-dependent diabetes have an increased risk of developing CRC and a poorer prognosis for survival than those without diabetes.[4]

Mortality

CRC is the third leading cause of cancer death in the United States.[1] An estimated 49,920 individuals will die from CRC in 2008. This accounts for 9% of all cancer-related deaths. The 5-year survival rate is 64%.[4] From 2000 to 2004, the median age at death for those with CRC was 75 years. CRC decreases life expectancy by an average of 13 years.[5] Over the past 20 years, the mortality rate from CRC for both women and men has declined, especially in recent years, most likely as a result of significant advances in treatment modalities and improved screening (Fig. 1-9). From 1985 to 2002, a 2% per year

decrease occurred compared with a 5% per year decrease from 2002 to 2004. Men are more likely to die from CRC than women (22.7 versus 15.9/100,000). This difference in survival has become less pronounced in recent years owing to a greater decline in mortality in men than in women.[4]

Mortality for all racial and ethnic groups has declined except in American-Indian and Alaskan natives. Blacks have a worse prognosis after diagnosis than do whites (see Fig. 1-8). Several studies have indicated that these findings are independent of socioeconomic status and stage, indicating that factors beyond health care access may account for these differences.[33-35] In rectal cancer, blacks have a 5-year survival rate of 41% compared with 50% in whites, and blacks are less likely to complete adjuvant therapy (49% versus 61%), which may contribute to their poorer prognosis.[23]

Disease stage directly affects mortality rate in CRC (Fig. 1-10). If the cancer is diagnosed while still localized or confined to the primary

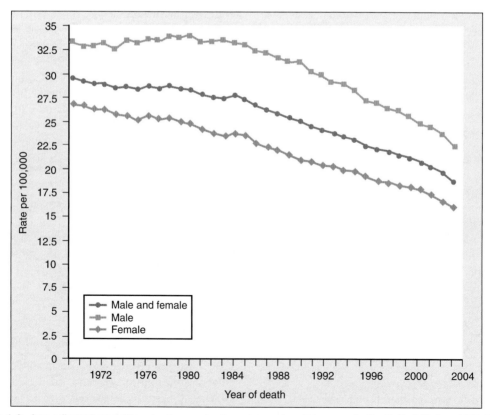

Figure 1-9. Age-adjusted mortality rates by gender for colon and rectal cancer in the United States, 1969–2004. (Data from the Surveillance, Epidemiology, and End Results Program. http://www.seer.cancer.gov. Accessed May 1, 2007.)

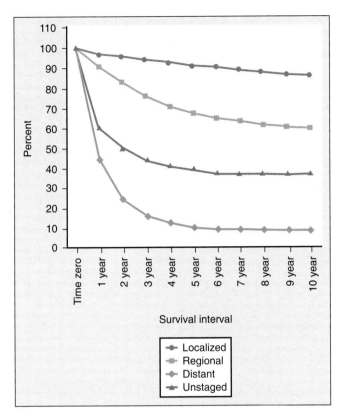

Figure 1-10. Relative survival rates by stage at diagnosis for colon and rectal cancer in the United States, 1988–2003. (Data from the Surveillance, Epidemiology, and End Results Program. http://www.seer.cancer.gov. Accessed May 1, 2007.)

site (stage I/IIa), survival rate is 90% at 5 years. However, only 39% of CRC is detected at an early stage. If the cancer has spread to regional lymph nodes (stage III) or directly beyond the primary site (stage IIb), the corresponding 5-year survival rate is 67%. If the cancer has already metastasized to distant sites (stage IV), the 5-year survival rate is 10%.[4]

Economic Burden of Disease

The costs of prevention, diagnosis, and treatment of CRC in the United States are significant. As the American population ages, the economic burden of CRC on the Medicare program and its beneficiaries will be substantial (Fig. 1-11). Estimated costs in 2000 for the initial diagnosis, ongoing treatment, and last year of life phases of care for CRC were approximately $3.2 billion, $1.7 billion, and $2.6 billion, respectively.[36] By the year 2020, under the "fixed" current incidence, survival rate, and cost scenario, projected costs for the initial diagnosis, ongoing treatment, and last year of life will be $4.7 billion, $2.6 billion, and $4.0 billion. Under the current trends

scenario (decreasing incidence, improving survival, and increasing costs), the annual costs are estimated to be $5.2 billion, $3.6 billion, and $5.3 billion, respectively. Therefore, at least a 50% increase in annual costs for CRC in patients 65 years and older is expected by the year 2020.[36]

Conclusion

Colorectal cancer is the third most common cancer in the United States today. However, the incidence of CRC has declined in the past two decades. This trend is likely to continue because of early detection and removal of polyps through screening colonoscopy. Survival rates are increasing because of earlier diagnosis and improved treatment modalities. Disparities in prognosis between racial and ethnic groups are attributed to complex socioeconomic and genetic factors as well as to differences in access to care. Further studies to better understand these differences are needed to decrease the burden of disease from CRC, particularly among the population's most disadvantaged groups.

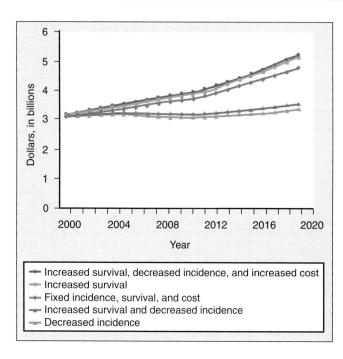

Figure 1-11. Projected costs of colorectal cancer in all phases of care (initial diagnosis, ongoing treatment, and last year of life) for 2000–2020 (sensitivity analysis). (From Yabroff R, Mariotto A, Feuer E, Brown M: Projections of the cost associated with colorectal cancer care in the US for 2000–2020. Health Econ 17(8):947–959, 2007.)

Legend for figure:
- Increased survival, decreased incidence, and increased cost
- Increased survival
- Fixed incidence, survival, and cost
- Increased survival and decreased incidence
- Decreased incidence

References

1. Corman M: Colon & Rectal Surgery, 4th ed. Philadelphia Lippincott-Raven, 1998, pp 884–888.
2. Burkitt DP: Epidemiology of cancer of the colon and rectum, 1971. Dis Colon Rectum 36(11):1071–1082, 1993.
3. Parkin DM, Bray F, Ferlay J, Pisani P: Global cancer statistics, 2002. CA Cancer J Clin 55:74–108, 2005.
4. Cancer Facts and Figures: 2009. Available at: http://www.cancer.org/downloads/STT/500809web.pdf. Accessed November 16, 2009.
5. Surveillance, Epidemiology, and End Results Program. Fast Stats: Colon and Rectum Cancer. Available at: http://seer.cancer.gov/. Accessed July 26, 2008.
6. Greene, F: AJCC Cancer Staging Manual, 6th ed. New York: Springer, 2002.
7. Paquette I, Finlayson SR: Rural versus urban colorectal and lung cancer patients: differences in stage at presentation. J Am Coll Surg 205(5):636–641, 2007.
8. Gross CP, Andersen MS, Krumholz HM, et al: Relation between Medicare screening reimbursement and stage at diagnosis for older patients with colon cancer. JAMA 296(23):2815–2822, 2006.
9. Wu XC, Chen VW, Steele B, et al: Subsite-specific incidence rate and stage of disease in colorectal cancer by race, gender, and age group in the United States, 1992–1997. Cancer 92:2547–2554, 2001.
10. Saltzstein SL, Behling CA, Savides TJ: The relation of age, race, and gender to the subsite location of colorectal carcinoma. Cancer 82:1408–1410, 1998.
11. Rabeneck L, Davila JA, El-Serag HB: Is there a true "shift" to the right colon in the incidence of colorectal cancer? Am J Gastroenterol 98(6):1400–1409, 2003.
12. Saltzstein S, Behling C: Age and time as factors in the left-to-right shift of the subsite of colorectal adenocarcinoma: a study of 213,383 cases from the California cancer registry. J Clin Gastroenterol 41:173–177, 2007.
13. Fuchs CS, Giovannucci EL, Colditz GA, et al: A prospective study of family history and the risk of colorectal cancer. N Engl J Med 331(25):1669–1674, 1994.
14. Schaffzin DM, Smith LE: Rectal cancer. In Cameron JL (ed): Current Surgical Therapy, 8th ed. Philadelphia: Elsevier Mosby, 2004, pp 216–223.
15. Jess T, Loftus EV Jr, Velayos FS, et al: Risk factors for colorectal neoplasia in inflammatory bowel disease: a nested case-control study from Copenhagen county, Denmark and Olmsted county, Minnesota. Am J Gastroenterol 102(4):829–836, 2007.
16. Loftus EV Jr: Epidemiology and risk factors for colorectal dysplasia and cancer in ulcerative colitis [review]. Gastroenterol Clin North Am 35(3):517–531, 2006.
17. Bernstein CN, Blanchard JF, Kliewer E, Wajda A: Cancer risk in patients with inflammatory bowel disease: a population-based study. Cancer 91(4):854–862, 2001.
18. Eaden JA, Abrams KR, Mayberry JF: The risk of colorectal cancer in ulcerative colitis: a meta-analysis. Gut 48(4):526–535, 2001.
19. Ekbom A, Helmick C, Zack M, Adami HO: Ulcerative colitis and colorectal cancer. A population-based study. N Engl J Med 323(18):1228–1233, 1990.
20. Fairley TL, Cardinez CJ, Martin J, et al: Colorectal cancer in U.S. adults younger than 50 years of age, 1998–2001. Cancer 1;107(5 Suppl):1153–1161, 2006.
21. McCashland TM, Brand R, Lyden E, de Garmo P; CORI Research Project: Gender differences in colorectal polyps and tumors. Am J Gastroenterol 96(3):882–886, 2001.
22. William, S: Who is more prone to develop colorectal cancer?. EzineArticles. July 14, 2005. Available at: http://ezinearticles.com/?Who-Is-More-Prone-To-Develop-Colorectal-Cancer?&id=51404. Accessed June 24, 2007.
23. Morris AM, Wei Y, Birkmeyer NJ, Birkmeyer JD: Racial disparities in late survival after rectal cancer surgery. J Am Coll Surg 203(6):787–794, 2006.
24. Maskarinec G, Noh JJ: The effect of migration on cancer incidence among Japanese in Hawaii. Ethn Dis 14(3):431–439, 2004.
25. Willett WC, Stampfer MJ, Colditz GA, et al: Relation of meat, fat, and fiber intake to the risk of colon cancer in a prospective study among women. N Engl J Med 323(24):1664–1672, 1990.
26. Baron JA: Dietary fiber and colorectal cancer: an ongoing saga. JAMA 294(22):2904–2906, 2005.
27. Park Y, Hunter DJ, Spiegelman D, et al: Dietary fiber intake and risk of colorectal cancer: a pooled analysis of prospective cohort studies. JAMA 294(22):2849–2857, 2005.
28. Bingham SA, Norat T, Moskal A, et al: Is the association with fiber from foods in colorectal cancer confounded by folate intake? Cancer Epidemiol Biomarkers Prev 14(6):1552–1556, 2005.
29. Larsson SC, Rutegard J, Bergkvist L, Wolk A: Physical activity, obesity, and risk of colon and rectal cancer in a cohort of Swedish men. Eur J Cancer 42(15):2590–2597, 2006.

30. Calton BA, James V, Lacey JV, et al: Physical activity and the risk of colon cancer among women: a prospective cohort study (United States). Int J Cancer 119(2):385–391, 2006.

31. Moore LL, Bradlee ML, Singer MR, et al: BMI and waist circumference as predictors of lifetime colon cancer risk in Framingham Study adults. Int J Obes Relat Metab Disord 28(4):559–567, 2004.

32. Pischon T, Lahmann PH, Boeing H, et al: Body size and risk of colon and rectal cancer in the European Prospective Investigation into Cancer and Nutrition (EPIC). J Natl Cancer Inst 98(13):920–931, 2006.

33. Morris AM, Billingsley KG, Baxter NN, Baldwin LM: Racial disparities in rectal cancer treatment: a population-based analysis. Arch Surg 139(2):151–155, 2004.

34. Dominitz J, Samsa G, Landsman P, Provenzale D: Race, treatment, and survival among colorectal carcinoma patients in an equal-access system. Cancer 82:2312–2320, 1998.

35. Ahuja N, Chang D, Gearhart S: Disparities in colon cancer presentation and in-hospital mortality in Maryland. A ten year review. Ann Surg Oncol 14(2):1507–1513, 2007.

36. Yabroff R, Mariotto A, Feuer E, Brown M: Projections of the cost associated with colorectal cancer care in the US for 2000–2020. Health Econ 17(8):947–959, 2007.

2 Presentation and Initial Evaluation of Colorectal Cancer

Susan Tsai and Susan L. Gearhart

KEY POINTS

- In the United States, nearly 85% of patients with colorectal cancer (CRC) are *symptomatic* from their tumors before a diagnosis is made.
- The most common symptoms of CRC include rectal bleeding, abdominal pain, and change in bowel habits.
- Accurate initial clinical staging allows for the selection of appropriate stage-specific therapy in the management of CRC.

Presentation

In the United States, colorectal cancer (CRC) is the third most common cancer diagnosis and the second leading cause of cancer death.[1] Because it is so prevalent, as early as 1980 the American Cancer Society issued guidelines for CRC screening in average-risk adults.[2] As a result, recent trends in the incidence of and mortality from CRC reveal declining rates, partly because of effective screening and prevention through polypectomy.[3] However, despite prospective randomized trials that have demonstrated decreased mortality rate with early detection of CRC,[4] most adults in the United States do not receive regular age- and risk-appropriate screening. Poor screening participation has been attributed to a variety of factors, including lack of health insurance and lower socioeconomic status.[5-7] However, even in the setting of universal health care, compliance with recommended screening remains low. A recent retrospective study from British Columbia, Canada, reported that out of 212 patients with CRC, less than 7% were diagnosed via a screening test, and only 15% of screening-eligible patients had been screened.[8] Similarly,

in the United States, nearly 85% of patients with CRC have symptoms from their tumors before a diagnosis is made.[9] Therefore, it remains especially important to recognize the clinical signs and symptoms of CRC and to appropriately initiate workup when necessary.

Symptoms

The symptoms of CRC are not inherently unique. Patients may present with occult or symptomatic anemia, bright red blood per rectum, abdominal pain, change in bowel habits, anorexia, weight loss, nausea, vomiting, or fatigue. Taken in isolation, most of these signs and symptoms are neither sensitive nor specific and may be present equally in benign and malignant diseases. However, the clustering of symptoms may be useful in identifying malignancies.

In a prospective study of 2268 patients in the United Kingdom with distal colonic symptoms, a questionnaire was developed to facilitate the prioritization of patients to be seen by a specialist. The questionnaire screened for primary symptoms and symptom complexes of CRC and was completed by the patients before seeing a specialist. A weighted numerical score was then derived from the questionnaire based on related symptoms (Fig. 2-1). The weighted numerical score is calculated by a computer based on a formula derived subjectively by weighting of symptoms and symptom complexes in relation to the likelihood of cancer outcome. The higher the numerical score, the greater are the odds that the patient has CRC, with scores higher than 70 associated with a 1 in 5 risk and scores lower than 40 associated with a risk of 1 in 967. Of the 2268 patients, 95 were found to have

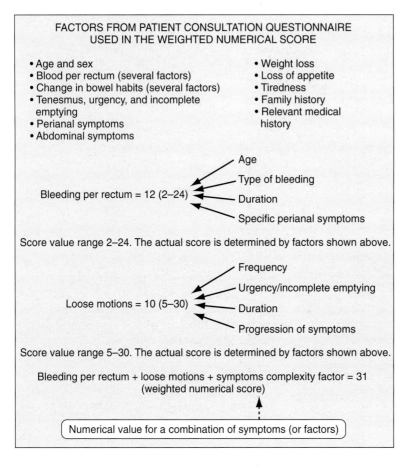

Figure 2-1. Principle of the weighted numerical score. (From Selvachandran SN, Hodder RJ, Ballal MS, et al: Prediction of colorectal cancer by patient consultation questionnaire and scoring system: a prospective study. Lancet 360:278–283, 2002.)

CRC, and the weighted numerical score was significantly higher for patients with cancer than for noncancer patients (mean 76.5 [95% confidence interval, CI, 72.2–80.9] compared with 44.5 [95% CI 43.6–45.4], $P < .0001$) (Fig. 2-2).[10] As with classic teaching, symptoms of bleeding per rectum, change in bowel habits to loose movements, and increased frequency of defecation were associated with the highest relative risk ratios. Although a computer-generated score may serve as a surrogate for experience-based clinical suspicion, it also demonstrates that it is possible to identify at-risk patients based on symptoms alone.

Another study that supports identifying symptom "clustering" was published by Majumdar and associates.[11] In classic teaching, the presentation of CRC may vary depending on the location of the tumor. Proximal colon cancers are more often occult and are more often associated with anemia, whereas distal cancers are more likely to demonstrate gross rectal bleeding or a change in stool caliber. A retrospective study of 194 consecutive patients with a known diagnosis of CRC identified distinct clustering of symp-

toms related to the location of the tumor.[11] In this study, 83% of patients were diagnosed with CRC based on investigation of related symptoms; the remaining 17% were detected by accident. Fifty-eight percent had distal tumors, and 48% had proximal tumors. The most common symptoms were rectal bleeding (58%), abdominal pain (52%), and a change in bowel habits (52%). On univariate analysis, patients who presented with a combination of anorexia, nausea, vomiting, abdominal pain, or fatigue were more likely to have a proximal CRC. Other symptoms such as diarrhea, mucus in stools, rectal pain, and tenesmus were associated with distal tumors. On multivariate analysis, independent predictors of a distal tumor included mild anemia, rectal bleeding, and constipation.

As the authors conclude, certain symptoms share common pathophysiology and therefore occur in clusters.[11] For example, patients with proximal tumors often present with symptomatic anemia without gross rectal bleeding, having generalized weakness or fatigue. Unlike more distal tumors, which manifest as rectal bleeding, proximal tumors may grow subclinically until

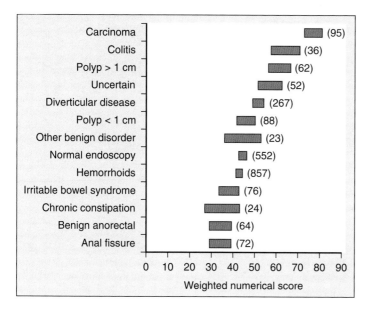

Figure 2-2. Disease outcome and 95% confidence interval of average weighted numerical score. (From Selvachandran SN, Hodder RJ, Ballal MS, et al: Prediction of colorectal cancer by patient consultation questionnaire and scoring system: a prospective study. Lancet 360:278–283, 2002.)

near obstruction, at which time patients present with nausea, vomiting, and abdominal pain. Another example is metastatic disease, which may manifest as right upper quadrant pain or constitutional symptoms, such as fevers, night sweats, and weight loss.

Signs

CRC is often difficult to establish based on physical examination alone. Infrequently, colon cancer may present as a palpable abdominal mass. In contrast, rectal cancer is often palpable on physical examination. In particular, several prognostic characteristics with regard to the primary rectal cancer have been identified. In a study of 769 patients with CRC who were undergoing preoperative radiation, the preoperative assessment of mobility of the tumor, the number of quadrants involved, as well as the distance of the tumor from the anal verge were identified in a multivariate analysis as being predictive of a curative resection.[12] Patients with tumors that were mobile regardless of the number of quadrants involved had a 78% to 84% curative resection rate. Those with tumors that were partially fixed and involved one quadrant had a 56% curative resection rate, whereas those with tumors that were partially fixed and involved more than one quadrant had a 39% curative resection rate. Although distance from the anal verge did not have an impact on resection rates, the 5-year survival rate was 42% for patients with tumors less than 5 cm from the

anal verge compared with 64% for those with tumors 10 to 15 cm from the anal verge.

In addition, anterior tumor location has been associated with a trend toward higher survival rates, although not statistically significant when compared with posteriorly located tumors.[13] Additional signs of CRC usually are associated with advanced disease. Anemia from gastrointestinal bleeding generally is associated with iron deficiency and may classically manifest as pallor, brittle spooned nails, and glossitis. Patients with hypoalbuminemia may present with ascites or anasarca. Hepatomegaly, supraclavicular lymphadenopathy, and cachexia may be indicative of metastatic disease.

Duration of Symptoms

There are several challenges in identifying patients with CRC. As previously discussed, the signs and symptoms of the disease may be misinterpreted as benign disease. Both patients and physician are influenced not only by the presence or absence of symptoms, but also by the severity, chronicity, and progressive nature of the symptoms. In a study of 294 CRC patients, symptoms that were unusual, severe, or of short duration were more likely to be reported by patients.[14] Majumdar and associates[11] reported median symptom durations of 3 months before diagnosis. This finding has been corroborated by other studies, which report durations of 2 to 4 months.[14,15] Symptoms such as obstruction or rectal bleeding had shorter duration, whereas

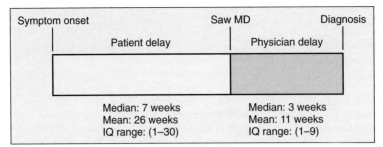

Figure 2-3. Duration of colorectal cancer symptoms: total, and relative contributions to delay by patients and physicians.   (From Majumdar SR, Fletcher RH, Evans AT: How does colorectal cancer present? Symptoms, duration, and clues to location. Am J Gastroenterol 94:3039–3045, 1999.)

more chronic symptoms such as weight loss had the longest duration (median 27 weeks). Moreover, patients and physicians contributed to delays in diagnosis[11] (Fig. 2-3). The median duration of symptoms before a patient sought medical care was 7 weeks. The median time to diagnosis after presentation to medical care was 3 weeks, and most cancers were diagnosed within 1 month of presentation. The study found no relation between duration of symptoms and the stage of cancer. The lack of association between duration of symptoms and cancer stage is counterintuitive but has been reported by previous studies as well.[15-17]

Clinical Presentation of Locally Advanced Colorectal Cancer

Patients with locally advanced CRC may present with obstruction, perforation, or fistulas. Obstruction is usually the result of tumor growth that has encroached on the bowel lumen and is less likely related to intussusception or volvulus. Patients may present with abdominal pain, nausea, vomiting, and abdominal distention. Obstruction may lead to perforation secondary to colonic ischemia and intraluminal pressure. Alternatively, the tumor itself may perforate through the colonic wall. In a report of 83 patients who presented with colonic perforation, 65% of patients had perforation at the tumor site and 35% had perforation at a more proximal site. Patients with perforation at a site proximal to the tumor had a higher operative mortality rate but a better cancer-related survival rate, with less peritoneal seeding, and there was a 5-year disease-related survival probability of 0.9 compared with 0.51 ($P = .049$) for patients who had a tumor perforating through the bowel wall.[18]

Colon cancer can also penetrate the bowel wall without frank perforation and invade adjacent structures, creating fistulas. Locally advanced rectal tumors may present as colovesical or colovaginal fistulas. In addition, locally advanced colonic tumors may also involve the duodenum, pancreas, stomach, or kidney, and the clinical presentation often reflects symptoms of the involved organ.

Initial Evaluation

For the newly diagnosed cancer patient, the initial visit to the surgeon's office can be an overwhelming experience. In this era of internet chat rooms and health care-oriented websites, prognostic information is readily available but often contradictory. It is paramount for the physician and the patient to establish a positive relationship and an open line of communication; the office visit provides an opportunity for the institution of both. Since anxieties around cancer diagnoses can often make discussion difficult, the focus of the office visit must first be to put the patient at ease. The presence of a family member to take notes or to just listen is usually beneficial for the patient. Furthermore, concerns regarding the effects of cancer treatment are best addressed early. Information about preparation for surgery and postoperative care should be discussed.

History and Physical

In addition to building a solid rapport with the patient and family, one of the primary objectives of the office visit is to record the patient's history. Aspects of the patient's history such as past disease and physical limitations may prove prohibitive to surgery or may signal the need for more acute perioperative care. Stratification of preoperative risk factors may be pursued along several courses. The most successful and complete assessments encompass the patient's cardiac health, pulmonary health, and potential for development of deep vein thrombosis (DVT).[19]

In conjunction with the medical history, the physical examination is the surgeon's primary tool for categorizing the patient's risk of developing postoperative complications. The preoperative evaluation is discussed further in Chapter 11. Furthermore, the link between CRC and a family history of the disease, especially among first-degree relatives, is well established.[20] Knowledge of how the disease has affected the patient's family can provide incentive to implement specific diagnostic procedures. Hereditary cancer syndromes are discussed further in Chapter 3. The location of the tumor within the bowel guides the clinician in determining what other studies should be carried out to evaluate the extent of the tumor.

Tumor Assessment

The next step in the treatment of a colorectal malignancy is to stage the tumor. Accuracy in the initial staging of CRC allows for the selection of appropriate stage-specific therapies. The most effective methods of tumor staging provide both the surgeon and the patient with the ability to make informed decisions regarding preoperative treatment. With the resources provided by these staging techniques, intraoperative options can be discussed and decided on before surgery. Perhaps most important is that long-term outcomes can be predicted. A review of current CRC staging is outlined in Chapter 1, Tables 1–1 and 1–2. Tumor staging and follow-up methods currently used include carcinoembryonic antigen (CEA) level, computed tomography (CT) scans, magnetic resonance imaging (MRI), transrectal ultrasonography (TRUS), and positron emission tomography (PET) imaging with or without combined CT.

Primarily used in the detection of cancer recurrence, CEA levels can also provide useful information in the process of initial tumor staging. Though not a complete diagnostic tool in and of itself, the measurement of CEA can be used to identify patients with a higher risk for developing metastatic disease.[21–23] In a 5-year study of CRC patients, Kanellos and associates[21] confirmed a correspondence between higher CEA levels in venous sampling performed at the time of surgery and advanced stages of the disease. Over an 8-year period, Dixon and colleagues[22] noted a significantly shorter survival time for CRC patients who originally presented with high CEA levels (defined as more than 5 ng/mL). Lower CEA levels were found to be indicative of favorable outcomes and accordingly supportive of more aggressive surgical intervention.

CT scans are used in the detection of hepatic and pulmonary metastases and in the delineation of regional tumor extension.[24] Although CT scans may be of limited value in certain circumstances, the implications of a raised CEA level argue for further exploration of the cancer's progression.[23] Information provided by preoperative tomography can have a direct impact on surgical planning, such as the decision to perform an open versus laparoscopic procedure, allowing for preparatory procedures such as the placement of ureteral stents, the involvement of appropriate support persons or systems, and/or the decision to pursue concurrent resection of other affected organs.[24,25] More complete knowledge of metastatic disease may also lead to alternative considerations of treatment, including the pursuit of more extensive preoperative therapy or palliative care.

MRI has proved to be highly accurate in predicting circumferential resection margin (CRM) in pelvic tumors.[26,27] Moreover, studies cite MRI findings as significant factors in treatment planning, affecting the decision to pursue preoperative neoadjuvant therapy as well as influencing the surgical procedure itself[27] (Fig. 2-4). Providing high-resolution images of the rectal wall, transrectal ultrasonography allows for efficient and accurate local staging of tumors[28] (Fig. 2-5). This technique for the staging of low rectal tumors has been shown to be comparable to results obtained from MRI. However, recently it has been suggested that the technique of transrectal ultrasonography is heavily operator-dependent, and it is recommended that this procedure be done only by an experienced clinician.[29]

The introduction of PET imaging provides a further diagnostic technique for the purposes of tumor staging. It has proved to be of value as an accurate predictor of metastasis and identifier of

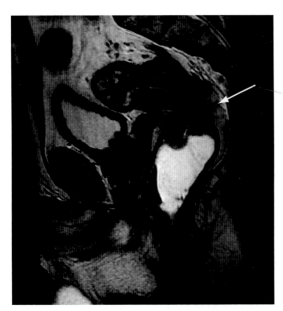

Figure 2-4. MRI of the pelvis (sagittal view) demonstrates a circumferential rectal cancer (*arrow*) with bowel wall invasion.

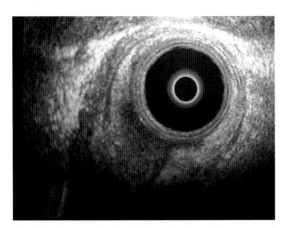

Figure 2-5. Local staging of rectal cancer with transrectal ultrasound demonstrates a clear plane between the tumor and the prostate.

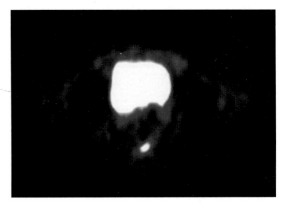

Figure 2-6. Positron emission tomography/computed tomography (PET/CT) of the pelvis demonstrates a fluorodeoxyglucose (FDG)-avid spot in the pelvis in a patient with rectal cancer.

previously unsuspected disease.[30] Its sensitivity in the determination of metastatic disease was found in several studies to be superior to that of CT scanning.[30] Bringing the two techniques together has provided physicians with one of the most effective staging instruments to date; hybrid PET/CT machines have shown increased accuracy in the detection of metastatic CRC[31] (Fig. 2-6). PET/CT scanning is also gaining momentum in the staging of primary disease. In a recent study, PET/CT imaging in primary rectal cancer altered both the initial staging and the initial treatment plan in nearly 30% of patients.[32] Currently, the role of PET/CT is being defined for radiation therapy treatment planning.[33]

Conclusion

Despite studies demonstrating the reduction in mortality associated with screening for CRC, symptomatic presentation remains the most common reason for diagnosis. The symptoms at presentation may vary depending on the location of the primary. Patients and physicians contribute to delay in diagnosis, 7 weeks and 3 weeks on average, respectively. The initial evaluation of a patient with CRC begins with an office visit in which the goal is to establish a rapport with the patient. Further investigations are aimed at staging the cancer clinically.

References

1. Jemal A, Siegel R, Ward E, et al: Cancer Statistics, 2008. CA Cancer J Clin 58:71–96, 2008.
2. Eddy D: ACS report on the cancer-related health checkup. CA Cancer J Clin 30:193–240, 1980.
3. Espey DK, Wu XC, Swan J, et al: Annual report to the nation on the status of cancer, 1975–2004. Cancer 110:2119–2152, 2007.
4. Hardcastle JD, Chamberlain JO, Robinson MH, et al: Randomized controlled trial of faecal-occult blood screening for colorectal cancer. Lancet 348:1472–1477, 1996.
5. Burack RC, Liang J: The early detection of cancer in the primary-care setting: factors associated with the acceptance and completion of recommended procedures. Prev Med 16:739–751, 1987.
6. Gordon NP, Rundal TG, Parker L: Type of health care coverage and the likelihood of being screened for cancer. Med Care 36:636–645, 1998.
7. Church TR, Yeazel MW, Jones RM: A randomized trial of direct mailing of fecal occult blood tests to increase colorectal cancer screening. J Natl Cancer Inst 96:770–780, 2004.
8. Smiljanic S, Gill S: Patterns of diagnosis for colorectal cancer: screening detected vs. symptomatic presentation. Dis Col Rec 51:573–577, 2008.

9. Speights VO, Johnson MW, Stoltenberg PH, et al: Colorectal cancer: current trends in initial clinical manifestations. South Med J 84:575–578, 1991.
10. Selvachandran SN, Hodder RJ, Ballal MS, et al: Prediction of colorectal cancer by patient consultation questionnaire and scoring system: a prospective study. Lancet 360:278–283, 2002.
11. Majumdar SR, Fletcher RH, Evans AT: How does colorectal cancer present? Symptoms, duration, and clues to location. Am J Gastroenterol 94:3039–3045, 1999.
12. Freedman LS, Macaskill P, Smith AN: Multivariate analysis of prognostic factors for operable rectal cancer. Lancet 29: 733–736, 1984.
13. Emslie J, Beart R, Mohiuddin M, Marks: Use of rectal cancer position as a prognostic indicator. Am Surg 10:958–961, 1998.
14. Funch DP: Predictors and consequences of symptom reporting behaviors in colorectal cancer patients. Med Care 26: 1000–1008, 1988.
15. Kyle SM, Isbister WH, Yeong ML: Presentation, duration of symptoms, and staging of colorectal carcinoma. Aust N Z J Surg 61:137–140, 1991.
16. Irvin TT, Greaney MG: Duration of symptoms and prognosis of carcinoma of the colon and rectum. Surg Gynecol Obstet 144:883–886, 1977.
17. Barillari P, de Angelis R, Valabrega S, et al: Relationship of symptom duration and survival in patients with colorectal carcinoma. Eur J Surg Oncol 15:441–445, 1989.
18. Carraro PG, Segala M, Orlotti C, Tiberio G: Outcome of large-bowel perforation in patients with colorectal cancer. Dis Colon Rectum 41:1421–1426, 1998.
19. Fleisher LA, Beckman JA, Brown KA, et al: ACC/AHA 2007 guidelines on perioperative cardiovascular evaluation and care for noncardiac surgery: a report of the American College of Cardiology/American Heart Association Task Force on Practice Guidelines (Writing Committee to Revise the 2002 Guidelines on Perioperative Cardiovascular Evaluation for Noncardiac Surgery). J Am Coll Cardiol 50:159–241, 2007.
20. Slattery ML, Levin TR, Ma K, et al: Family history and colorectal cancer: predictors of risk. Cancer Causes Control 14(9): 879–887, 2003.
21. Kanellos I, Zacharakis E, Kanellos D, et al. Prognostic significance of CEA levels and detection of CEA mRNA in draining venous blood in patients with colorectal cancer. J Surg Oncol 94:3–8, 2006.
22. Dixon M, Haukoos JS, Udani SM, et al: Carcinoembryonic antigen and albumin predict survival in patients with advanced colon and rectal cancer. Arch Surg 138:962–966, 2003.
23. Holt AD, Kim JT, Murell Z, et al: The role of carcinoembryonic antigen as a predictor of the need for preoperative computed tomography in colon cancer patients. Am Surg 72(10):897–901, 2006.
24. Mauchley D, Lynge DC, Langdale LA, et al: Clinical utility and cost-effectiveness of routine preoperative computed tomography scanning in patients with colon cancer. Am J Surge 189(5):512–517, 2005.
25. Zbar AP, Rambarat C, Shenoy RK: Routine preoperative abdominal computed tomography in colon cancer: a utility study. Tech Coloproctol 11:105–109, 2007.
26. Videhult P, Smedh K, Lundin P, Kraaz W: Magnetic resonance imaging for preoperative staging of rectal cancer in clinical practice: high accuracy in predicting circumferential margin with clinical benefit. Colorectal Dis 9(5):412–419, 2007.
27. Mathur P, Smith JJ, Ramsey C, et al: Comparison of CT and MRI in the pre-operative staging of rectal adenocarcinoma and prediction of circumferential resection margin involvement by MRI. Colorectal Dis 5:396–401, 2003.
28. Ptok H, Marusch F, Meyer F, et al: Feasibility and accuracy of TRUS in the pre-treatment staging for rectal carcinoma in general practice. Eur J Surg Oncol 32(4);420–425, 2006.
29. Rao SX, Zeng MS, Xu JM, et al: Assessment of T staging and mesorectal fascia status using high-resolution MRI in rectal cancer with rectal distention. World J Gastroenterol 13(30): 4141–4146, 2007.
30. Llamas-Elvira JM, Rodríguez-Fernández A, Gutiérrez-Sáinz J, et al: Fluorine-18 fluorodeoxyglucose PET in the preoperative staging of colorectal cancer. Eur J Nucl Med Mol Imaging 34:859–867, 2007.
31. Even-Sapir E, Parag Y, Lerman H, et al: Detection of recurrence in patients with cancer: PET/CT after abdominoperineal or anterior resection. Radiology 232(3):815–822, 2004.
32. Gearhart SL, Frassica D, Rossen R, et al: Improved staging with pretreatment positron emission tomography/computed tomography in low rectal cancer. Ann Surg Oncol 13(3):397–404, 2006.
33. Gregoire V, Haustermans K, Xavier G, et al: PET-based treatment planning in radiotherapy: a new standard. J Nucl Med 48:68S–77S, 2007.

3

Hereditary Colorectal Cancer and Polyp Syndromes

Francis M. Giardiello

KEY POINTS

- Hereditary colorectal cancer accounts for 3% to 5% of all cases of colorectal cancer.
- The well-described forms of hereditary colorectal cancer include hereditary nonpolyposis colorectal cancer (HNPCC) and familial adenomatous polyposis (FAP).
- Other inherited syndromes that carry an increased risk of colorectal cancer and neoplasm include *MYH*-associated polyposis (MAP), juvenile polyposis, Cowden syndrome, Bannayan-Ruvalcaba-Riley syndrome, and Peutz-Jeghers syndrome.
- Specific germline mutations cause hereditary colorectal cancer.
- The application of genetic testing, commercially available for many forms of hereditary colorectal cancer, is the standard of care in the management of these disorders.
- Vigilant screening of those at risk and surveillance for those affected are imperative in patients with hereditary colorectal cancer.

Introduction

Colorectal adenocarcinoma is a major human health problem. This malignancy affects 1 million individuals per year worldwide, causing 500,000 deaths annually.[1] In the United States, each person has a 6% lifetime risk of colorectal cancer, and colorectal adenocarcinoma is the second leading cause of cancer-related death.

In the majority of patients, colorectal cancer results from a complex interaction between environmental factors and genetic predisposition. However, in a minority of cases, perhaps 3% to 5%, the occurrence of colorectal adenocarcinoma is directly attributable to a molecularly definable, usually inherited, cause.

This chapter discusses the two well-described forms of hereditary colorectal cancer: hereditary nonpolyposis colorectal cancer (HNPCC) and familial adenomatous polyposis (FAP). Also, other syndromes caused by germline mutations that increase the risk of colorectal cancer are reviewed (Table 3-1).

Hereditary Nonpolyposis Colorectal Cancer

Hereditary nonpolyposis colorectal cancer (HNPCC) is a syndrome known by other appellations including Lynch syndrome and cancer family syndrome.[2] More recently, this condition has been designated HNPCC, unlike FAP, in which colorectal cancer arises from colorectal adenomatous *polyposis*. In hereditary *nonpolyposis* colorectal cancer, colon malignancies usually occur from a single or a few adenomas—hence the term *nonpolyposis*.

Characteristics

HNPCC is an autosomal dominant condition caused by mutation of one of the mismatch repair (MMR) genes.[3] These genes are responsible for maintaining the fidelity of DNA by correcting base-pair mismatches that occur during cell replication. HNPCC accounts for about 1% to 3% of all colorectal cancer. The lifetime risk of colorectal cancer in persons with an MMR gene mutation approaches 80%, and the mean age at diagnosis of colorectal cancer in this syndrome is 44 years old. However, a wide range of age at diagnosis is noted; patients not infrequently present with colorectal malignancy in the second or third decade of life. Most tumors in HNPCC (60% to 80%) are found in the right colon defined as proximal to the splenic

Table 3-1. Inherited Disorders Causing Colorectal Cancer

Inherited Condition	Genes Mutated
Hereditary nonpolyposis colorectal cancer (HNPCC)	Mismatch repair (MMR) genes (*MLH1*, *MSH2*, *MSH6*, *PMS2*)
Muir-Torre syndrome	MMR (usually *MSH2*)
Attenuated HNPCC	*MSH6*
Trimbath syndrome	MMR biallelic mutation
Turcot syndrome	MMR
Familial adenomatous polyposis (FAP)	*APC*
Attenuated FAP	*APC* 5′,3′ mutation
Crail syndrome	*APC*
MYH-associated polyposis (MAP)	*MYH* biallelic mutation
MYH-associated colon cancer	*MYH* monallelic mutation
I1307K mutation of *APC* gene	*APC I1307K* mutation
Juvenile polyposis	*SMAD4*, *BMPR1A*
Cowden syndrome	*PTEN*
Bannayan-Ruvalcaba-Riley syndrome	*PTEN*
Peutz-Jeghers syndrome	*STK11/LKB1*

flexure.[4] Histologically, HNPCC is more likely to be poorly differentiated, abundant in extracellular mucin, and distinguished by a lymphoid (peritumoral lymphocytes) host response to the tumor.[4] Some investigators report that patients with HNPCC have an improved 5-year survival rate, compared stage for stage with individuals with sporadic (noninherited) colorectal malignancy.

HNPCC patients and family members can develop a wide range of extracolonic malignancies.[5] The highest risk for other tumors is that for endometrial cancer (40% to 70% lifetime risk). Also, these patients can have adenocarcinomas of the stomach, small bowel, biliary tract, or ovary; glioblastoma of the brain; and transitional cell carcinoma of the ureter, urethra, bladder, or renal pelvis. The lifetime risks for these cancers range between 2% and 13%. Also, lung, breast, hemopoietic, and prostate and larynx cancers have been reported in HNPCC kindreds, but most studies have not noted increased relative risks for these malignancies. Café-au-lait spots, sebaceous gland tumors, and keratoacanthomas (the latter two are stigmata of the Muir-Torre variant of HNPCC) are the only reported clinical signs in HNPCC patients.

In 1990, the International Collaborative Group (ICG) on Hereditary Nonpolyposis Colorectal Cancer established research criteria for HNPCC[6] (Box 3-1). Known as the Amsterdam I criteria, these guidelines are used for the clinical diagnosis of HNPCC. Some experts felt

Box 3-1. Amsterdam I and II Criteria for Diagnosis of Hereditary Nonpolyposis Colorectal Cancer (HNPCC)

Amsterdam I Criteria

1. Three or more relatives with histologically verified colorectal cancer, one of whom is a first-degree relative of the other two: Familial adenomatous polyposis should be excluded
2. Colorectal cancer involving at least two successive generations
3. One or more colorectal cancer cases diagnosed before age 50

Amsterdam II Criteria

1. Three or more relatives with histologically verified HNPCC-associated cancer (colorectal, endometrial, small bowel, ureter, or renal pelvis), one of whom is a first-degree relative of the other two: Familial adenomatous polyposis should be excluded
2. HNPCC-associated cancer involving at least two successive generations
3. One or more cancer cases diagnosed before age 50

these standards were too stringent for clinical application, and alternative criteria (Amsterdam II criteria) were proposed[7] (see Box 3-1).

Genetics

HNPCC is caused by mutation in one of four DNA MMR genes: *MSH2*, *MLH1*, *PMS2*, and *MSH6*. The germline mutations of *MSH2* and *MLH1* account for more than 90% of the mutations found in HNPCC families.

Microsatellite instability (MSI) is an event noted in the colorectal cancer DNA of individuals with germline mismatch repair gene mutations but not in the patient's adjacent normal colorectal mucosa. MSI is found in 90% of colon tumors of HNPCC patients diagnosed by Amsterdam I criteria.[8] In comparison, MSI is noted in 15% to 20% of individuals with sporadic colorectal cancers. MSI is typified by expansion or contraction of short, repeated DNA sequences (microsatellites) due to insertion or deletion of repeated units. The revised Bethesda criteria are clinical indications for obtaining MSI testing on patients with colorectal cancer[9] (Box 3-2).

Several genotype-phenotype correlations are known in HNPCC as follows: (1) Muir-Torre syndrome, a rare variant of HNPCC, is defined as the association of HNPCC with skin sebaceous gland neoplasms (adenomas, epithelioma, carcinomas) and/or keratoacanthomas.[10] In Muir-Torre patients with identified germline alterations of the MMR genes, *MSH2* mutations are most often found. (2) Those with mutation of the *MSH6* gene have an "attenuated" form of HNPCC.[11] *MSH6* carriers have less risk for all HNPCC-related tumors (except for one) than patients with alterations of the *MLH1* or *MSH2* genes. In *MSH6* carriers, the cumulative risk for colorectal cancer is lower than other MMR gene mutations—69% in males and 30% in females (80% in other MMR gene mutation carriers) at 70 years of age. However, endometrial cancer risk is higher (71%) in those with *MSH6* mutations (40% in other MMR gene carries). (3) Homozygous mutations of the MMR genes, such as *PMS2* and *MLH1*, result in pedigrees typified by cutaneous café-au-lait spots, early onset of colorectal neoplasia, oligopolyposis (5 to 100 adenomas of the colon), glioblastoma at young age, and lymphoma. This constellation of findings is known as Trimbath syndrome.[12] (4) Turcot syndrome describes patients with HNPCC and a glioblastoma brain tumor as an extracolonic manifestation.

Screening

Recommendations for colorectal screening in HNPCC have been generated by consensus opinion.[13] Without genetic testing, first-degree relatives of affected individuals are recommended to have a colonoscopy every 1 to 2 years, starting between 20 and 30 years of age and continuing annually after 40 years of age, or alternatively every 1 to 2 years, beginning at age 20 to 25 or 10 years younger than the age of the person with the earliest colorectal cancer diagnosis in the family—whichever comes first. (Individuals with germline mutations are recommended to have an annual colonoscopy.). Because of the associated risk for endometrial and ovarian cancer, annual screening in women beginning at age 25 to 35 is recommended with consideration of transvaginal ultrasound (with or without CA-125 testing) and endometrial biopsy. In families with a predilection for gastric or urologic tumors, upper endoscopy or urinalysis and urine cytology, respectively, should be included in the surveillance protocol.

When possible, genetic testing for HNPCC is recommended for screening first-degree relatives of HNPCC patients who are over age 18. Screening begins by testing an affected member of the family to identify the pedigree mutation. Microsatellite testing and/or immunohistochemistry testing is indicated for patients who meet the Revised Bethesda Criteria. Germline testing for mutations of *MSH2*, *MLH1*, and *MSH6* is

---

Box 3-2. Revised Bethesda Guidelines for Microsatellite Instability Testing of Colorectal Tumors

1. Colorectal cancer diagnosed in a patient <age 50.
2. Presence of synchronous, metachronous colorectal, or other HNPCC-associated tumors,* regardless of age.
3. Colorectal cancer with the MSI-H[†] histology[‡] diagnosed in a patient <age 60.
4. Colorectal cancer diagnosed in one or more first-degree relatives with an HNPCC-related tumor, with one of the cancers being diagnosed <age 50.
5. Colorectal cancer diagnosed in two or more first- or second-degree relatives with HNPCC-related tumors, regardless of age.

*Colorectal, endometrial, stomach, small bowel, ovarian, pancreas, ureter and renal pelvis, biliary tract, and brain (usually glioblastoma) cancers, and sebaceous gland neoplasms (carcinomas adenomas) and keratoacanthomas

[†]MSI-H, microsatellite instability—high; tumors with changes in two or more of the five National Cancer Institute-recommended panels of microsatellite markers.

[‡]Presence of tumor infiltrating lymphocytes, Crohn-like lymphocytic reaction, mucinous/signet-ring differentiation, or medullary growth pattern.

Adapted from Umar A, Boland CR, Terdiman JP, et al: Revised Bethesda Guidelines for hereditary nonpolyposis colorectal cancer (Lynch syndrome) and microsatellite instability. J Natl Cancer Inst 96:261–268, 2004.

also commercially available. For details of genetic testing in HNPCC, see Chapter 4.

Treatment

Because of the high rate of metachronous colorectal cancer, subtotal colectomy with ileorectal anastomosis and postsurgical endoscopic rectal surveillance are recommended when colorectal cancer develops in the setting of HNPCC.[14] There is no consensus regarding prophylactic surgery of the colon, uterus, and ovaries for MMR gene mutation carriers, but it should be considered on an individual patient basis.

Familial Adenomatous Polyposis

Familial adenomatous polyposis (FAP) is an autosomal dominant syndrome caused by a germline mutation of the *APC* (adenomatous polyposis coli) gene.[15] This disorder occurs in 1 in 10,000 to 14,000 live births, affects both sexes equally, and has worldwide distribution.

Characteristics

Patients with FAP characteristically develop colorectal adenomatous polyposis (i.e., ≥100 colorectal adenomas) in teenage years (Fig. 3-1). The mean age of polyposis development is 15. If colectomy is not performed, the lifetime risk of colorectal cancer is virtually 100% and occurs at an average age of 35 to 43 years.[16]

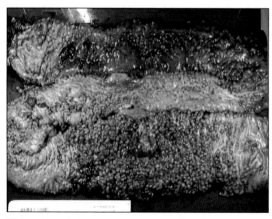

Figure 3-1. Colectomy specimen of familial adenomatous polyposis.   Patient had several hundred adenomatous polyps scattered diffusely throughout the colorectal mucosa.

In addition to colorectal adenomatous polyposis, patients with FAP can develop a variety of benign extracolonic manifestations.[17] These include cutaneous lesions (lipomas, fibromas, and sebaceous and epidermoid cysts), desmoid tumors, osteomas, occult radiopaque jaw lesions, dental abnormalities, pigmented ocular fundic lesions (congenital hypertrophy of the retinal pigment epithelium), and nasopharyngeal angiofibroma. Patients can also have extracolonic polyps, including adenomas of the small intestine and stomach and fundic gland retention polyps of the stomach. Extracolonic malignancies can occur in those affected with FAP. These malignancies comprise hepatoblastoma, upper gastrointestinal tract malignancies (duodenum and periampullary area, very rarely jejunum), and thyroid gland, biliary tree, pancreas, and brain malignancies.

Genetics

Mutations in the *APC* gene, located on chromosome 5q21, account for about 95% of all cases of colorectal adenomatous polyposis.[18] The *APC* gene is a tumor suppressor gene comprising 15 exons encoding a 2843 amino acid protein. *APC* gene protein functions include cell adhesion, signal transduction, and transcriptional activation. Ten percent of FAP patients have a mutation in codon 1309, although more than 300 mutations of the *APC* gene causing FAP have been reported. The test of choice for confirming the diagnosis of FAP and screening family members for this syndrome is *APC* gene testing for deleterious mutations.

Attenuated Familial Adenomatous Polyposis

Mutations between codon 169 and 1393 result in classic FAP, as previously described. However, mutations in the very 5′ and 3′ regions of the gene (at the extremes of the coding region) cause a milder disorder called *attenuated familial adenomatous polyposis* (AFAP). Several genotype-phenotype correlations occur in FAP, but the most important is AFAP.[19] AFAP is characterized by oligopolyposis (fewer than 100 adenomatous polyps) rather than polyposis at clinical presentation, but marked phenotypic variation in polyp number can exist within a pedigree. Also, AFAP patients have a delayed onset of colorectal cancer—about 12 years later than in classic FAP. In addition, a plethora of upper tract lesions has been noted in some patients with AFAP. Of note, *Crail syndrome* is the term applied to patients with FAP and brain tumor, usually medulloblastoma.

Screening

The screening test of choice for at-risk individuals (i.e., first-degree relatives of those affected with FAP) in classic or attenuated FAP families is genetic testing of the *APC* gene for mutations. When genetic testing is not feasible, at-risk individuals in classic FAP families should undergo screening with yearly sigmoidoscopy starting at age 12 years, then every 2 years after age 25 and every 3 years after age 35. After age 50, patients are recommended to follow the Multi-Society Task Force–American Cancer Society guideline for colorectal cancer screening of average-risk individuals. In AFAP pedigrees, at-risk individuals should have a colonoscopy at ages 12, 15, 18, and 21 and every 2 years after.

Treatment

Colectomy continues to be the only effective treatment for reducing the ineluctable risk of colorectal cancer in FAP patients. In general, surgery is recommended at the time of diagnosis to minimize any risk of colorectal cancer. Surgical options include colectomy with ileorectal anastomosis, total protocolectomy with Brooke ileostomy, and total protocolectomy with ileo-anal pouch procedure. For patients with classic FAP, most authorities recommend removal of the entire colorectum, if possible. In AFAP, the option of colectomy with ileorectal anastomosis should be considered. Because cancer can occur in the rectum, patients with retained rectal segment should have biannual endoscopic evaluation of this area. In those with ileal pouches, endoscopic surveillance should occur on a biennial basis, since neoplasia has been seen in the pouch.

Duodenal and periampullary carcinoma occurs in 4% to 5% of FAP patients.[20] Therefore, most experts recommend upper endoscopic surveillance of the stomach, duodenum, and periampullary area every 1 to 3 years, depending on the findings. Gastrectomy is usually not indicated in patients with FAP, even those with multiple gastric fundic gland polyps.

FAP patients also have an increased risk for neoplasms of the thyroid, usually in women in the third decade of life.[21] A high index of suspicion should be maintained for this tumor with annual physical examination of the thyroid and consideration for ultrasound screening.

Hepatoblastoma occurs in 1 in 300 at-risk persons under age 7 years and 1 in 150 in offspring who are determined by genetic testing to have FAP.[22] Because of the magnitude of hepatoblastoma risk and the potential curability with early surgical intervention, consideration for ultrasound testing should be given in at-risk youngsters between birth and 7 years old.

MYH-Associated Polyposis

MYH-associated polyposis (MAP) is a recently described cause of colorectal adenomatous polyposis and oligopolyposis.[23] MAP is an autosomal recessive syndrome caused by biallelic germline mutation of the *MYH* gene, the human homolog *Mut Y* gene, located on chromosome 1p35. The *MYH* gene acts in the base excision repair (BER) pathway to remove adenine bases that mispair with 8-oxoguanine during oxidation of DNA. Failure to correct these mispairings leads to $G:C \rightarrow T:A$ transversion mutations that are typical of oxidative DNA damage. Germline *MYH* mutations inhibit the BER pathway and prevent the repair of somatic *APC* mutations, leading to the FAP phenotype (similar to FAP caused by germline mutations within the *APC* gene).

MAP accounts for 1% of all cases of adenomatous polyposis but up to 30% of cases of oligopolyposis. The highest incidence of biallelic *MYH* mutations is in patients with 15 to 100 colorectal adenomas. The most common pathogenic mutations of the *MYH* gene in the Caucasian population are *Y165C* and *G382D*. Two other protein truncating mutations, *E466X* and *Y90X*, are founder mutations in Indian and Pakistani descendants, respectively. Most other changes found in the *MYH* gene are classified as variants of uncertain significance, since limited data exist regarding the effects these changes have on the function of this newly discovered gene.

Affected individuals develop colorectal adenomatous polyposis or oligopolyposis (i.e., less than 100 adenomas at presentation) at a young age, with phenotypes indistinguishable from classic or attenuated FAP. Also, extracolonic manifestations like those in FAP/AFAP can be noted in these patients. Biallelic mutations of the *MYH* gene may also be a rare cause of early-onset colorectal cancer in the absence of multiple colorectal adenomas.

Although increased risk of colorectal cancer and multiple adenomas is known to occur in patients with biallelic *MYH* gene mutations, the risk of colorectal neoplasia among monoallelic carriers is unclear. Recently, a Canadian population-based series of 1238 colorectal cancer patients and 1255 healthy controls noted a mild increased risk of colorectal cancer in monoallelic carriers (relative risk 1.54; 95% CI 1.10–2.16).[24]

Screening

First-degree relatives of patients with MAP are at risk for inheriting this autosomal recessive disorder. Offspring of affected individuals are at least monoallelic *MYH* mutation carriers. These individuals should consider starting colorectal cancer screening at a younger age—perhaps at 40 years old—rather than age 50, as recommended for the average-risk population. Also, MAP patients should consider genetic testing to determine whether biallelic mutation is present, as described in detail in Chapter 4.

Treatment

The treatment of patients with biallelic mutation of the *MYH* gene should be the same as that described for patients with FAP and AFAP.

APC I1307K Mutation

Discovered in 1997, *I1307K* of the *APC* gene causes familial colorectal cancer.[25] This mutation forms an unstable polyadenine tract in the *APC* gene, which confuses the DNA replication machinery and results in susceptibility to additional somatic mutations elsewhere on the same allele of the *APC* gene during cell division. Found in 6% to 8% of the Ashkenazi and 1% to 4.7% of non-Ashkenazi Jews, this mutation doubles the lifetime risk of colorectal cancer in gene mutation carriers. Contrary to findings in patients with other germline *APC* gene mutations, extracolonic malignancies have not been found to carry excess risk in individuals with

APC I1307K mutation. Colonoscopy every 2 to 3 years has been suggested for those with this mutation. This is an autosomal dominant condition, and screening first-degree relatives of affected individuals can be done by commercial genetic testing.

Juvenile Polyposis Syndrome

Juvenile polyps are histologically distinct gastrointestinal polyps that can manifest as sporadic juvenile polyps or as juvenile polyposis syndrome. Sporadic juvenile polyps are not infrequently encountered. Most affected individuals present to medical attention in infancy or early childhood (average age of presentation 4 years) with *one* or *two* juvenile polyps in the rectosigmoid colon. The usual symptoms are rectal bleeding or anal prolapse of a polyp. Sporadic juvenile polyps are a noninherited condition without an increased risk of colorectal cancer.

Familial/Juvenile Polyposis Coli

Juvenile polyposis can be strictly defined as five or more juvenile polyps.[26] Affected individuals can have from five to hundreds of polyps occurring primarily in the colorectum, but in some patients polyps are noted in the small intestine and stomach. Juvenile polyps are hamartomas with edematous mucosa and dilated mucus-filled cysts. Juvenile polyposis is an autosomal dominant syndrome caused in 24% of cases by mutation of *BMPR1A* (*b*one *m*orphogenetic *p*rotein *r*eceptor 1A) gene on chromosome 10q22-23, and in 17% by mutation of the *SMAD4/MADH4* (small mothers against decapentaplegic deleted in pancreatic carcinoma locus 4) gene on chromosome 18q21, also known as *DPC4* (deleted in pancreatic carcinoma locus 4).[27] Whether *PTEN* germline mutations are present in these patients is unclear. Patients typically present to medical attention in late childhood or early adolescence (but can be preschoolers) with anemia, rectal bleeding, failure to thrive, hypoalbuminemia, and/or abdominal pain. Other individuals, with less polyp burden, can be asymptomatic.

A high incidence of colorectal neoplasia (dysplasia and adenocarcinoma) is noted in individuals affected with juvenile polyposis, with lifetime estimates of 38%.[28] Colorectal cancer occurs at a young age (average 37 years), but dysplasia has been found in the colectomy specimens of children less than 5 years of age. Gastric, small bowel, and pancreatic cancers also have been reported to occur in these patients, but the true risk of these tumors is unclear. Arteriovenous and other cardiovascular malformations are associated manifestations in patients with *SMAD4/MADH4* mutations (alterations in *SMAD4* have recently been implicated as the cause of hereditary hemorrhagic telangiectasia, also known as Osler-Weber-Rendu syndrome).

Screening

If possible, screening should be carried out in at-risk persons with genetic testing for *SMAD4* or *BMPR1A* mutations after first identifying the pedigree mutation in an affected family member. If genetic testing is not available, an initial screening of first-degree relatives at 12 years of age with colonoscopy should be considered. Some authorities recommended subsequent screening with endoscopy every 3 to 5 years.

Treatment

Sporadic juvenile polyps should be removed. In patients with a solitary juvenile polyp and no family history, the lifetime risk of colorectal cancer is equal to that of the general population. In contrast, patients with multiple juvenile polyps (five or more rectosigmoid polyps) or with a family history of juvenile polyps should have complete upper and lower endoscopy and small bowel radiography examination to determine whether juvenile polyps exist. In those affected, periodic colorectal surveillance by endoscopy with multiple random biopsies of both polyps and flat mucosa every 1 to 3 years is recommended. The upper tract should probably also be surveyed. Removal of dysplastic juvenile polyps should be attempted by endoscopic polypectomy. Colectomy, with consideration for total proctocolectomy, is indicated in those in whom surveillance is not feasible and in those with persistent rectal bleeding or refractory protein loss. Postoperatively, remaining colorectal requires vigilant surveillance owing to the risk of metachronous neoplasia. Screening for arteriovenous and cardiovascular malformations in patients with *SMAD4/MADH4* mutations should be considered.

Cowden Syndrome

Characteristics

Cowden syndrome (CS) is a very rare autosomal dominant syndrome with variable hamartomatous involvement of the skin, mucous membranes, thyroid, breast, gastrointestinal tract, and adnexa.[26] Germline mutations of the *PTEN* (phosphatase and tensin) gene on chromosome 10q are found in 80% of these patients. The characteristic feature of this condition on physical examination is multiple facial trichilemmomas occurring around the mouth, nose, and eyes noted in more than 90% of patients. Also, verrucous skin lesions of the face and limbs and cobblestone-like papules of the gingiva and buccal mucosa and tongue can be seen.

About 35% of patients with CS have gastrointestinal hamartomatous polyps. These polyps can occur throughout the intestinal tract including the esophagus. The histopathology of these lesions can be variable with gastrointestinal lipomas, juvenile polyps, inflammatory polyps, ganglioneuromas, and lymphoid hyperplasia.

Extragastrointestinal lesions in affected individuals include adenomas and cysts of the thyroid (70%), thyroid cancer (3%), fibrocystic disease and fibroadenomas of the breast (52%) in women, and breast cancer (28%). In 60% of patients, genitourinary disease (carcinoma of the ovary, uterus, and cervix and ovarian cysts) is noted. Central nervous system, eye, craniofacial, and skeletal abnormalities have also been reported. An association between CS and Lhermitte-Duclos disease, a hamartomatous condition of the cerebellum, has been noted.

Treatment

Recognition of CS provides the opportunity to screen for thyroid and breast cancer. Males and females should have surveillance with annual physical examinations and attention to the thyroid examination instituted at age 18 years or 5 years younger than the age of the person with the earliest cancer in the family. For women, a clinical breast examination starting at 25 years with mammography at 30 years or 5 years younger than the age of the person with the earliest breast cancer in the family is recommended. Also, women should consider endometrial biopsies at 35 years or 5 years younger than the age of the person with the earliest uterine cancer in the family and a urinanalysis annually. If gastrointestinal symptoms are not present, investigation of the gastrointestinal tract is not necessary.

Bannayan-Riley-Ruvalcaba Syndrome (Bannayan-Zonana Syndrome)

Bannayan-Riley-Ruvalcaba syndrome (BRRS) is known by several names including Bannayan-Zonana syndrome and Bannayan–Ruvalcaba-Myhre-Smith syndrome. BRRS is an ill-defined, very rare, and probably autosomal dominant condition that seems to be a variant of CS.[26]

Characteristics

BRRS patients can have manifestations of CS as previously described. However, craniofacial abnormalities, developmental delay, and lipid storage myopathy can distinguish this condition from CS. Characteristic findings in BRRS (not noted in CS) on physical examination are macrocephaly and pigmented macules on the shaft and glans of the penis. In addition, affected patients can have hamartomatous polyps of the colon including juvenile polyps. The rate of gastrointestinal malignancy in these patients appears to be no greater than in the general population but depends on the type of gastrointestinal polyps discovered. Germline mutations of the PTEN (phosphatase and tensin) gene on chromosome 10q are found in 50% to 60% of BRRS patients.

Treatment

The conservative recommendations for BRRS patients include screening in a similar manner to those with CS.

Peutz-Jeghers Syndrome

Peutz-Jeghers syndrome (PJS) is an autosomal dominant condition caused by mutation of the STK11 (serine threonine kinase 11) gene (also known as the LKB1 gene) on chromosome 19p.[29]

Characteristics

PJS polyps occur primarily in the small intestine but can also be noted in the colon and stomach.

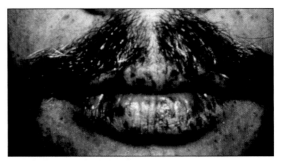

Figure 3-2. Labial pigmentation in patient with Peutz-Jeghers syndrome.

Polyps number 1 to 20 per intestinal segment. Histopathologically, the PJS polyp has epithelium supported by an arborizing framework of smooth muscle. Patients with PJS characteristically have brown macular melanin pigmentation measuring 1 to 5 mm on the lips and buccal mucosa (Fig. 3-2), and occasionally on the digits of hands, feet, and above the eyelashes. These cutaneous lesions are most pronounced in childhood and often fade in teenage years.

The primary complication of PJS patients in childhood is small intestine intussusception; intestinal bleeding can also occur.[30] Neoplastic transformation of the Peutz-Jeghers polyp is rare but can happen. Adults have a strikingly increased risk for colon cancer with a lifetime risk of 34%. Other cancers that occur very frequently are cancers of the breast, pancreas, stomach, ovary, lung, small intestine, uterus, and esophagus.[31] Unusual tumors noted in patients with PJS are sex cord tumors of the ovary and adenoma malignum of the cervix in women and testicular tumors in prepubescent boys.

Screening

Screening at-risk individuals (i.e., those who are first-degree relatives of PJS patients) beginning at birth with annual history and physical examination and evaluation for melanotic spots, precocious puberty, and testicular tumors is recommended.[31] At-risk individuals who are asymptomatic and without stigmata at age 8 should be offered genetic testing for mutation of the STK11/LKB1 gene (see Chapter 4). If genetic testing is not feasible, then at-risk members should have upper endoscopy, colonoscopy, and small bowel series at ages 12, 18, and 24.

Table 3-2. Recommendations for Peutz-Jeghers Syndrome Surveillance by Age and Sex

Age (years)	Males	Females
From birth to 12 years	History and physical exam with examination of testicles and routine blood tests annually (consider ultrasound of the testicles every 2 years until age 12)	History and physical exam with routine blood tests annually
At age 8	Upper endoscopy and small bowel series.* If positive, continue every 2–3 years	Upper endoscopy, and small bowel series.* If positive, continue every 2–3 years
Age 18 on	Colonoscopy, upper endoscopy, and small bowel series* every 2–3 years	Colonoscopy, upper endoscopy, and small bowel series* every 2–3 years Breast self-exam monthly
Age 21 on	—	Pelvic exam with Pap smear annually
Age 25 on*	Endoscopic ultrasound every 1–2 years (consider CT scan and/or CA 19-9 as options)	Endoscopic ultrasound every 1–2 years (consider CT scan and/or CA 19-9 as options) Clinical breast exam semiannually Mammography† annually (MRI offered as alternative) Transvaginal ultrasound and serum CA-125 annually

*Consider capsule endoscopy intermittently to limit radiation exposure.
†Mammography may begin earlier based on earliest age of onset in family.

Treatment

Authorities recommend polypectomy for polyps in the stomach or colon that are larger than 1 cm noted during endoscopic surveillance. Surgery or endoscopic removal has been recommended for symptomatic or rapidly growing small intestinal polyps or asymptomatic polyps larger than 1 to 1.5 cm. Recently, the use of double-balloon enteroscopy for removal of small bowel PJS polyps has been reported and may decrease the need for laparotomy.

Surveillance

As noted, individuals affected with PJS have a high risk at a young age for colorectal cancer as well as for a wide variety of other malignancies. Consequently, a series of surveillance studies are recommended.[31] See Table 3-2 for surveillance guidelines for patients with PJS according to age and sex.

References

1. Ferlay J, Bray F, Pisani P, Parkin DM: Globocan 2000: Cancer Incidence, Mortality and Prevalence Worldwide, Version 1.0. IARC CancerBase No. 5. Lyon, IARC, 2001.
2. Lynch HT, Shaw MW, Magnuson CW, et al: Hereditary factors in two large midwestern kindreds. Arch Intern Med 117: 206–212, 1966.
3. Annie Yu HJ, Lin KM, Ota DM, Lynch HT: Hereditary nonpolyposis colorectal cancer: preventive management. Cancer Treat Rev 29(6):461–470, 2003.
4. Smyrk TC, Lynch HT, Watson PA, Appelman HD: Histologic features of hereditary nonpolyposis colorectal carcinoma. In

Utsunomiya J, Lynch HT (eds): Hereditary Colorectal Cancer. Tokyo: Springer-Verlag, 1990, pp 357.
5. Aarnio M, Sankila R, Pukkala E, et al: Cancer risk in mutation carriers of DNA-mismatch-repair genes. Int J Cancer 81: 214–218, 1999.
6. Vasen HF, Mecklin JP, Meera Khan P, Lynch HT: The International Collaborative Group on Hereditary Non-Polyposis Colorectal Cancer (ICG-HNPCC). Dis Colon Rectum 34: 424–425, 1991.
7. Vasen HF, Watson P, Mecklin JP, Lynch HT, the ICG-HNPCC: New criteria for hereditary non-polyposis colorectal cancer (HNPCC, Lynch syndrome) proposed by the International Collaborative Group on HNPCC (ICG-HNPCC). Gastroenterology 116:1453, 1999.
8. Aaltonen LA, Salovaara R, Kristo P, et al: Incidence of hereditary nonpolyposis colorectal cancer and the feasibility of molecular screening for the disease. N Engl J Med 338:1481–1487, 1998.
9. Umar A, Boland CR, Terdiman JP, et al: Revised Bethesda Guidelines for hereditary nonpolyposis colorectal cancer (Lynch syndrome) and microsatellite instability. J Natl Cancer Inst. 96(4):261–268, 2004.
10. Mangold E, Pagenstecher C, Leister M, et al: A genotype-phenotype correlation in HNPCC: strong predominance of MSH2 mutations in 41 patients with Muir-Torre syndrome. J Med Genet 41(7):567–572, 2004.
11. Hendriks YM, Wagner A, Morreau H, et al: Cancer risk in hereditary nonpolyposis colorectal cancer due to MSH6 mutations impact on counseling and surveillance. Gastroenterology 127:17–25, 2004.
12. Trimbath JD, Petersen GM, Erdman SH, et al: Cafe-au-lait spots and early onset colorectal neoplasia: a variant of HNPCC? Fam Cancer 1:101–105, 2001.
13. NCCN Colorectal Cancer Screening Practice Guidelines. National Comprehensive Cancer Network. Oncology CSCR16, 2005.
14. Burke W, Petersen G, Lynch P, et al: Recommendations for follow-up care of individuals with inherited predisposition to cancer. I. Hereditary nonpolyposis colon cancer. JAMA 277:915–919, 1997.
15. Kinzler KW, Nilbert MC, Su LK, et al: Identification of FAP locus genes from chromosome 5q21. Science 253:661–665, 1991.
16. Bussey HJR: Familial Polyposis Coli. Family Studies, Histopathology, Differential Diagnosis, and Results of Treatment. Baltimore: Johns Hopkins University Press, 1975.
17. Trimbath JD, Giardiello FM: Genetic testing and counseling for hereditary colorectal cancer. Aliment Pharmacol Ther 16: 1843–1857, 2002.

18. Laken SJ, Papadopoulos N, Petersen G, et al: Analysis of masked mutations in familial adenomatous polyposis. Proc Natl Acad Sci 96:2322–2326, 1999.
19. Brensinger JD, Laken SJ, Luce MC, et al: Variable phenotype of familial adenomatous polyposis in pedigrees with 3′ mutations in the *APC* gene. Gut 43:548–552, 1998.
20. Offerhaus GJA, Giardiello FM, Krush AJ, et al: The risk of upper gastrointestinal cancer in familial adenomatous polyposis. Gastroenterology 102:1980–1982, 1992.
21. Giardiello FM, Offerhaus GJA, Lee DH, et al: Increased risk of thyroid and pancreatic carcinoma in familial adenomatous polyposis. Gut 34:1394–1396, 1993.
22. Giardiello FM, Offerhaus GJA, Krush AJ, et al: The risk of hepatoblastoma in familial adenomatous polyposis. J Pediatr 119:766–788, 1991.
23. Sieber OM, Lipton L, Crabtree M, et al: Multiple colorectal adenomas, classic adenomatous polyposis, and germ-line mutations in MYH. N Engl J Med 348:791–799, 2003.
24. Croitoru ME, Cleary SP, Di Nicola N, et al: Association between biallelic and monoallelic germline MYH gene mutations and colorectal cancer risk. J Natl Cancer Inst 96:1631–1634, 2004.
25. Laken SJ, Petersen GM, Gruber SB, et al: Familial colorectal cancer in Askenazim due to a hypermutable tract in APC. Nature Genet 17:79–83, 1997.
26. Burt RW, Jacoby RF: Polyposis syndromes. In Yamada T, Alpers DH, Kaplowitz N, et al (eds): Textbook of Gastroenterology, 4th ed. Philadelphia: Lippincott Williams & Wilkins, 2003.
27. Howe JR, Sayed MG, Ahmed AF, et al: The prevalence of MADH4 and BMPR1A mutations in juvenile polyposis and absence of BMPR2, BMPR1B, and ACVR1 mutations. J Med Genet 41:484–491, 2004.
28. Coburn MC, Pricolo VE, DeLuca FG, Bland KI: Malignant potential in intestinal juvenile polyposis syndromes. Ann Surg Oncol 2:386–391, 1995.
29. Jenne DE, Reimann H, Nezu J, et al: Peutz-Jeghers syndrome is caused by mutations in a novel serine threonine kinase. Nature Genet 18:38–43, 1998.
30. Utsunomiya J, Gocho H, Miyanaga T, et al: Peutz-Jeghers syndrome: its natural course and management. Johns Hopkins Med J 136:71–82, 1975.
31. Giardiello FM, Trimbath JD: Peutz-Jeghers syndrome and management recommendations. Clin Gastroenterol Hepatol 4:408–415, 2006.

4

Genetic Screening

Cheryl J. Pendergrass

KEY POINTS

- Genetic testing is an important part of the clinical care of patients with colorectal cancer.
- Prior to genetic testing, patients should have genetic counseling to learn about the benefits and potential risks associated with testing.
- As our understanding increases regarding hereditary conditions, the role of genetic testing in the clinical management of this disease will be further defined.

Introduction

Over the past 20 years, tremendous strides have been made in understanding the molecular mechanisms of hereditary colorectal cancer syndromes. Genetic testing for many inherited colorectal cancer syndromes is clinically available and is becoming the standard of care in the management of these disorders. When used appropriately, genetic testing can provide opportunities for patients and at-risk family members to confirm a diagnosis, modify screening strategies, and adopt effective coping and management skills. Genetic testing also provides physicians with information regarding prognosis, surgical management, and the likelihood of response to chemotherapeutic agents. There are several hereditary colorectal cancer syndromes, and it is crucial to identify individuals who are at risk and who are appropriate for genetic testing (Table 4-1).

Proper Use of Clinical Genetic Testing

The annual incidence of colorectal cancer in the United States is approximately 146,970, causing 49,920 deaths per year.[1] Most colorectal cancers—70% to 80%—are sporadic, meaning that they are caused by numerous environmental factors as well as genetic influences. About 10% to 20% of colorectal cancers are familial, meaning that affected individuals have two or more first- or second-degree relatives with colorectal cancer. Unfortunately, the cause of most familial colorectal cancers is not understood, and no clinically useful genetic testing is available.[2] Only 5% to 10% of all colorectal cancers are hereditary and associated with a known gene(s) mutation. Therefore, most persons diagnosed with colorectal cancer are not appropriate for genetic testing.

Several organizations have policy statements concerning genetic testing, including the American Society of Clinical Oncology (ASCO), the National Advisory Council of Human Genome Research, and the American Gastroenterological Association (AGA).[3-5] Genetic testing is appropriate only for individuals who meet the following five criteria: (1) the family history or clinical history is suspicious for a hereditary cancer syndrome; (2) the person has a reasonable likelihood of carrying an altered cancer susceptibility gene; (3) the genetic test result is interpretable; (4) the genetic test result will influence medical management of the patient or the patient's family members or is integral to reproductive decision making; and (5) the patient wants the information.

Genetic testing is a complex process, and the organizations producing policy statements on this topic emphasize the need for in-person pre- and post-test genetic counseling because of the clinical, psychosocial, and ethical issues raised throughout the testing process. Studies show that, without consultation with a genetic counselor or physician experienced with genetic testing, predictive and diagnostic genetic testing

Table 4-1. Hereditary Colorectal Cancer Syndromes

Disease	Gene(s) (Cost)	Inheritance Pattern	Clinical Manifestations (% lifetime risk) (average age at diagnosis)
Lynch syndrome	MLH1 MSH2 MSH6 PMS2 ($800–2000)	Autosomal dominant	Colorectal cancer (80%) (age 44) Endometrial cancer (40–70%) Ovarian cancer (10–12%) Small bowel cancer, stomach cancer, transitional cell cancer of ureter, urethra, bladder, renal pelvis, and biliary tract cancer (2–13%) Sebaceous adenomas/carcinomas (Muir-Torre variant, <1%) Glioblastoma (Turcot variant, <1%)
FAP/AFAP	APC MYH ($1400–1800)	Autosomal dominant (20–30% de novo) Autosomal recessive	Colorectal cancer (100%) (FAP late 30s) (AFAP 50s) Duodenal cancer (4–12%) Thyroid cancer (2%) Pancreas cancer (1–2%) Hepatoblastoma (1%) (age 0–7) Medulloblastoma (Turcot variant, <1%) FAP, >100 colorectal adenomas (100%) (teens) AFAP, <100 colorectal adenomas (90%) (40s) Upper GI tract adenomas (50–90%) Fundic gland polyps (50%) Osteomas, dental abnormalities, nasopharyngeal angiofibromas, CHRPE, desmoid tumors, cutaneous lesions
I1307K (Ashkenazi Jewish)	APC ($400–600)	Autosomal dominant	Colorectal cancer (10–20%) (late 50s) <10 Colorectal adenomas
Juvenile polyposis syndrome	BMPR1A SMAD4 ($1000–2000)	Autosomal dominant (25% de novo)	Small bowel cancer (9–50%) Colorectal cancer (38%) (37 years) Stomach cancer Pancreatic cancer Colorectal hamartomatous polyps (98%) Upper GI tract hamartomatous polyps (2–13%) Arteriovenous malformations (SMAD4) Hemorrhagic telangectasia (SMAD4)
Peutz-Jeghers syndrome	STK11 ($900–1500)	Autosomal dominant (50% de novo)	Breast cancer (54%) Colorectal cancer (39%) Pancreas cancer (36%) Stomach cancer (29%) Ovarian cancer (21%) Lung cancer (15%) Small intestine cancer (13%) Cervical cancer (10%) Endometrial cancer (9%) Testicular cancer (9%) Esophageal cancer (0.5%) Melanin pigmentation of lips, buccal mucosa, fingers, and toes and above eyelashes GI hamartomatous polyps Small bowel intussusception
Cowden syndrome	PTEN ($900–1200)	Autosomal dominant	GI hamartomatous polyps (35%) Facial trichilemmomas: mouth, eyes, nose (90%) Verrucous skin lesions of face and limbs Adenomas and cysts of thyroid (70%) Follicular thyroid cancer (3%) Fibrocystic breasts and fibroadenomas of breast (53%) Breast cancer (28%) Genitourinary disease: ovarian cancer, endometrial cancer, cervical cancer, ovarian cysts (60%) Papillomatous papules: face, lips, tongue, oral mucosa
Bannayan-Riley-Ruvalcaba syndrome (BRRS)	PTEN ($900–1200)	Autosomal dominant	Cowden syndrome manifestations Developmental delay Lipid storage myopathy Pigmented macules on the penis

CHRPE, congenital hypertrophy of the retinal pigmented epithelium; FAP/AFAP, familial adenomatous polyposis/attenuated familial adenomatous polyposis.

is often ordered and interpreted inappropriately.[6] The National Society of Genetic Counselors maintains a directory of genetic counselors listed by geographic location, institution, and specialty (Box 4-1).

The Genetic Counseling Process

Several components of the genetic counseling process should be discussed in person with patients who are considering genetic testing. The genetic counseling session should include discussion of risk stratification and risk assessment, genetic syndrome education, genetic testing strategy, choosing a laboratory, cost and insurance coverage, psychosocial issues, resources, genetic discrimination, informed consent, follow-up, and disclosure.

Risk stratification and risk assessment involve (a) constructing a pedigree to view the cancer pattern in the family, (b) obtaining medical records on the patient and as many affected family members as possible, (c) developing an overall assessment of the family to recognize a hereditary syndrome, (d) identifying at-risk individuals, (e) determining the patient's risk perceptions and expectations, and (f) establishing the patient's motivation for gathering information and genetic testing. The most important step in the diagnosis of a hereditary colorectal

cancer syndrome is a detailed cancer family history. A detailed pedigree history determines a true suspicion for a hereditary cancer syndrome, whether genetic testing is appropriate, and who is the most appropriate family member to begin the genetic testing process. Without a comprehensive cancer family history, the likelihood of misdiagnosis or nondiagnosis of a syndrome is high.

Patient education on the genetic syndrome involves the general characteristics of hereditary cancer syndromes and the specific features of the disorder suspected in the patient. A discussion of the inheritance pattern for the suspected syndrome, including a description of basic genetics and the gene(s) associated with the syndrome, is given. Also, a physical examination may be performed to look for characteristic signs of a hereditary cancer syndrome along with the provision of management recommendations.

The genetic testing strategy may be complex or very straightforward. If genetic testing involves a stepwise process, this should be explained along with a discussion of testing type, whether the test is for screening or diagnostic purposes, the timelines, and the cost. Also, identification of the most appropriate family member to begin testing should be determined. Genetic testing is most informative when starting with an affected family member to identify the specific family mutation. This strategy is important because most genetic tests are not 100% sensitive, and therefore the mutation search should start in an individual who appears affected. Once the family mutation is identified, this person serves as the positive control, and other family members can have predictive testing. Findings suggest that most individuals who undergo genetic testing had a previous diagnosis of cancer and are likely motivated to undergo testing to allow unaffected relatives predictive testing.[7] If a specific mutation cannot be identified in an affected family member, the results are considered inconclusive and other unaffected at-risk family members cannot undergo genetic testing for the suspected syndrome.

Choosing a laboratory for genetic testing can be a complicated process, since most genetic tests are performed at only a few laboratories. Several aspects should be considered when choosing a laboratory. Most important, the laboratory should be Clinical Laboratory Improvement Amendments (CLIA)–certified.

This organization continues to monitor quality control and reliability. Also, researching the laboratory's testing options is necessary to determine whether the specific type of genetic testing essential to answering your patient's clinical question is offered. Often, several methodologies are available for genetic testing of a particular gene. Some tests can be performed on only one type of sample (i.e., blood, tissue, amniotic fluid); other methods require the initial identification of the family mutation. Also, turnaround time and cost are of concern because some patients need the results quickly for medical management, whereas others, whose testing is not covered by insurance, would rather have testing at a slower, less expensive laboratory. Finally, support services offered by the laboratory, including interpretation of results, insurance billing, and insurance preauthorization should be understood.

Cost and insurance coverage for genetic testing always concern patients, since genetic testing is expensive. Full gene sequencing with large rearrangement, the gold standard for most hereditary cancer syndromes, ranges from $1000 to $3000. Once a family mutation is identified, genetic testing for at-risk family members is much less expensive, ranging from $250 to $500 (testing relatives for only the known family mutation). Many insurance companies cover at least a portion of the cost, but an understanding of the patient's insurance plan is essential. Most laboratories offer an insurance preauthorization process, allowing patients to know their out-of-pocket costs before testing. Preauthorization often requires a letter of medical necessity with diagnostic testing codes from the health care provider.

Psychosocial issues vary from one patient to another, but the amount of patient distress usually depends on his or her motivation for testing. Research shows that the greatest distress occurs when testing is undertaken to help guide personal screening and surgical management.[8] Some patients who test positive for a deleterious gene mutation are relieved to know the cause of their condition and thankful to be able to provide other at-risk family members with informative test results. Others are scared, angry, depressed, in denial, shocked, or feeling guilty about the potential of passing the mutation to the next generation. Patients who test negative usually feel relief and happiness; however, others may have survivor's guilt, for being the family member pardoned from the disease, or mutation regret, the sense of lost opportunities by having lived life as though affected. Patients who receive inconclusive results (i.e., "no mutation found" in absence of a family mutation) are usually unsatisfied, whereas others have a false sense of security because a definitive mutation was not identified. Genetic testing also has health implications for other family members. Therefore, this issue should be addressed in detail with patients, noting the possibility of changing family dynamics.

Providing resources for families undergoing genetic testing affords patients with further support and information to cope with a diagnosis, decide about genetic testing, and select a management plan that works best for their personal situation. Genetic counselors often facilitate the patient's entry into clinical trials, research studies, and support groups, and even connect them with other patients in similar situations. Numerous organizations are available to provide patient resources regarding cancer diagnosis, hereditary cancer syndromes, genetic testing, and research opportunities (see Box 4-1).

Genetic discrimination, though not seen frequently, can occur with health, life, or disability insurance and in the workplace. In 1997, the Health Insurance Portability and Accountability Act (HIPAA) was established to protect the patient's personal information. HIPAA also has a provision against genetic discrimination. The law states that as long as the patient is part of a group health insurance plan he or she cannot be dropped from health insurance because of personal genetic test results, and individual insurance premiums cannot be increased because of genetic test results. Also, many states have supplemental laws governing genetic discrimination and health insurance. HIPAA does not provide protection for health insurance purchased in the individual market, small group plans (fewer than 50 individuals and self-administered), life, or disability insurance. Some states have legislation governing genetic discrimination of life, disability, and long-term care insurance. Most recently, the Genetic Information Nondiscrimination Act (GINA) of 2008 (P.L. 110–233, 122 Stat. 881), was signed into law. GINA is a federal law that prohibits discrimination in health coverage and employment based on genetic information (Box 4-2). GINA, together with HIPAA, prohibits health

---

Box 4-2. Genetic Discrimination Resources

National Conference of State Legislatures
Genetic and Health Insurance State Anti-Discrimination
  Laws
www.ncsl.org/program/health/genetics/ndishlth.htm

National Conference of State Legislatures
Genetics and Life, Disability and Long-term Care
  Insurance
www.ncsl.org/program/health/genetics/ndislife.htm

**United States Department of Health and
  Human Services**
Health Insurance Portability and Accountability Act
  (HIPAA)
www.hhs.gov/ocs/hipaa
The Genetic Information Nondiscrimination Act of 2008
  (GINA)
http://frwebgate.access.gpo.gov/cgi-bin/getdoc.
cgi?dbname=110_cong_public_laws&docid=f:
publ233.110.pdf

Box 4-4. General Risks, Benefits, and Limitations
of Genetic Testing

Risks
Psychological distress
Loss of privacy
False sense of security/reassurance
Guilt or worry about children
Change in family dynamics
Possible lifestyle changes
Discrimination by insurers and/or employer
Stigmatization

Benefits
Improved cancer risk management and surgical
  options
Relief from uncertainty and anxiety regarding cancer
  risk
Decreased health care screening costs based on risk
  stratification
Early detection of malignancies or other sequelae
Availability of predictive information for family members

Limitations
Not all mutations are detectable
Uncertain significance of some test results
Inconclusive test results
Ineffective screening for certain malignancies
Ambiguity of developing cancer based on penetrance

---

insurers from requiring genetic information of an individual or the individual's family members or using it for decisions regarding coverage, rates, or preexisting conditions. The law also prohibits most employers from using genetic information for hiring, firing, or promotion decisions and for any decisions regarding terms of employment.

Informed consent is one of the most important aspects of genetic testing. ASCO created 12 aspects of informed consent that must be achieved before genetic testing (Box 4-3). Most important, the risks, benefits, and limitations of the test must be described to the patient, including the potential implications of a positive, nega-

---

Box 4-3. American Society of Clinical Oncology
(ASCO): Basic Elements of Informed Consent for
Cancer Susceptibility Testing

1. Information on the specific test being performed
2. Implications of a positive and negative result
3. Possibility that the test will not be informative
4. Options for risk estimation without genetic testing
5. Risk of passing mutation to children
6. Technical accuracy of test
7. Fees involved in testing and counseling
8. Psychological implications of test results (benefits
   and risks)
9. Risks of insurance or employee discrimination
10. Confidentiality issues
11. Options and limitations of medical surveillance and
    strategies for prevention following testing
12. Importance of sharing genetic test results with at-
    risk relatives so that they may benefit from this
    information

---

tive, or inconclusive test result and alternatives to genetic testing (Box 4-4). Written informed consent is obtained from adults or parents for their children. Genetic testing of individuals under age 18 is performed only when the hereditary cancer syndrome suspected requires screening and management before age 18.

Follow-up after the genetic counseling session varies among providers, but usually a written summary of the counseling session is sent to the patient and the referring physician. Other follow-up duties include obtaining samples for genetic testing (i.e., tissue, blood), managing insurance issues such as letters of medical necessity, and coordinating genetic counseling for other family members.

In-person disclosure of test results is imperative. This session should focus on patient psychosocial implications and medical management. Correct interpretation of genetic test results is vital, since several possible genetic test results can occur including positive, negative, variant of uncertain significance, and neutral polymorphisms. A positive result occurs when a deleterious, cancer-causing mutation is found. The risk of cancer with a positive mutation depends on the specific gene mutation and penetrance of the

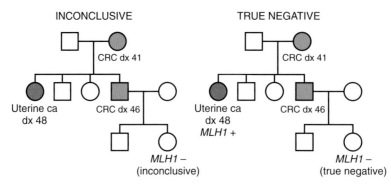

Figure 4-1. Interpretation of genetic test results. Affected with syndrome does not guarantee the development of cancer. Penetrance determines the risk of cancer. Obligate carrier is an individual known to possess a gene with a mutation based on the genetic information of successive generations. Ca, cancer; CRC, colorectal cancer; dx, diagnosis.

gene. A negative genetic test result can be confusing, since the result can be termed negative because no mutation was found (inconclusive) or because it is a true negative (Fig. 4-1). If no mutation is previously known in the family and the patient's results are "no mutation found," this is an inconclusive test result because no positive control exists in the family. The literature suggests that some patients are falsely reassured by inconclusive results and may need additional follow-up.[7] If a family mutation is known and an individual tests negative for the known mutation, this person has a true negative result. Test results reported as variants of uncertain significance also confuse patients. A variant of uncertain significance means a gene change was found, but insufficient information exists to determine whether this change is deleterious (causes disease). A neutral polymorphism is a change in the gene of interest, but it is not a deleterious change. After discussing test results, the counselor should have a conversation with other family members to share these results. Often the genetic counselor writes a letter that the patient can disseminate to family members explaining the hereditary cancer syndrome, genetic test results, family members appropriate for genetic testing, and information on location of genetic services for other family members.

Genetic Testing for Colorectal Cancer Syndromes

Lynch Syndrome

Lynch syndrome, also known as hereditary non-polyposis colorectal cancer (HNPCC), is a condition characterized by an excess of early-onset colorectal cancer and a defined spectrum of extracolonic malignancies with the most prevalent being endometrial and ovarian cancer (see Chapter 6). Lynch syndrome is an autosomal dominant condition, affecting males and females equally, and offspring of an affected individual are at 50% risk of inheriting the condition (Fig. 4-2). Lynch syndrome results from germline mutations in one of the mismatch repair (MMR) genes: *MLH1* on chromosome 3p21, *MSH2* on chromosome 2p16, *MSH6* on chromosome 2p15 and infrequently *PMS2* on chromosome 7p22. The MMR genes act as "spell checker" genes to correct DNA mismatches that occur during cell division. The normal function of MMR genes is imperative for DNA repair and the maintenance of genomic integrity. More than 90% of Lynch syndrome individuals with a detectable mutation have mutations in the *MLH1* and *MSH2* genes, which leads to classic Lynch syndrome. Individuals with mutations in the *MSH6* gene have a milder version of Lynch

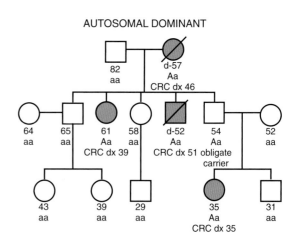

a = normal gene   aa = unaffected
A = gene with mutation   Aa = affected with syndrome

Figure 4-2. Autosomal dominant inheritance.
Ca, cancer; CRC, colorectal cancer; dx, diagnosis.

syndrome with lower lifetime risks of colorectal cancer than individuals with other MMR gene mutations, but a higher lifetime risk of endometrial cancer (see Chapter 6). Also, a majority of individuals with MMR germline mutations causing the Muir-Torre variant of Lynch syndrome (individuals with sebaceous gland neoplasms of the skin as well as Lynch syndrome) have *MSH2* mutations.

Several layers of complexity exist with genetic testing for Lynch syndrome. First, approximately 45% to 64% of families meeting the Amsterdam criteria have an identifiable MMR gene mutation, and up to 47% of Amsterdam-negative families have detectable MMR gene mutations.[9] Also, MMR genes may have variants of uncertain significance detected, meaning it is unclear whether or not these variations are deleterious. In addition, mild genetic modifier genes, *EXO1* and *MLH3*, have been discovered, which may account for some families with Lynch syndrome.

Families meeting the Amsterdam I or II criteria are considered to be clinically affected with Lynch syndrome, and individuals meeting the revised Bethesda criteria evoke suspicion for this disorder (see Tables 6-2 and 6-3). Individuals fulfilling either the Amsterdam or Bethesda criteria are appropriate for genetic testing. However, testing is not performed on those younger than age 18, since usually screening and management for this syndrome begin at age 20.

Genetic testing for Lynch syndrome usually proceeds in a stepwise fashion because of the numerous genes involved and the moderate rate of mutation detectability (Figs. 4-3 and 4-4). The revised Bethesda guidelines were created to identify individuals suspicious for having Lynch syndrome and candidates for genetic screening, which currently involves microsatellite instability (MSI) testing and immunohistochemistry (IHC) testing. MSI-IHC testing is usually the first step in the genetic testing process for Lynch syndrome. MSI refers to alterations in the length of short repeated DNA sequences, microsatellite repeats. DNA mismatches occur more frequently in these microsatellite repeats, and therefore MSI in colorectal tumor tissue indicates possible MMR gene defects. MSI testing involves screening the DNA of colorectal tumor tissue with a consensus panel of microsatellite markers and comparing the results with the DNA in the adjoining normal tissue. Tumor tissue with two or more markers showing instability is deemed microsatellite instability high (MSI-H) and is likely associated with Lynch syndrome. Approximately 90% of Lynch syndrome–associated colorectal tumors exhibit MSI compared with only 12% to 18% of sporadic colorectal tumors.[10]

IHC testing examines the protein products of the MMR-associated genes in tumor tissue. Loss of an MMR gene protein in tumor tissue results from either a germline mutation or a somatic event. The loss of protein expression through IHC suggests which MMR gene should be screened for germline mutation, therefore providing more targeted, less expensive gene sequencing. Frequently, when loss of MSH2 or MSH6 protein is observed in tumor tissue, the cause is a germline mutation, whereas loss of MLH1 protein often occurs by somatic hypermethylation of the *MLH1* gene.[11] Studies show that combination MSI-IHC tumor tissue testing is needed to identify individuals with Lynch syndrome.[12] MSI-IHC testing costs approximately $700 to $900 and takes about 4 to 6 weeks. Most laboratories offering MSI-IHC testing allow insurance billing and perform insurance preauthorization.

If MSI-IHC testing reveals MSI-H and loss of a specific MMR gene, target gene sequencing and deletion/duplication studies (if available) are the next step. Clinical sequencing is available for *MLH1*, *MSH2*, *MSH6*, and *PMS2*, costs approximately $800 to $2000, and takes 1 to 2 weeks for results. Deletion/duplications studies of *MLH1*, *MSH2*, and *MSH6* are part of clinical genetic testing for these two genes and are included in the cost of sequencing. Most laboratories offering these studies of MMR genes allow insurance billing and perform insurance preauthorization.

If a specific mutation is identified, targeted genetic testing for the known mutation is offered to other family members at $350 to $500. If MSI-IHC testing reveals MSI-H and abnormal MLH1 protein expression and genetic testing reveal no mutation found, MLH1 promoter methylation testing is appropriate to determine the cause of the abnormal MSI-IHC test result. If MSI-IHC testing reveals a microsatellite-stable (MSS) tumor and normal protein expression of all four MMR gene proteins, no further genetic testing is recommended and management guidelines are based on personal and family history.

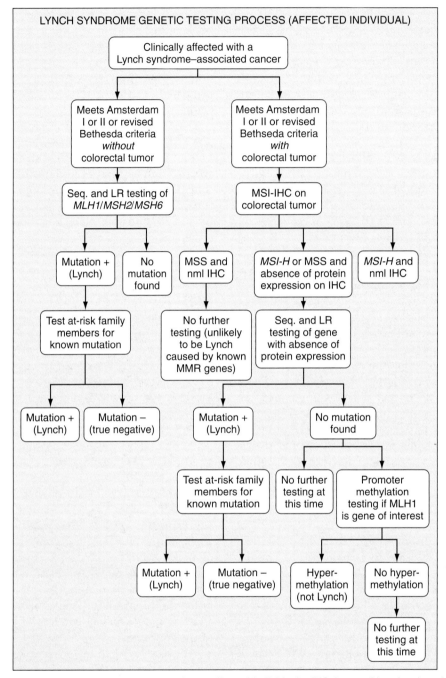

Figure 4-3. Genetic testing for Lynch syndrome in an affected individual. IHC, immunohistochemistry; LR, large rearrangement (deletion/duplication) testing; MMR, mismatch repair; MSI-H, microsatellite instability high; MSI-IHC, microsatellite instability and immunohistochemistry testing; MSS, microsatellite-stable; nml, normal; Seq., sequencing.

Although the detectability of MMR gene mutations causing Lynch syndrome is less than perfect, detection of mutations facilitates at-risk relatives' education about cancer risk and provides benefits through intensive screening and management proven to reduce overall mortality by 65%.[13]

Familial Adenomatous Polyposis

Classic familial adenomatous polyposis (FAP) is a distinct syndrome clinically diagnosed by the presence of 100 adenomatous colorectal polyps in teenage years and colorectal cancer development in the third decade of life if colectomy

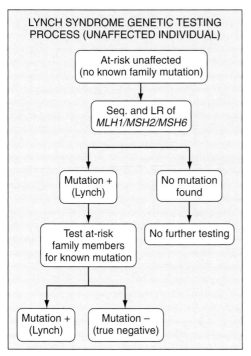

LYNCH SYNDROME GENETIC TESTING
PROCESS (UNAFFECTED INDIVIDUAL)

At-risk unaffected
(no known family mutation)

↓

Seq. and LR of
MLH1/MSH2/MSH6

Mutation +
(Lynch)

No mutation
found

Test at-risk
family members
for known mutation

No further testing

Mutation +
(Lynch)

Mutation −
(true negative)

**Figure 4-4. Genetic testing for Lynch syndrome in an
unaffected individual.** LR, large rearrangement
(deletion/duplication) testing; Seq., sequencing.

is not performed. Individuals with FAP also
present with upper gastrointestinal polyps, cutaneous lesions, dental abnormalities, jaw cysts,
desmoid tumors, osteomas, and congenital
hypertrophy of the retinal pigmented epithelium (CHRPE) (see Chapter 6). Attenuated
familial adenomatous polyposis (AFAP) is a less
severe version of FAP clinically defined by oligopolyposis (less than 100 adenomatous colorectal polyps) developing in the third decade of life
with a tendency toward rectal sparing and later
age at onset of colorectal cancer than in FAP
(i.e., in the fourth and fifth decades).

FAP/AFAP is a well-described autosomal
dominant condition with high penetrance. Autosomal dominant conditions affect males and
females equally, and all offspring of an affected
individual have a 50% risk of inheriting the disorder (see Fig. 4-2). Moreover, virtually all individuals who inherit this condition develop
polyposis. FAP/AFAP is predominantly caused
by germline mutations in the APC gene, a tumor
suppressor or "gatekeeper" gene. Up to 30% of
individuals affected with FAP have no family
history of the disease and represent the first

pedigree member with a mutation (de novo
mutation). The APC gene located on chromosome 5q21 has a large coding region composed
of 15 exons that produce a 2843-amino acid
protein. The APC gene protein functions in
regulating cell adhesion, transcriptional activation, and signal transduction. Most APC gene
mutations cause protein truncation through
deletions, insertions, and nonsense mutations
that lead to frameshifts or premature stop
codons. Variants of uncertain significance are
not frequently found in the APC gene, since
nearly all variations discovered are clearly inac-
tivating mutations associated with disease.

Genetic testing of the APC gene was originally performed through protein truncation
testing. The current gold standard for testing the
APC gene is sequence analysis of the entire
coding region and deletion/duplication analysis
(Figs. 4-5 to 4-7). Routine screening techniques
fail to detect deleterious APC germline mutations in 10% to 30% of classic FAP patients and
up to 90% of AFAP patients.[14] The most commonly occurring mutation in the APC gene is a
deletion of AAAAG in codon 1309.

The cost of gold standard APC genetic testing
is approximately $1300 to $1900, and the turn-
around time is 4 to 8 weeks. Most laboratories
allow insurance billing, and several offer insurance preauthorization before testing. Genetic
testing for the APC gene is expensive, and most
insurance companies cover some portion of
the cost in affected individuals or at-risk
individuals in a family with a known mutation.
Once a mutation is identified in a pedigree,
at-risk family members need only specific
genetic testing that searches for the known
family mutation ($350 to $500). Genetic
testing is recommended in at-risk individuals
between the ages of 10 and 12, since endoscopic
screening of the colorectum in affected individuals is suggested to commence at this time.
Some affected parents choose to have their children gene-tested very early, since affected individuals are at risk for hepatoblastoma from birth
to age 7 and because semiannual screening is
recommend until age 7 if risk status is not
known.

Several genotypic/phenotypic correlations
have been discovered through various research
studies. Mutations in the 5′ and 3′ ends of the
gene and mutations in the alternatively spliced
region of exon 9 are associated with AFAP,

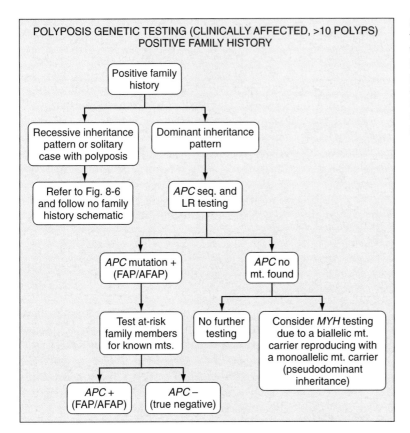

POLYPOSIS GENETIC TESTING (CLINICALLY AFFECTED, >10 POLYPS) POSITIVE FAMILY HISTORY

Figure 4-5. Polyposis genetic testing for an affected individual with a positive family history. FAP/AFAP, familial adenomatous polyposis/attenuated familial adenomatous polyposis; LR, large rearrangement (deletion/duplication) testing; mt, mutation; seq., sequencing.

whereas mutations in the center of the gene, between codons 169 and 1393, are associated with classic FAP.[15,16] Other observations include desmoid tumors with mutations between codons 1445 and 1580[17] and copious polyposis, especially rectal polyposis in individuals with mutations between codon 1250 and 1464.[18] Correlations between CHRPE and mutations between codons 463 and 1444 have been delineated.[19] Although genotype phenotype correlations have been discovered, FAP/AFAP is heterogeneous with intra- and interfamilial phenotypic variation.

APC I1307K Mutation

The *I1307K* missense mutation of the *APC* gene is found in individuals of Ashkenazi Jewish descent. This condition, like other hereditary cancer syndromes, is inherited in an autosomal dominant manner (see Fig. 4-2). This mutation is found in 6% to 8% of the Ashkenazi Jewish population and is associated with familial colorectal cancer. Unlike other changes in the *APC* gene that result in inactivation of the gene protein, the

I1307K change forms an unstable polyadenine tract immediately flanking codon 1307. This unstable tract causes the DNA replication machinery to act with less efficiency, allowing further somatic mutations on the same allele of the *APC* gene during cell division. Therefore, the *I1307K* mutation is not the change that disrupts the normal APC tumor suppressor function; rather, it is the additional somatic mutations that disrupt the *APC* gene function and cause the increased risk for cancer.

Genetic testing for the *APC I1307K* mutation is clinically available at a cost of approximately $200 to $500. Although available, genetic testing for the *APC I1307K* mutation in an Ashkenazi Jewish individual may not be the most appropriate gene test performed. Evaluation of the pedigree may reveal a strong family history of early-onset colorectal cancer and, although the *APC I1307K* mutation is prevalent in the Ashkenazi Jewish population, it confers only a 10% to 20% lifetime risk of late-onset colorectal cancer. Therefore, if an Ashkenazi Jewish individual presents with a high family penetrance of early-onset colorectal cancer,

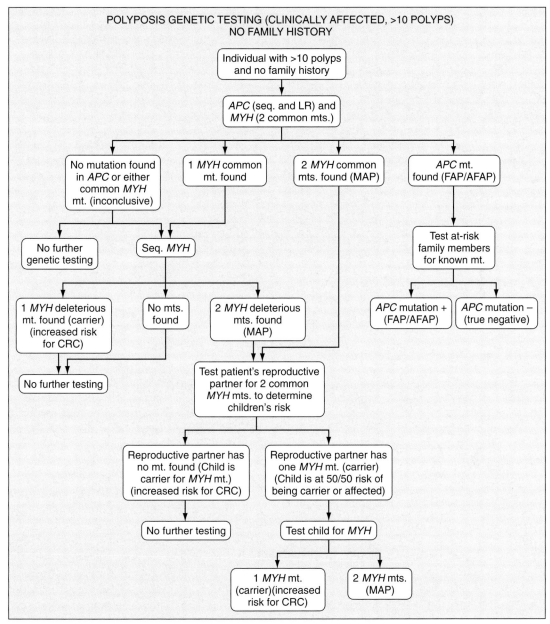

Figure 4-6. Polyposis genetic testing for an affected individual with a negative family history. CRC, colorectal cancer; FAP/AFAP, familial adenomatous polyposis/attenuated familial adenomatous polyposis; LR, large rearrangement (deletion/duplication) testing; MAP, *MYH*-associated polyposis; mt, mts, mutation(s); Seq., sequencing.

Lynch syndrome may be a more appropriate genetic syndrome to consider. A comprehensive cancer family history often helps to determine which route to pursue.

MYH-Associated Polyposis

MYH-associated polyposis (MAP) is a recently described syndrome of multiple colorectal adenomatous polyps and carcinoma (see Chapter 6). Individuals with MAP develop colorectal adenomatous polyposis or oligopolyposis (less than 100 adenomas) at a young age. The clinical presentation is indistinguishable from FAP/AFAP with regard to the number of colorectal adenomas or extracolonic manifestations.

MAP is the only autosomal recessive inherited colorectal cancer syndrome (Fig. 4-8). Individuals have two copies of every gene, and those affected with an autosomal recessive condition

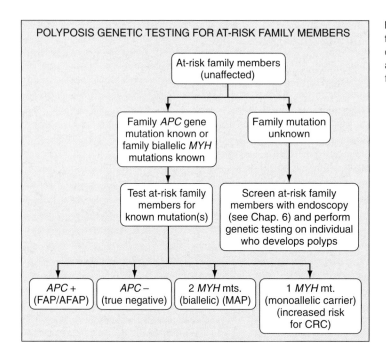

POLYPOSIS GENETIC TESTING FOR AT-RISK FAMILY MEMBERS

Figure 4-7. Polyposis genetic testing for an affected individual. CRC, colorectal cancer; FAP/AFAP, familial adenomatous polyposis/attenuated familial adenomatous polyposis.

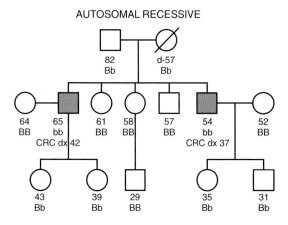

AUTOSOMAL RECESSIVE

b = gene with mutation
B = normal gene
bb = affected with syndrome
Bb = carrier
BB = unaffected with syndrome

Figure 4-8. Autosomal recessive inheritance. CRC, colorectal cancer; dx, diagnosis.

have mutations in both copies. Since individuals pass down 50% of their genetic material to offspring, an affected individual with MAP passes one mutated *MYH* gene to every child. Therefore, the offspring of all affected individuals are at least carriers of MAP, meaning that one copy of their *MYH* gene has a mutation and the other copy is normal. If an individual affected with an autosomal recessive condition reproduces with a carrier of the same condition, the offspring has a 50% chance of being affected (mutation in both genes) and a 50% risk of being a carrier for the condition (one gene with a mutation and one normal gene). If this occurs, the inheritance pattern appears to be autosomal dominant, but is really pseudodominant (Fig. 4-9).

MAP is caused by biallelic germline mutations in the *MYH* gene, the human homologue *Mut Y* gene, located on chromosome 1p35. The *MYH* gene acts in the base excision repair (BER) pathway to remove adenine bases that mispair with 8-oxoguanin during oxidation of DNA. Failure to correct these mispairings leads to $G:C \rightarrow T:A$ transversion mutations that are typical of oxidative DNA damage.[20] Germline *MYH* mutations inhibit the BER pathway and prevent the repair of somatic *APC* mutations, which leads to the FAP phenotype (similar to FAP caused by germline mutations within the *APC* gene). MAP accounts for 1% of all adenomatous polyposis cases but up to 30% of oligopolyposis cases. The highest incidence of biallelic *MYH* mutations is in patients with 15 to 100 colorectal adenomas.[21] The most frequent pathogenic mutations of the *MYH* gene in the Caucasian population are *Y165C* and *G382D*.[22] Two other protein truncating mutations, *E466X* and *Y90X*, are founder mutations in Indian and Pakistani descendants, respec-

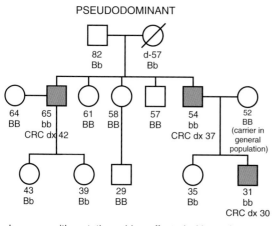

PSEUDODOMINANT

b = gene with mutation   bb = affected with syndrome
B = normal gene   Bb = carrier
                         BB = unaffected with syndrome

Figure 4-9. Autosomal recessive inheritance with a pseudodominant presentation. Inheritance appears to be autosomal dominant, although it is an autosomal recessive condition. The transmission appears dominant owing to a carrier in the general population reproducing with an individual affected with the same syndrome. CRC, colorectal cancer; dx, diagnosis.

tively. Most other changes found in the *MYH* gene are classified as variants of uncertain significance, since limited data exist about the effects these changes have on the function of this newly discovered gene.

Genetic testing for the *MYH* gene is clinically available. Usually, testing of the two common *MYH* mutations, *Y165C* and *G382D*, is performed first. Currently, some laboratories perform analysis of two common *MYH* mutations along with sequencing and deletion/duplication studies of the *APC* gene in patients with polyposis. The cost of testing only the two common *MYH* mutations is approximately $200 to $400 and takes 4 to 8 weeks. In the Caucasian population, up to 90% of individuals with biallelic mutations have at least one of the two common *MYH* mutations.[21] If one of the two common mutations is detected, full sequencing of the *MYH* coding region is recommended, since another discovered change in the *MYH* gene may be classified as a variant of uncertain significance. Full sequencing costs approximately $1000 to $1200 and takes approximately 6 to 8 weeks. If an individual is not Caucasian, full sequencing is recommended owing to ancestry-specific mutations outside the two common mutations. Again, variants of uncertain signifi-

cance are common and patients need to be aware of the likelihood of inconclusive results. Most laboratories offering *MYH* testing allow insurance billing and perform insurance pre-authorization. Many insurance companies cover testing of the two common *MYH* mutations, since this test is performed with *APC* gene analysis.

Genetic Testing for Juvenile Polyposis

Juvenile polyposis is a rare autosomal dominant condition defined by five or more histologically discrete juvenile polyps (see Fig. 4-2). Individuals with juvenile polyposis may have hundreds of polyps, and pathologic determination of polyp type is necessary to confirm the diagnosis before genetic testing is offered. Approximately 40% of juvenile polyposis cases can be attributed to a single gene defect, whereas the cause in the other 60% of patients is unknown. Also, 25% of patients with juvenile polyposis have de novo mutations, meaning that neither of their parents is affected with the condition and they are the first to have the gene mutation. Mutation in the *BMPR1A* gene located on chromosome 10q22-23 is detectable in approximately 24% of juvenile polyposis patients, and alteration in the *SMAD4/MADH4* gene located on chromosome 18q21 is detectable in approximately 17%. *SMAD4/MADH4* is involved in the mediation of cellular responses to transforming growth factor-beta (TGF-β) and prevention of cellular proliferation and neoplasia. *BMPR1A* is part of the TGF-β family and is involved with *SMAD4/MADH4* in mediating bone morphogenic protein intracellular signaling.

Individuals clinically affected with the syndrome are the most appropriate to begin testing. Also, genetic testing for juvenile polyposis is permitted before age 18, since clinical management and presentation occur in adolescence and teenage years. Genetic testing of both *BMPR1A* and *SMAD4/MADH4* is clinically available at only one laboratory in the United States, Ohio State University Molecular Pathology Laboratory. Currently, the cost is $1030 per gene, and the laboratory performs sequential testing. One gene is tested and if no mutation is found, the second gene is tested. The turn-around time for this clinical testing is approximately 12 weeks. This laboratory does not bill insurance companies, requiring patients to pay in advance for genetic testing and seek later reimbursement from their insurance company.

Although a minority of patients with juvenile polyposis have detectable mutations, a positive gene test result can alter surveillance recommendations. Individuals with *SMAD4/MADH4* gene mutations have clinical manifestations of juvenile polyposis and can develop additional manifestations including arteriovenous and other cardiovascular malformations. Therefore, juvenile polyposis patients with *SMAD4/MADH4* mutations require cardiovascular as well as gastrointestinal screening.

Bannayan-Riley-Ruvalcaba Syndrome and Cowden Syndrome

Bannayan-Riley-Ruvalcaba syndrome (BRRS) and Cowden syndrome are two rare autosomal dominant syndromes associated with hamartomatous polyposis (see Chapter 6; Fig. 4-2). Cowden syndrome has multiple manifestations with some of the most prevalent including hamartomatous polyps of the gastrointestinal tract, facial trichilemmomas, and a high risk of breast and thyroid cancer. BRRS is not well defined, but seems to be a variant of Cowden syndrome. BRRS patients may present with Cowden-like sequelae as well as developmental delay, lipid storage myopathy, and pigmented macules on the penis. Both Cowden syndrome and BRRS are caused by mutations in the *PTEN* gene located on chromosome 10q. *PTEN* is a tumor suppressor gene that inhibits growth by acting like a check and balance system on cell growth through the protein tyrosine kinase. Approximately 80% of individuals clinically diagnosed with Cowden syndrome have a detectable mutation in *PTEN*, whereas only 50% to 60% of BRRS patients have a detectable mutation in *PTEN*. The majority of patients with Cowden syndrome and BRRS do not have affected parents, but these syndromes are underdiagnosed.

Genetic testing for *PTEN* is clinically available and consists of sequence analysis of the coding region. The test costs approximately $900 to $1200, and it takes 6 to 12 weeks to perform. Deletion and promoter analysis of *PTEN* is conducted on a research basis and may detect another 11% of BRRS and 10% of Cowden cases, respectively. Most laboratories performing testing allow insurance billing and provide insurance preauthorization. Detection of a *PTEN* mutation confirms the diagnosis and provides support for the screening recommendations for these syndromes.

Peutz-Jeghers Syndrome

Peutz-Jeghers syndrome (PJS) is characterized by Peutz-Jeghers polyps in the small bowel, melanin pigmentation of the lips, buccal mucosa, fingers, toes, and above the eyelashes, as well as other malignancies (see Table 6-4). PJS is an autosomal dominant condition with variable expression due to mutations in the *STK11/LBK1* gene on chromosome 19p13.3 (see Fig. 4-2). *STK11/LBK1* acts as a tumor suppressor gene encoding a protein involved in the transduction of intracellular growth signals. Up to 70% of individuals with familial PJS have a detectable mutation, and 30% to 67% of sporadic cases have a detectable mutation.[23,24] Approximately 50% of individuals with PJS have a de novo mutation (i.e., neither parent is affected). Genetic testing should be performed on an individual affected with PJS to determine the family mutation. The gold standard for PJS testing is sequencing the entire coding region of the *STK11/LBK1* gene. Clinical genetic testing for *STK11/LBK1* is available at a cost of $900 to $1500, and the turn-around time is 6 to 12 weeks. Most laboratories performing testing allow insurance billing and provide insurance preauthorization so the patient is aware of the out-of-pocket expense before testing is started. Unaffected at-risk individuals in a family with a known mutation should undergo genetic testing at around 8 years of age to help determine management.

Conclusion

When performed appropriately genetic testing has the ability to provide patients, family members, and health care providers with vital information that can help individuals cope with a diagnosis and prepare for the future. Genetic testing for hereditary colorectal cancer syndromes may provide a concrete diagnosis that would allow comprehensive medical management as well as identification of affected relatives. All patients deserve access to cancer risk assessment and should benefit from this information.

References

1. American Cancer Society Cancer statistics, 2009.
2. Vasen HF: Clinical diagnosis and management of hereditary colorectal cancer syndromes. J Clin Oncol 18(21 Suppl): 81S–92S, 2000.
3. American Society of Clinical Oncology Policy Statement Update: genetic testing for cancer susceptibility. J Clin Oncol 21:2397–2406, 2003.
4. National Advisory Council for Human Genome Research Statement on use of DNA testing for presymptomatic identification of cancer risk. JAMA 271:785, 1994.
5. American Gastroenterology Association Medical Position Statement: hereditary colorectal cancer and genetic testing. Gastroenterology 121:195–197, 2001.
6. Giardiello FM, Brensinger JD, Peterson GM, et al: The use and interpretation of commercial APC genetic testing for familial adenomatous polyposis. N Engl J Med 336(12):823–827, 1997.
7. Meiser B: Psychological impact of genetic testing for cancer susceptibility: an update of the literature. Psychooncology 14(12):1060–1074, 2005.
8. Frost CJ, Venne V, Cunningham D, et al: Decision making with uncertain information: learning from women in a high risk breast cancer clinic. J Genet Couns 13(3):221–236, 2004.
9. Giardiello FM, Brensinger JD, Peterson GM: AGA technical review on hereditary colorectal cancer and genetic testing. Gastroenterology 12(1):198–213, 2001.
10. Thibodeau SN, Bren G, Schaid D: Microsatellite instability in cancer of the proximal colon. Science 260:816–819, 1993.
11. Arnold CN, Goel A, Compton C, et al: Evaluation of microsatellite instability, hMLH1 expression and hMLH1 promoter hypermethylation in defining the MSI phenotype of colorectal cancer. Cancer Biol 3(1):73–78, 2004.
12. Engel C, Forberg J, Holinski-Feder E, et al: Novel strategy for optimal sequential application of clinical criteria, immunohistochemistry and microsatellite analysis in the diagnosis of hereditary nonpolyposis colorectal cancer. Int J Cancer 118(1):115–122, 2006.
13. Jarvinen HJ, Aarnio M, Mustonen H, et al: Controlled 15-year trial on screening for colorectal cancer in families with hereditary nonpolyposis colorectal cancer. Gastroenterology 188(5): 829–834, 2000.
14. Armstrong JG, Davies DR, Guy SP, et al: APC mutations in familial adenomatous polyposis families in the Northwest of England. Hum Mutat 10(5):376–380, 1997.
15. Leggett B: When is molecular genetic testing for colorectal cancer indicated? J Gastroenterol Hepatol 17:389–393, 2002.
16. Fearnhead NS, Britton MP, Bodmer WF: The ABC of APC. Hum Mol Genet 10(7):721–733, 2001.
17. Friedl W, Caspari R, Sengteller M, et al: Can APC mutation analysis contribute to therapeutic decisions in familial adenomatous polyposis? Experience from 680 FAP families. Gut 48(4): 515–521, 2001.
18. Bertario L, Russo A, Radice P, et al: Genotype and phenotype factors as determinants for rectal stump cancer in patients with familial adenomatous polyposis. Hereditary Colorectal Tumors Registry. Ann Surg 231(4):538–543, 2000.
19. Giardiello FM, Peterson GM, Piantadosi S, et al: APC gene mutations and extraintestinal phenotype of familial adenomatous polyposis. Gut 40(4):521–525, 1997.
20. Thomas D, Scot AD, Barbey R, et al: Inactivation of OGG1 increases the incidence of G : C → T : A transversions in *Saccharomyces cerevisiae*: evidence for endogenous oxidative damage to DNA in eukaryotic cells. Mol Gen Genet 254(2):171–178, 1997.
21. Sieber OM, Lipton L, Crabtree M, et al: Multiple colorectal adenomas, classic adenomatous polyposis, and germline mutations in MYH. N Engl J Med 348(9):791–799, 2003.
22. Al-Tassan N, Chmiel NH, Maynard J, et al: Inherited variants of MYH associated with somatic G : C → T : A mutations in colorectal tumors. Nat Genet 30(2):227–232, 2002.
23. Amos CI, Bali D, Thiel TJ, et al: Fine mapping of genetic locus for Peutz-Jeghers syndrome on chromosome 19p. Cancer Res 57(17):3653–3656, 1997.
24. Boardman LA, Couch FJ, Burgart LJ, et al: Genetic heterogeneity in Peutz-Jeghers syndrome. Hum Mutat 16(1):23–30, 2000.

5 Behavior and Dietary Modification in the Prevention of Colon Cancer

Stephanie R. Downing, Emmanouil P. Pappou,* and Nita Ahuja

KEY POINTS

- Several dietary and lifestyle factors are likely to have an impact on the development of colorectal cancer. Focus on primary prevention, in combination with screening and surveillance, is the best strategy against this common yet highly preventable disease.
- Diets high in red and processed meat are associated with a higher risk of colorectal cancer.
- The data on fiber and colon cancer prevention are still inconclusive but lean toward a protective effect.
- Several micronutrients and vitamins, including calcium, vitamin D, folate, and selenium may reduce the risk of colorectal cancer, but most of the data so far do not conclusively support this view.
- Physical inactivity and, to some extent, obesity have consistently been shown to be risk factors for colon cancer.
- Exposure to tobacco products for an extended period of time and excess alcohol consumption are associated with an increased risk of colorectal cancer.

Introduction

Colorectal cancer is found throughout the world (Fig. 5-1). In the United States, it is the second leading cause of cancer. In addition to genetics, environment and lifestyle play important roles in the development of colorectal cancer. The effects of environmental influences on human cancer became evident when early epidemiologic studies showed that cancer rates vary strikingly among countries—by five- to tenfold—and that immigrants moving from low-risk to high-risk countries adopt the rates of the new country.[1,2] Moreover, Burkitt's hypothesis in the 1970s that colon cancer rates of European lineage populations in South Africa were much higher than those of the native Bantu populations—theoretically because of an increased intake of refined cereals, protein, fat, and sugar—added further interest in diet as a possible etiologic factor of malignancy.[3] By comparing rates of cancer mortality around the world, Doll and Peto[4] in 1981 "guesstimated" that approximately 90% of colon cancers in the United States could be attributed to environmental factors and therefore could have been avoided. Although this theoretical maximum was an obvious overestimate, the analysis provided an important starting point for subsequent studies on environmental causes of cancer and strategies for cancer prevention.

In the past 30 years, many epidemiologic studies have tried to identify environmental factors related to colon carcinogenesis, including (1) ecologic studies, in which rates of consumption of dietary components are compared among different populations or countries; (2) case-control studies, in which the diet and lifestyle factors of people with colon cancer are compared with those without cancer; and (3) prospective cohort studies, in which groups of people are observed over a period of time to determine the new incidence of colon cancer and its association with environmental exposures. Nevertheless, all these epidemiologic studies must be read critically, since they have many weaknesses and the possibility of confounding selection and information biases is great.

Beginning in the 1980s, randomized controlled trials of nutritional supplementation were used in an effort to isolate individual components of foods that could be responsible for the effect of diet on colon cancer. However,

---

*The authors contributed equally to this manuscript.

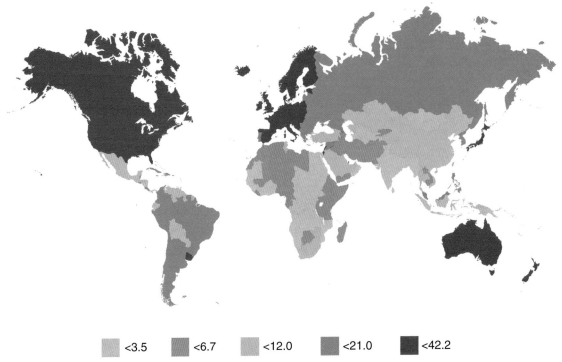

| <3.5 | <6.7 | <12.0 | <21.0 | <42.2 |

Figure 5-1. Distribution of colon cancer worldwide, 2002. (From GLOBOcon 2002.)

intervention trials have their own challenges as well, because the timing of intervention, duration of the trial, and compliance of the subjects can greatly influence the results.

In this chapter, we review the scientific evidence on dietary and lifestyle factors that are related to primary prevention of colorectal cancer. Chemoprevention of colorectal cancer is discussed in Chapter 6.

Macronutrients

Red Meat: Intake and Cooking

Reports from the World Cancer Research Fund, the Chief Medical Officer's Committee on Medical Aspects of Food, and a World Health Organization consensus statement all reached similar conclusions regarding a possible increased risk of colorectal cancer associated with high intake of red meat.[5–7] The bulk of evidence supports this view, but the data are not entirely consistent. Epidemiologic studies show conflicting results, with countries such as Greece having an increasing meat intake and low colorectal cancer rates and with Australia and the United Kingdom having decreasing meat intake but increasing colorectal cancer rates.[8] Most case-

control studies, however, have shown a positive association between red meat intake and colon cancer, with a few exceptions.[9–14] Cohort studies have also shown a statistically significant association between processed meat and risk of colorectal cancer.[15–17] Other cohort studies have not confirmed this finding, however.[18] The Nurses' Health Study, which is one of the largest and longest-running studies on factors affecting women's health and which comprises a cohort of about 90,000 nurses in the United States, identified consumption of red meat as a colon cancer risk factor.[19] However, in the Polyp Prevention Trial (PPT), a randomized controlled trial that included 1905 subjects followed up for approximately 4 years, the adoption of a diet that de-emphasized red meat did not decrease the recurrence of colorectal adenomas.[20] It has been suggested that poor adherence to the diet and the short duration of the trial might be reasons that this study did not support the findings of observational studies.

A meta-analysis of 34 case-control studies and 14 cohort studies conducted in 2002 concluded that high intake of red meat, and particularly processed meat, was associated with a moderate but significant increase in colorectal cancer risk.[21] Average relative risk (RR) and 95%

confidence interval (CI) for the highest quantile of consumption of red meat were 1.35 (CI 1.21–1.51) and of processed meat 1.31 (CI 1.13–1.51). A recent meta-analysis of prospective studies published through March 2006, which included 15 prospective studies on red meat (involving 7367 cases) and 14 prospective studies on processed meat consumption (7903 cases), showed that consumption of red meat and processed meat was positively associated with an increased risk of both colon and rectal cancer, although the association with red meat appeared to be stronger for rectal cancer.[22] The estimated summary relative risks were 1.28 (95% CI 1.18–1.39) for an increase of 120 g/day of red meat and 1.09 (95% CI 1.05–1.13) for an increase of 30 g/day of processed meat. Specifically, the relative risk for colon cancer was 1.21 (1.05–1.40) and for rectal cancer 1.56 (1.25–1.95). The evidence that prolonged high consumption of red and processed meat may increase the risk of cancer in the distal portion of the large intestine as opposed to the proximal colon has been somewhat consistent.[15,16,22]

The mechanism by which high red or processed meat intake might increase the risk of colorectal cancer is entirely unclear. Some experimental data suggest that protein escapes digestion in the small intestine and is degraded by the colonic microflora, giving rise to a number of products that may promote colorectal cancer (ammonia, phenols, indoles, amines). Processed meat may also contribute to high colonic nitrosamine concentrations or may be a source of heme iron, which can act as a peroxidant. Recent studies have focused on the role of cooking methods of meat in the increased risk. Heterocyclic amines (HCAs), which are formed on the surface of heavily cooked meats exposed to high temperatures, are potent mutagens. Some studies have reported that increased consumption of well-done or fried red meat with a heavily browned surface is associated with an increased risk of colorectal cancer, but the risk is not increased among those who consume meat with a medium or lightly browned surface.[9,23,24] Not all studies have confirmed this finding, however.[25,26] It has also been suggested that acetylation polymorphisms can influence the risk of colorectal neoplasia and that subjects with a fast acetylator status (i.e., increased activity of the N-acetyltransferase enzymes), who would readily activate aromatic and heterocyclic amine carcinogens within the colon to their ultimate carcinogenic forms, are especially sensitive to brown meat and exhibit a greater colorectal cancer risk.[27]

These findings have not been replicated by more recent studies.[28] Future investigations should further determine the role of heterocyclic amines in colorectal carcinogenesis and whether genetic polymorphisms influence susceptibility to their adverse effects. The role of chemicals derived from cooked meat in colorectal neoplasia has not yet been clearly defined.

Dietary Fat

Data from earlier epidemiologic studies had generally shown an association between risk of colon cancer and fat intake.[29–31] Rates of colorectal cancer in various countries were strongly associated with per-capita consumption of animal fat.[1,32] The incidence of colorectal cancer in Japan began rising steeply after World War II, and this coincided with a 2.5-fold increase in fat intake.[33] These data led to the hypothesis that dietary fat increases excretion of bile acids, which can be converted to carcinogens. The combined epidemiologic and experimental evidence led the Committee on Diet, Nutrition, and Cancer of the National Research Council in 1986 to recommend a reduction in dietary fat from 40% to 30% of calories as a possible means of reducing cancer risk.[34] However, more recent studies have suggested that this is not supported by strong evidence and that the association seen between colorectal cancer and animal fat might be explained by factors in red meat other than its fat content. A meta-analysis of data from 13 case-control studies conducted in populations with differing colorectal cancer rates and dietary practices found a significant association between total energy intake and colon cancer but no association between dietary fat intake and risk of colorectal cancer independent of total energy.[35] The Nurses' Health Study, one of the best cohort studies of diet and colon cancer, showed a positive association between animal fat intake and the risk of colon cancer.[19] The relative risk for the women in the highest quintile compared with that in the lowest quintile was 1.89 (95% CI 1.13–3.15). Nevertheless, a subsequent multivariate analysis of these data, which included red meat and animal fat intakes in the same model, showed no association with animal fat, whereas red meat intake remained significantly predictive of colon cancer.[36] Similarly, other large cohort studies from the United States and the Netherlands found no direct relation between fat intake and mortality due to colon cancer.[17,37,38] Four randomized controlled trials that investigated the usefulness of low-fat diets in colorectal adenoma and cancer prevention failed to show protection.[20,39-41] As previously mentioned, results of the Polyp Prevention Trial (PPT) showed no reduction in the risk of colorectal adenoma recurrence over approximately 4 years.[20] Similarly, in the Women's Health Initiative (WHI), a large randomized controlled trial involving 36,282 postmenopausal women followed up for 7 years, a low-fat dietary pattern did not affect colorectal cancer risk.[41] Potential reasons for the null results in these trials may reflect the complex multistage process of colorectal carcinogenesis, timing of dietary change, duration of the study, as well as poor dietary adherence among participants in these trials. It is interesting that a recent subset analysis of the PPT trial identified a group of the most adherent subjects to a low-fat, high-fiber, high-fruit and high-vegetable diet, defined as "super compliers" ($n = 210$). The authors observed 35% reduced odds of adenoma recurrence and nearly 50% lower odds of multiple and advanced adenoma recurrence among super compliers compared with controls, suggesting that consistent adherence to a low-fat, high-fiber, high-fruit and high-vegetable diet may be effective in preventing recurrence of colorectal adenomas and possibly in preventing colorectal cancer.[42] Furthermore, although increased total fat and animal fat intake may increase the risk of colorectal carcinogenesis, increased consumption of polyunsaturated fats such as fatty acids found in fish oils may conversely decrease the risk of colorectal cancer.[7,43] Ongoing and future investigations are warranted to determine the exact relation between fat and the risk of colon cancer.

Fiber

Increased dietary fiber has long been postulated as a protective factor against the development of colorectal cancers (Box 5-1). However, a consensus has yet to be reached owing to wide differences in study results over the past 30 years.

Box 5-1. Examples of High-Fiber Foods

Eating 30 to 40 grams of fiber each day is very important for good health and may help prevent colorectal cancer. Here are some examples of high-fiber foods that could be included in a daily diet.

Fruits

Raspberries
Pears, with skin
Apples, with skin
Strawberries
Bananas
Oranges
Figs, dried
Raisins

Grains, Cereal, and Pasta

Spaghetti, whole wheat
Barley, pearl
Bran flakes
Oat bran
Oatmeal
Popcorn
Brown rice
Bread, rye
Bread, whole wheat or multigrain

Legumes, Nuts, and Seeds

Pistachios
Pecans

Vegetables

Artichokes
Peas
Broccoli
Turnip greens
Sweet corn
Brussels sprouts
Potatoes, baked
Carrots

Adapted from Mayo Clinic E-Newsletter, Available at www.mayoclinic.com/health/high-fiber-foods/NU00582.

Strong evidence from both animal and human studies has shown that consumption of a diet high in fiber can reduce the risk of colorectal cancers by several mechanisms, including increase in stool bulk and decrease in stool transit time, increased binding of potential mutagens, fermentation of fiber into short-chain fatty acids (SCFA), and reduction of luminal pH. An increase in dietary fiber and a subsequent increase in stool bulk were the first of these factors shown to be inversely linked to the risk of colorectal cancers and were thought to act by reducing transit time and thus the amount of time that the colonic mucosa is exposed to other diet carcinogens.[44,45] This increase in bulk may also provide a chemical or physical barrier for the colonic mucosa to known carcinogens in the diet, such as high concentrations of the secondary bile salts lithocholic and deoxycholic acids.[46,47] In addition, some fiber types are fermented by large bowel bacteria into short-chain fatty acids, particularly butyrate, which has been shown to inhibit the growth of hyperproliferative epithelium in the case of ulcerative colitis and bile salt exposure.[48–52] Furthermore, butyrate has been shown to inhibit histone deacetylase, causing histone hyperacetylation and thus disinhibition of gene expression and leading to cell apoptosis and unresponsiveness to local growth factors.[48,53,54] This colonic fermentation further reduces colonic pH, which has been shown to reduce secondary bile salt solubility and is associated with lower cancer risk in humans.[46,47,55] Furthermore, reduction in colonic pH has been shown to shift gut flora away from a more anaerobic mix that is associated with an increased risk of colorectal cancer. This action is thought to be through the production of carcinogens such as heterocyclic amines and phenolic compounds by anaerobic bacteria of *Clostridia* and *Bacteroides* species.[46,55]

Investigations of large international, population-based data, such as one by Bingham and associates,[61] have shown a strong inverse correlation between fiber consumption and colorectal cancer; furthermore, most case-control studies have shown that increased dietary fiber has a protective effect against the development of colorectal cancers.[1,11,56–71] However, a few case-control studies have failed to show this protective effect; moreover, all of these case-control and population-based studies are plagued by confounding factors such as inconsistent estimation of portion sizes and sources of fiber in the diet.[72–75]

To help elucidate the impact of these seemingly contrary results, Howe and associates[35] pooled the data from 13 case-control studies regarding the influence of dietary fiber on colorectal cancer development and found that, in aggregate, the relative risk of cancer in the highest quintile of fiber consumption compared with that in the lowest was 0.53 (95% CI 0.47–0.61), a figure similar to other large studies and pooled results. However, these results were highly criticized because they did not take into account the quality of individual studies. Although Howe's study[35] showed serious methodologic concerns, the study of Friedenreich and associates[76] showed that using a random-effects or fixed-effects model to account for differences in the quality of the same 13 studies did not drastically change the odds ratio for the interquintile range (random effects: odds ratio [OR] 0.46, 95% CI 0.34–0.64; fixed-effects: OR 0.51, 95% CI 0.44–0.59), indicating that the variability in case-control results could not be attributed to quality of study design.

Buoyed by these results, several interventional trials have been undertaken to elucidate the effect of dietary fiber on subsequent colorectal polyp development. However, these were generally of very short duration (2 to 4 years), examined only high-risk populations (personal history of polyps or cancer, familial adenomatous polyposis), and, because of a short follow-up, looked only at polyp development, not cancer development. Consequently, there has been little to no indication that the supplementation of fiber over a short period of time reduces the risk of polyp development in these high-risk populations.[20,39,40,77–81] There is one exception to this trend: Alberts and associates[82] showed in a randomized, double-blind, placebo-controlled trial that wheat bran fiber significantly reduced fecal bile acid content.

Overall, most studies have shown an inverse relationship between dietary fiber and colorectal cancer risk, but clearly proving such an interaction has been difficult owing to challenges in measurement, control, and type of fiber intake.

Vegetables and Fruits

Adding some confusion to the fiber debate is the inclusion of dietary fiber from vegetables and fruits, which may have additional dietary micronutrients that also may influence the development of colorectal cancer. For instance, Negri and associates[65] have shown that fiber intake from a vegetable source had the greatest reduction of associated colorectal cancer risk in Italian patients. The majority of studies have shown a reduction of colorectal cancer risk with the consumption of vegetables, fruits, or both.[57,65–67,69,71,73,83–87] Of note, some studies have shown no association for all patients or for selected populations, such as cigarette smokers.[17,88,89]

Of particular interest is consumption of members of the *Allium* genus of plants such as garlic, onions, shallots, chives, and leeks. Compounds found in these vegetables, such as diallyl sulphide, flavonols quercetin, and kaempferol and glutathione, have been implicated as anticarcinogens.[90] Consumption of *Allium* vegetables have been shown to be associated with a decreased risk of colorectal cancer, particularly distal cancer in 9 of the 16 published studies on the topic, including the only two randomized controlled trials in the group.[17,31,66,67,71,84,85,89–96] Furthermore, a meta-analysis by Fleischauer and associates,[97] including seven of these studies, and a review of the quality of literature by Ngo and colleagues[98] both showed a preponderance of quality evidence in favor of an inverse association between *Allium* genus plant consumption and colorectal cancer.

On balance, most experts agree that vegetables and fruits, especially of the *Allium* genus, are protective against colorectal cancers.

Insulin and Glycemic Load

Risk factors for colorectal cancer and insulin resistance syndromes show considerable overlap, such as central obesity and low physical activity (discussed elsewhere in this chapter), leading some experts to postulate that increased insulin levels promote colorectal cancers.[99–101] For instance, several researchers have shown that non–insulin-dependent diabetes mellitus is an independent risk factor for colorectal cancer even when controlling for their joint risk factors.[102–104] This was clearest in the Iowa Women's Health Study, which showed a link between those with recently diagnosed type 2 diabetes but not for those with a longstanding diabetes diagnosis, the latter of which would presumably not be associated with elevated insulin levels.[38]

In addition, high consumption of foods that cause a dramatic spike in postprandial insulin, so-called *high glycemic load* foods such as sugar or sugar-dense foods, has been shown to correlate with the development of colorectal cancer in several population-based and case-control studies.[38,83,86,105–112] Notably, several other studies have shown no significant risk increase for those with high sugar consumption but have shown a correlation between high overall energy intake and colorectal cancers.[1,10,14,69,84,85,113–117] Furthermore, Ma and associates[118] showed with prospective collected data that, even in nondiabetic

men, circulating levels of plasma C-peptide correlated with the development of colorectal cancer (risk ratio for the highest quintile to the lowest = 3.4, $P = .02$), a finding previously shown in elderly men and in women.[104,119]

The association of both peripheral insulin resistance and the consumption of high glycemic load foods lends strength to the hypothesis that insulin plays a significant role in the development of colorectal cancer. Furthermore, this may lend further strength to the actions of dietary fiber, which has been shown to reduce the glycemic load of other foods by sequestering simple sugars in the gut. However, further research is needed in this area to determine the impact of insulin on the development of colorectal cancers.

Coffee and Tea

Several studies have examined the impact of coffee and tea drinking on the development of colorectal cancers. Coffee drinking has been shown to be associated with a lower risk of colorectal cancer in several studies,[10,14,91,106,113,120–124] but several other studies showed no association.[125–131] One review article has shown a protective effect of coffee consumption against the development of colorectal cancers.[132] In contrast to the consumption of black teas, which seems to have no association with the development of colorectal cancers in several studies,[133–135] green teas have been shown to have anticancer effects, primarily through a compound called *epigallocatechin gallate*.[136] Furthermore, green teas have been shown to be associated with reduced colorectal cancer risk, including in a review paper by Bushman.[137–140]

Dairy Foods and Probiotics

It is not surprising that attempts to compare dairy products with the risk of colorectal cancer have resulted in extremely varied results owing to the fact that dairy foods tend to contain high levels of both dietary fat and calcium (discussed later in this chapter). Most studies have shown that the consumption of dairy foods has a nonsignificant protective effect on the development of colorectal cancer.[38,73,130,141,142] However, the consumption of milk products significantly reduced the risk of colorectal cancers in two pooled datasets.[143,144] Furthermore, in one study that has examined skim and whole milks separately, it was found that skim milk consumption was associated with reduced colorectal cancer risk but whole milk consumption was not.[145] Finally, consumption of milk was shown to be protective against colorectal cancer in male smokers in Finland.[146]

In addition, the impact of fermented milk products (yogurt, buttermilk, and cheeses) and unpasteurized milk has been investigated in association with colorectal cancers. For the former, there is some evidence that lactic acid bacteria such as *Lactobacillus* and *Bifidobacterium* can reduce cell proliferation, urinary mutagenicity, and bacterial enzyme activity that can produce carcinogens.[147,148] Although no evidence has been seen from cohort studies of protective benefits from fermented milk products, three of the larger case-control studies have shown a protective benefit even when controlling for other factors.[149–153] It has been hypothesized that unpasteurized milk, in contrast, increases colorectal cancer risk through exposure to bovine pathogens, particularly bovine leukemia virus.[154,155] However, using data from the Iowa Women's Health Study, Sellers and colleagues[156] actually found a protective benefit in the consumption of unpasteurized milk with regard to the development of colorectal cancer, which became nonsignificant after controlling for other factors.

Vitamins and Micronutrients

Calcium

A possible protective effect of calcium on colorectal cancer was suggested primarily from results of in vitro animal studies. It has been hypothesized that dietary calcium provides protection from colon cancer by binding with fat and reducing the concentrations of free fatty acids and bile in the lumen of the bowel, thus reducing their proliferative influence on the colon mucosa.[157] It has also been proposed that calcium can directly reduce mucosal proliferation.[158] The epidemiologic evidence, however, has been inconsistent. Several, but not all, studies showed a weak inverse association of calcium intake with risk of colorectal adenoma or cancer.[159] Pooled results from two large prospective cohorts, the Nurses' Health Study (NHS) and the Health Professionals Follow-up

Study (HPFS), with a follow-up of at least 10 years, showed an inverse association between calcium intake and distal but not proximal colon cancer. Furthermore, the authors showed that the benefit of calcium intake has a threshold effect, in that intake beyond approximately 700 mg/day appeared to have minimal additional effect, suggesting that calcium intake beyond moderate levels may not be associated with a further risk reduction.[160] Another cohort of 35,216 women from Iowa showed that calcium intake was associated with a significantly reduced risk of colon cancer (RR 0.5, CI 0.3–0.7) among women with a negative family history but not among women with a positive family history.[161]

Several randomized controlled trials have tested the protective role of calcium supplementation against adenoma recurrence and colorectal cancer.[80,162–165] The trial reported by Baron and colleagues[162] found that calcium supplementation at 1200 mg/day for 4 years reduced adenoma recurrence by 15%. This effect was shown to extend as long as 5 years after cessation of supplementation.[166] Bonithon-Kopp and colleagues[80] reported a 34% reduction in the recurrence rate of adenomas after taking 2000 mg calcium per day for 3 years, but the result did not reach statistical significance. In the WHI, the latest and largest placebo-controlled randomized trial, which involved 36,282 postmenopausal women, daily supplementation with a combination of 1000 mg calcium and 400 units of vitamin D for 7 years had no effect on the incidence of colorectal cancer.[41] However, one of the major criticisms of this study was that the mean baseline calcium intake in these women was 1151 mg/day, resulting in a total calcium intake of approximately 2150 mg/day, levels that, based on the prospective cohort study data, are consistent with no effect. As a result, the WHI did not test whether calcium supplementation would convey protection among individuals with low or moderately low baseline intakes of this nutrient.[167]

On the whole, the literature supports a moderate protective effect of calcium against colorectal cancer. A recent summary of systematic reviews from the World Cancer Research Fund concluded that there is a modest, significant inverse association between calcium intake and colorectal cancer.[168] The latest American Cancer Society Guidelines on Nutrition and Cancer

Prevention also recommend 1000 mg calcium per day for adults up to age 50 years and 1200 mg/day for those older than 50 years.[169]

Vitamin D

Vitamin D was proposed as a potential protective factor against colon cancer in the 1980s, when correlational studies revealed that colon cancer mortality rates in the United States were highest in places where populations were exposed to the least amounts of natural light, including major cities and rural areas in high latitudes.[170] Vitamin D is a fat-soluble vitamin that can be obtained from fatty fish, fish oil, and fortified dairy products, or it can be synthesized endogenously in the skin after exposure to ultraviolet light. Its primary role is in the regulation of calcium homeostasis in the body. Putative biologic activities related to the presumable protective effects of vitamin D in colon neoplasia include its pro-differentiating and antiproliferative effects through induction of cell-cycle arrest and apoptosis.[171-173] Four prospective cohort studies have reported inverse associations between dietary vitamin D and colorectal cancer, but this was significant only in the Western Electric Study, a study of men only.[174] In the Iowa Women's Health Study and the Health Professionals Follow-up Study, a significant inverse relation was observed for vitamin D intake and risk of colon cancer, although this was attenuated and was no longer significant after multivariate adjustment.[175,176] Secondary analysis of the data from the prospective Nurses' Health cohort study showed an inverse association between intake of vitamin D and risk of colorectal cancer.[177] Some case-control studies have shown a decreased risk of colorectal cancer with higher levels of dietary vitamin D, whereas others have not.[83,152,178,179] However, a recently published meta-analysis of 17 epidemiologic studies demonstrated an inverse association between vitamin D and colorectal adenoma incidence and recurrence. The highest quintile of vitamin D intake was associated with an 11% decreased risk of colorectal adenomas compared with low vitamin D intake (OR 0.89, 95% CI 0.78–1.02).[180] Moreover, further analysis of the data from the randomized trial of Baron and colleagues[184] showed that higher serum 25-(OH) vitamin D levels were associated with a reduced risk of adenoma recurrence among subjects receiving calcium supplements. This suggests that calcium supplementation and vitamin D status act largely synergistically to reduce the risk of colorectal adenoma recurrence.

The largest randomized trial of combined calcium and vitamin D is the WHI.[41] In this trial, 18,716 women were randomized to receive both 1000 mg/day of elemental calcium and 400 IU/day of vitamin D while 18,106 women received matching placebo. After a mean follow-up of 7 years, the combination of calcium and vitamin D had no effect on the incidence of colorectal cancer. This study had several potential limitations. Only a single regimen was evaluated, and it is therefore unknown whether other formulations would have changed the results. The calcium as well as vitamin D doses that were used might have been insufficient to demonstrate a protective effect, particularly given the percentage of participants who were not fully compliant throughout the study. A larger dose of vitamin D than that used in the WHI trial may be necessary for any measurable chemopreventive effect. Therefore, the relation among vitamin D status, dose of vitamin D supplements, and colon cancer incidence or recurrence still remains unknown.

Folate

Folate is a water-soluble B vitamin common in legumes and dark-green leafy vegetables that functions as an important cofactor in single-carbon transfer. It is essential to numerous bodily functions, including DNA synthesis and repair, DNA methylation, modulation of cell proliferation, and protein metabolism. Experimental studies have shown that folate deficiency can lead to incorporation of uracil into genomic DNA and to increased chromosomal breaks, which can be reversed with folic acid supplementation.[182] In addition to animal data, a number of case-control and cohort studies have suggested that folate intake may be inversely related to colon cancer risk.[161,183,184] The Nurses' Health Study (NHS) cohort showed a significant 75% reduction of colon cancer among women who used folate supplements for at least 15 years, after adjusting for many factors including other vitamins and minerals (RR 0.25, 95% CI 0.13–0.51).[185] A meta-analysis of seven cohort and nine case-control studies, which included the data of the NHS study, showed a significantly lower risk of colorectal cancer among those in the highest category of dietary folate intake compared with those in the lowest category.[186] Nonetheless, clinical trials of folate have not confirmed these results. One of the most important randomized trials by Cole and associates[187] found that 1 mg/day of folic acid supplementation for 3 years in subjects with a history of colorectal adenoma did not prevent metachronous adenoma risk but in fact increased it. A proposed mechanism to explain these results is that the impact of folate may be bimodal, depending on timing and dosage.[188] Folate deficiency could increase the risk of mutation and thus tumorigenesis, but supplementation with high levels of folate may increase the survival and replication of already existing mutated cells by facilitating DNA replication or methylation of CpG islands of tumor-suppressor genes.[189] A recent meta-analysis of five randomized controlled trials testing folic acid supplementation failed to show any potential benefit.[190] Future trials with different dosages and duration are needed to further examine the possible protective effect of folic acid on colorectal neoplasia.

Furthermore, it is important to note that a relation between a common polymorphism of the methylenetetrahydrofolate reductase (MTHFR) gene with folate intake and the risk of colorectal neoplasia has been described. MTHFR is an enzyme that regulates folate metabolism and methionine synthesis. An estimated 10% to 15% of the population has a homozygous mutant, which reduces the enzyme activity by approximately 30%.[191] Studies that have examined the interaction of folate and MTHFR have shown that people with low folate intake and the homozygous mutant MTHFR gene have the highest risk of adenomas and colorectal cancer. This suggests that the effect of the enzyme in folate metabolism may play a role in the etiology of colorectal neoplasia via effects on DNA methylation and nucleotide synthesis.[192–194] More studies are warranted to establish the exact role of folate metabolism and MTHFR polymorphism in colorectal cancer.

Selenium

Selenium is a trace element naturally found in cereal, plants, seafood, and meat. Its concentration in the soil and therefore in food varies widely by geographic location. It is an important cofactor of glutathione peroxidase, an enzyme whose main biologic role is to protect the organism from oxidative damage. This antioxidant effect may prevent DNA damage caused by peroxidation. Epidemiologic studies have indicated that regions in the United States with low selenium in the soil have higher cancer mortality rates.[195–197] In a secondary analysis of a randomized clinical trial by Clark and colleagues,[198] which was initially conducted to determine whether selenium could prevent the recurrence of skin cancer, supplementation with 200 µg selenium per day reduced colorectal cancer incidence by 58%. However, a subsequent analysis with longer follow-up revealed that these results were attenuated and the result was no longer significant.[199] Additional clinical trials evaluating the role of selenium supplementation in colorectal cancer are currently in progress.

Other Vitamins and Antioxidants

Several other vitamins with antioxidant properties, including vitamins C, E, and carotenoids, have been thought to protect against oxidative stress and thereby decrease colon cancer risk. An important randomized clinical trial of 864 patients followed up for 4 years showed no efficacy of beta carotene, vitamins C and E, or their combination in preventing colorectal adenomas.[200] Compliance with study medications was high in this trial. The lack of efficacy of these vitamins argues against the use of supplemental beta carotene and vitamins C and E to prevent colorectal cancer.

Lifestyle

A number of lifestyle decisions have been associated with increased risk of cancer in general. The American Cancer Society's recommendations for a healthy lifestyle are given in Box 5-2. Although the relation between these factors and the development of colorectal cancer may not be fully proven, few could argue with the advice to lead a healthy lifestyle.

Tobacco

Beyond those tissues in direct contact with cigarette smoke, several other cancers have been linked with cigarette use, including stomach,

Recommendations for Individual Choices

Maintain a healthy weight throughout life.

Balance calorie intake with physical activity.

Avoid excessive weight gain throughout life.

Achieve and maintain a healthy weight if currently overweight or obese.

Adopt a physically active lifestyle.

   Adults: Engage in at least 30 minutes of moderate to vigorous physical activity, above usual activities on 5 or more days of the week; 45 to 60 minutes of intentional physical activity are preferable.

   Children and adolescents: Engage in at last 60 minutes per day of moderate to vigorous physical activity at least 5 days per week.

Eat a healthy diet, with an emphasis on plant sources.

   Choose foods and drinks in amounts that help achieve and maintain a healthy weight.

   Eat 5 or more servings of a variety of vegetables and fruits every day.

   Choose whole grains over processed (refined) grains.

   Limit intake of processed and red meats.

If you drink alcoholic beverages, limit your intake.

   Drink no more than 1 drink per day for women or 2 per day for men.

kidney, bladder, and pancreas.[201] Some of the earliest reports examining cigarette use and the incidence of colorectal cancers have shown no association,[92,94,111,126,202–212] but as pointed out in a review by Giovannucci,[201] the majority of these studies had a follow-up period in the 1950s and 1960s. Since smoking cigarettes became popular in the 1920s in the United States, this was enough time only for the heaviest of smokers to reach a 30 to 40 pack-year history.[201] As the majority of the population reached this 40 pack-year threshold in the late 1980s and 1990s, smoking was first strongly linked to colonic adenoma formation[11,72,213–229] and then to colon cancer formation.[38,125,142,230–248] Exceptions that prove this rule are Peters and associates,[111] who investigated only young men (under 45 years old) and Kono and colleagues,[206] who, after re-examining the same population with a longer follow-up period, subsequently found a significant risk of colorectal cancers among Japanese smokers. It is interesting that in a case-control study of Canadian men by Sharpe and associates,[212] smokers were shown to have

an increased risk (though nonsignificant) of proximal colon cancers only. These authors postulate that this could be a contributing factor to the increasing incidence of proximal colon cancers compared with distal colon cancers in Western nations.

Alcohol

Alcohol consumption has long been linked to cancers of the upper digestive tract such as the oral cavity, pharynx, hypopharynx, and esophagus. However, the direct association between alcohol consumption and colorectal cancers has been somewhat tenuous, with some studies proving no association[10,13,14,85,94,106,113,115,125,126,207,237,249,250] and others showing a strong association.[30,86,116,128,206,251–262] To clarify the interaction, several pooled analyses and meta-analyses were performed, including those by Bagnardi and associates[263] and Longnecker and associates,[227] which showed that with increased alcohol consumption, colorectal cancer risk increased. Furthermore, studies highly controlled for other patient dietary factors have shown a small but significant increase in colorectal cancer risk.[241,264,265] Possible causative mechanisms of the impact of alcohol on the development of colorectal cancers include the immunosuppressive effects of alcohol, liver enzyme and bile composition changes, and the nitrosamine content of alcoholic drinks.

Physical Activity

Multiple retrospective and prospective epidemiologic studies have consistently shown an inverse association between physical activity and risk of colon but not rectal cancer (Fig. 5-2). A recent meta-analysis of 52 studies confirmed this by showing that individuals can likely reduce their risk of colon cancer overall by 24% through participation in physical activity (RR 0.76, 95% CI 0.72–0.81).[266] If a causal relationship between physical activity and colon cancer exists, the mechanisms are poorly understood. Physical activity is thought to stimulate intestinal transit, decrease the colon prostaglandin content, and thus reduce inflammation and prevent hyperinsulinemia. The intensity and duration of physical activity that offer the greatest risk reduction and the period of life during which physical activity

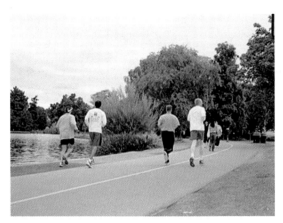

Figure 5-2. Regular physical activity has been shown to be an important factor in overall health and may be a factor in the prevention of colorectal cancer. (Photo by Stephanie Cartier.)

may have the greatest impact have not been determined.

Excess Weight

Obesity has reached epidemic proportions in the United States and is a major contributor to the burden of chronic disease and disability. Findings from numerous studies have shown a positive association between obesity and risk of colon cancer. Published meta-analyses of prospective and retrospective studies show that higher body mass index is associated with a modest increased risk of developing colon cancer in men and women and rectal cancer in men.[267-269] The association is seen for both adenomas and colorectal cancer. Plausible mechanisms linking excess weight and colorectal neoplasia risk are not fully understood, particularly because important confounding factors (e.g., physical activity and total energy intake) may not have been measured with sufficient precision. Several mechanisms have been proposed, including excess secretion of insulin, free insulin-like growth factor (IGF), and adiponectin, which could act mitogenically and may directly contribute to the development of colorectal cancer.

Immigration

The fact that the risk of colorectal cancer is greatly influenced by environmental change is evident from studies in immigrant populations who moved from low- to high-risk areas and vice versa. Data from various countries have shown

that over time migrant groups tend to assume a risk of colon cancer similar to that of the native population, implying that dietary and other environmental factors constitute a major component of risk.[270,271] For example, although colon cancer is still relatively uncommon in Japan, the incidence among Japanese in the United States is currently higher than that in both U.S. whites and blacks. This suggests that, as the genetic composition of the migrants had not changed, their risk was influenced by the new environment.[2] Studies have shown similar results of a shifting pattern of cancer incidence among other migrant Asian-American populations such as the Chinese, Koreans, and Filippinos.[272-274] Migration of blacks from Africa to the United States also led to a dramatic increase in the incidence of colorectal cancers among this group. According to one study, 75% of African Americans are believed to have come from West Africa, with 40% being ethnologically related to present-day Nigerians.[275] The incidence of colorectal cancer in African-American males and females far exceeds that among Nigerian people, providing further support that as groups of people move to a new land, their risks of cancer shift away from the pattern prevailing in their country of origin toward that of the host country[276] (Fig. 5-3). Similarly, migration to low-risk regions has been shown to decrease colon cancer risk. Migrants from the British Isles to Australia had

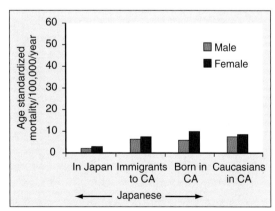

Figure 5-3. Mortality rates from colon cancer comparing Japanese in their homeland with those immigrating to or born in California. Note the similarity in rates between Japanese born in California and native white Californians. (From Mortality for Colon Cancer (Japan and California) from Public Health Toxicology. Available at http://ocw.jhsph.edu. Copyright © Johns Hopkins Bloomberg School of Public Health. Creative Commons BY-NC-SA.)

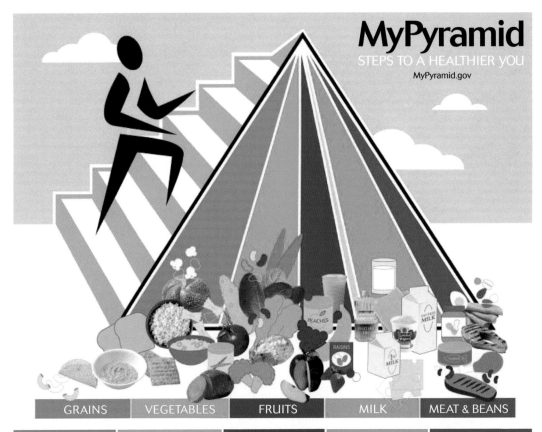

Figure 5-4. Current version of the USDA MyPyramid, showing steps to a healthy lifestyle. Note that physical activity is emphasized along with healthy eating habits. (From U.S. Department of Agriculture, Center for Nutrition Policy and Promotion, April 2005.)

a decreased risk of colorectal cancer.[277] This is even more evident in a study of Italians immigrating to South America, which showed that rates of colon cancer decreased in the low-risk area of São Paulo and increased in the high-risk area of Argentina.[278]

Conclusion

Several modifiable risk factors for colorectal cancer have been identified, including a diet high in red and processed meats, physical inactivity, and long exposure to tobacco or alcohol. Although not all studies have shown a significant association, diets high in fiber—particularly vegetable fiber—low in fat, and containing probiotics, combined with physical activity, may decrease the risk of colorectal cancer (Fig. 5-4). Furthermore, a diet high in vitamins and micronutrients such as folate and selenium is thought to decrease the risk of colorectal cancer, although this has not been resolutely proved by epidemiologic studies. Unfortunately, interventional studies in dietary modifications to prevent colorectal cancers have met with little success largely because of poor compliance with study design and small differences among study groups.

Despite the limitations of the data available, most experts agree that diets high in fiber and vitamins and low in red meats and fats are beneficial with regard to the development of colorectal cancer, although the precise interaction and mechanisms are not yet known.

References

1. Armstrong B, Doll R: Environmental factors and cancer incidence and mortality in different countries, with special reference to dietary practices. Int J Cancer 15(4):617–631, 1975.
2. Haenszel W, Kurihara M: Studies of Japanese migrants. I. Mortality from cancer and other diseases among Japanese in the United States. J Natl Cancer Inst 40(1):43–68, 1968.
3. Burkitt DP: Epidemiology of cancer of the colon and rectum. Cancer 28(1):3–13, 1971.
4. Doll R, Peto R: The causes of cancer: quantitative estimates of avoidable risks of cancer in the United States today. J Natl Cancer Inst 66(6):1191–1308, 1981.
5. Scheppach W, Bingham S, Boutron-Rouault MC, et al: WHO consensus statement on the role of nutrition in colorectal cancer. Eur J Cancer Prev 8(1):57–62, 1999.
6. Nutritional aspects of the development of cancer. Report of the Working Group on Diet and Cancer of the Committee on Medical Aspects of Food and Nutrition Policy. Rep Health Soc Subj (Lond) 48:i–xiv, 1–274, 1998.
7. Glade MJ: Food, nutrition, and the prevention of cancer: a global perspective. American Institute for Cancer Research/World Cancer Research Fund, American Institute for Cancer Research, 1997. Nutrition 15(6):523–526, 1999.
8. Jacobs ET, Thompson PA, Martinez ME: Diet, gender, and colorectal neoplasia. J Clin Gastroenterol 41(8):731–746, 2007.
9. Gerhardsson de Verdier M., Hagman U, Peters RK, et al: Meat, cooking methods and colorectal cancer: a case-referent study in Stockholm. Int J Cancer 49(4):520–525, 1991.
10. La Vecchia C, Negri E, Decarli A, et al: A case-control study of diet and colo-rectal cancer in northern Italy. Int J Cancer 41(4):492–498, 1988.
11. Lee HP, Gourley L, Duffy SW, et al: Colorectal cancer and diet in an Asian population—a case-control study among Singapore Chinese. Int J Cancer 43(6):1007–1016, 1989.
12. Young TB, Wolf DA: Case-control study of proximal and distal colon cancer and diet in Wisconsin. Int J Cancer 42(2):167–175, 1988.
13. Berta JL, Coste T, Rautoureau J, et al: [Diet and rectocolonic cancers. Results of a case-control study]. Gastroenterol Clin Biol 9(4):348–353, 1985.
14. Macquart-Moulin G, Riboli E, Cornée J, et al: Case-control study on colorectal cancer and diet in Marseilles. Int J Cancer 38(2):183–191, 1986.
15. Chao A, Thun MJ, Connell, CJ, et al: Meat consumption and risk of colorectal cancer. JAMA 293(2):172–182, 2005.
16. English DR, Macinnis RJ, Hodge AM, et al: Red meat, chicken, and fish consumption and risk of colorectal cancer. Cancer Epidemiol Biomarkers Prev 13(9):1509–1514, 2004.
17. Giovannucci E, Rimm EB, Stampfer MJ, et al: Intake of fat, meat, and fiber in relation to risk of colon cancer in men. Cancer Res 54(9):2390–2397, 1994.
18. Thun MJ, Calle EE, Namboodiri MM, et al: Risk factors for fatal colon cancer in a large prospective study. J Natl Cancer Inst 84(19):1491–1500, 1992.
19. Willett WC, Stampfer MJ, Colditz GA, et al: Relation of meat, fat, and fiber intake to the risk of colon cancer in a prospective study among women. N Engl J Med 323(24):1664–1672, 1990.
20. Schatzkin A, Lanza E, Corle D, et al: Lack of effect of a low-fat, high-fiber diet on the recurrence of colorectal adenomas. Polyp Prevention Trial Study Group. N Engl J Med 342(16):1149–1155, 2000.
21. Norat T, Lukanova A, Ferrari P, Riboli E, et al: Meat consumption and colorectal cancer risk: dose-response meta-analysis of epidemiological studies. Int J Cancer 98(2):241–256, 2002.
22. Larsson SC, Wolk A: Meat consumption and risk of colorectal cancer: a meta-analysis of prospective studies. Int J Cancer 119(11):2657–2664, 2006.
23. Schiffman MH, Felton JS: Re: "Fried foods and the risk of colon cancer." Am J Epidemiol 131(2):376–378, 1990.
24. Murtaugh MA, Ma KN, Sweeney C, et al: Meat consumption patterns and preparation, genetic variants of metabolic enzymes, and their association with rectal cancer in men and women. J Nutr 134(4):776–784, 2004.
25. Lyon JL, Mahoney AW: Fried foods and the risk of colon cancer. Am J Epidemiol 128(5):1000–1006, 1988.
26. Muscat JE, Wynder EL: The consumption of well-done red meat and the risk of colorectal cancer. Am J Public Health 84(5):856–858, 1994.
27. Lang NP, Butler MA, Massengill J, et al: Rapid metabolic phenotypes for acetyltransferase and cytochrome P4501A2 and putative exposure to food-borne heterocyclic amines increase the risk for colorectal cancer or polyps. Cancer Epidemiol Biomarkers Prev 3(8):675–682, 1994.
28. Chen J, Stampfer MJ, Hough HL, et al: A prospective study of N-acetyltransferase genotype, red meat intake, and risk of colorectal cancer. Cancer Res 58(15):3307–3311, 1998.
29. Jain M, Cook GM, Davis FG, et al: A case-control study of diet and colo-rectal cancer. Int J Cancer 26(6):757–768, 1980.
30. Potter JD, McMichael AJ: Diet and cancer of the colon and rectum: a case-control study. J Natl Cancer Inst 76(4):557–569, 1986.
31. Graham S, Marshall J, Haughey B, et al: Dietary epidemiology of cancer of the colon in western New York. Am J Epidemiol 128(3):490–503, 1988.
32. Rose DP, Boyar AP, Wynder EL: International comparisons of mortality rates for cancer of the breast, ovary, prostate, and colon, and per capita food consumption. Cancer 58(11):2363–2371, 1986.
33. Honda T, Kai I, Ohi G: Fat and dietary fiber intake and colon cancer mortality: a chronological comparison between Japan and the United States. Nutr Cancer 33(1):95–99, 1999.

34. Palmer S: Dietary considerations for risk reduction. Cancer 58(8 Suppl):1949–1953, 1986.
35. Howe GR, Aronson KJ, Benito E, et al: The relationship between dietary fat intake and risk of colorectal cancer: evidence from the combined analysis of 13 case-control studies. Cancer Causes Control 8(2):215–228, 1997.
36. Willett WC: Dietary fat intake and cancer risk: a controversial and instructive story. Semin Cancer Biol 8(4):245–253, 1998.
37. Goldbohm RA, van den Brandt PA, van 't Veer P, et al: A prospective cohort study on the relation between meat consumption and the risk of colon cancer. Cancer Res 54(3):718–723, 1994.
38. Bostick RM, Potter JD, Kushi LH, et al: Sugar, meat, and fat intake, and non-dietary risk factors for colon cancer incidence in Iowa women (United States). Cancer Causes Control 5(1):38–52, 1994.
39. MacLennan R, Macrae F, Bain C, et al: Randomized trial of intake of fat, fiber, and beta carotene to prevent colorectal adenomas. J Natl Cancer Inst 87(23):1760–1766, 1995.
40. McKeown-Eyssen GE, Bright-See E, Bruce WR, et al: A randomized trial of a low fat high fibre diet in the recurrence of colorectal polyps. Toronto Polyp Prevention Group. J Clin Epidemiol 47(5):525–536, 1994.
41. Wactawski-Wende J, Kotchen JM, Anderson GL, et al: Calcium plus vitamin D supplementation and the risk of colorectal cancer. N Engl J Med 354(7):684–696, 2006.
42. Sansbury LB, Wanke K, Albert PS, et al: The effect of strict adherence to a high-fiber, high-fruit and -vegetable, and low-fat eating pattern on adenoma recurrence. Am J Epidemiol 170(5):576–584, 2009.
43. Franceschi S, LaVecchia C, Russo A, et al: Macronutrient intake and risk of colorectal cancer in Italy. Int J Cancer 76(3):321–324, 1998.
44. Sengupta S, Tjandra JJ, Gibson PR: Dietary fiber and colorectal neoplasia. Dis Colon Rectum 44(7):1016–1033, 2001.
45. Lupton JR, Turner ND: Potential protective mechanisms of wheat bran fiber. Am J Med 106(1A):24S–27S, 1999.
46. Chaplin MF: Bile acids, fibre and colon cancer: the story unfolds. J R Soc Health 118(1):53–61, 1998.
47. Breuer N, Goebell H: The role of bile acids in colonic carcinogenesis. Klin Wochenschr 63(3):97–105, 1985.
48. Archer S, Meng S, Wu J, et al: Butyrate inhibits colon carcinoma cell growth through two distinct pathways. Surgery 124(2):248–253, 1998.
49. Marchetti C, Migliorati G, Moraca R, et al: Deoxycholic acid and SCFA-induced apoptosis in the human tumor cell-line HT-29 and possible mechanisms. Cancer Lett 114(1–2):97–99, 1997.
50. Bartram HP, Englert S, Scheppach W, et al: Antagonistic effects of deoxycholic acid and butyrate on epithelial cell proliferation in the proximal and distal human colon. Z Gastroenterol 32(7):389–392, 1994.
51. Hague A, Elder DJ, Hicks DJ, Paraskeva C: Apoptosis in colorectal tumour cells: induction by the short chain fatty acids butyrate, propionate and acetate and by the bile salt deoxycholate. Int J Cancer 60(3):400–406, 1995.
52. Scheppach W, Sommer H, Kirchner T, et al: Effect of butyrate enemas on the colonic mucosa in distal ulcerative colitis. Gastroenterology 103(1):51–56, 1992.
53. McBain JA, Eastman A, Nobel CS, Mueller GC: Apoptotic death in adenocarcinoma cell lines induced by butyrate and other histone deacetylase inhibitors. Biochem Pharmacol 53(9):1357–1368, 1997.
54. Archer SY, Hodin RA: Histone acetylation and cancer. Curr Opin Genet Dev 9(2):171–174, 1999.
55. Fadden K, Hill MJ, Owen RW: Effect of fibre on bile acid metabolism by human faecal bacteria in batch and continuous culture. Eur J Cancer Prev 6(2):175–194, 1997.
56. McKeown-Eyssen GE, Bright-See E: Dietary factors in colon cancer: international relationships. Nutr Cancer 6(3):160–170, 1984.
57. Trock B, Lanza E, Greenwald P: Dietary fiber, vegetables, and colon cancer: critical review and meta-analyses of the epidemiologic evidence. J Natl Cancer Inst 82(8):650–661, 1990.
58. Liu K, Stamler J, Moss D, et al: Dietary cholesterol, fat, and fibre, and colon-cancer mortality. An analysis of international data. Lancet 2(8146):782–785, 1979.
59. Irving D, Drasar BS: Fibre and cancer of the colon. Br J Cancer 28(5):462–463, 1973.
60. Caygill CP, Charlett A, Hill MJ: Relationship between the intake of high-fibre foods and energy and the risk of cancer of the large bowel and breast. Eur J Cancer Prev 7(Suppl 2):S11–S17, 1998.
61. Bingham SA, Day NE, Luben R, et al: European Prospective Investigation into Cancer and Nutrition. Dietary fibre in food and protection against colorectal cancer in the European Prospective Investigation into Cancer and Nutrition (EPIC): an observational study. Lancet 361(9368):1496–1501, 2003.
62. Freudenheim JL, Graham S, Horvath PJ, et al: Risks associated with source of fiber and fiber components in cancer of the colon and rectum. Cancer Res 50(11):3295–3300, 1990.
63. Arbman G, Axelson O, Ericsson-Begodzki AB, et al: Cereal fiber, calcium, and colorectal cancer. Cancer 69(8):2042–2048, 1992.
64. Kune S, Kune GA, Watson LF: Case-control study of dietary etiological factors: The Melbourne Colorectal Cancer Study. Nutr Cancer 9(1):21–42, 1987.
65. Negri E, Franceschi S, Parpinel M, La Vecchia C: Fiber intake and risk of colorectal cancer. Cancer Epidemiol Biomarkers Prev 7(8):667–671, 1998.
66. Levi F, Pasche C, La Vecchia C, et al: Food groups and colorectal cancer risk. Br J Cancer 79(7–8):1283–1287, 1999.
67. Le Marchand L, Hankin JH, Wilkens LR, et al: Dietary fiber and colorectal cancer risk. Epidemiology 8(6):658, 1997.
68. Iscovich JM, L'Abbe KA, Castelleto R, et al: Colon cancer in Argentina. II: risk from fibre, fat and nutrients. Int J Cancer 51(6):858–861, 1992.
69. Bidoli E, Franceschi S, Talamini R, et al: Food consumption and cancer of the colon and rectum in north-eastern Italy. Int J Cancer 50(2):223–229, 1992.
70. West DW, Slattery ML, Robison LM, et al: Dietary intake and colon cancer: sex- and anatomic site-specific associations. Am J Epidemiol 130(5):883–894, 1989.
71. Witte JS, Longnecker MP, Bird CL, et al: Relation of vegetable, fruit, and grain consumption to colorectal adenomatous polyps. Am J Epidemiol 144(11):1015–1025, 1996.
72. Giovannucci E, Rimm EB, Stampfer MJ, et al: A prospective study of cigarette smoking and risk of colorectal adenoma and colorectal cancer in U.S. men. J Natl Cancer Inst 86(3):183–191, 1994.
73. Pietinen P, Malila N, Virtanen M, et al: Diet and risk of colorectal cancer in a cohort of Finnish men. Cancer Causes Control 10(5):387–396, 1999.
74. Platz EA, Giovannucci E, Rimm EB, et al: Dietary fiber and distal colorectal adenoma in men. Cancer Epidemiol Biomarkers Prev 6(9):661–670, 1997.
75. Fuchs CS, Giovannucci EL, Colditz GA, et al: Dietary fiber and the risk of colorectal cancer and adenoma in women. N Engl J Med 340(3):169–176, 1999.
76. Friedenreich CM, Brant RF, Riboli E: Influence of methodologic factors in a pooled analysis of 13 case-control studies of colorectal cancer and dietary fiber. Epidemiology 5(1):66–79, 1994.
77. DeCosse JJ, Miller HH, Lesser ML: Effect of wheat fiber and vitamins C and E on rectal polyps in patients with familial adenomatous polyposis. J Natl Cancer Inst 81(17):1290–1297, 1989.
78. Alberts DS, Martinez ME, Roe DJ, et al: Lack of effect of a high-fiber cereal supplement on the recurrence of colorectal adenomas. Phoenix Colon Cancer Prevention Physicians' Network. N Engl J Med 342(16):1156–1162, 2000.
79. Almendingen K, Trygg K, Hofstad B, et al: Results from two repeated 5 day dietary records with a 1 y interval among patients with colorectal polyps. Eur J Clin Nutr 55(5):374–379, 2001.
80. Bonithon-Kopp C, Kronborg O, Giacosa A, et al: Calcium and fibre supplementation in prevention of colorectal adenoma recurrence: a randomised intervention trial. European Cancer Prevention Organisation Study Group. Lancet 356(9238):1300–1306, 2000.
81. Alberts DS, Einspahr J, Rees-McGee S, et al: Effects of dietary wheat bran fiber on rectal epithelial cell proliferation in patients with resection for colorectal cancers. J Natl Cancer Inst 82(15):1280–1285, 1990.
82. Alberts DS, Ritenbaugh C, Story JA, et al: Randomized, double-blinded, placebo-controlled study of effect of wheat

bran fiber and calcium on fecal bile acids in patients with resected adenomatous colon polyps. J Natl Cancer Inst 88(2):81–92, 1996.

83. Benito E, Cabeza E, Moreno V, et al: Diet and colorectal adenomas: a case-control study in Majorca. Int J Cancer 55(2):213–219, 1993.

84. Iscovich JM, L'Abbe KA, Castelleto R, et al: Colon cancer in Argentina. I: Risk from intake of dietary items. Int J Cancer 51(6):851–857, 1992.

85. Manousos O, Day NE, Trichopoulos D, et al: Diet and colorectal cancer: a case-control study in Greece. Int J Cancer 32(1):1–5, 1983.

86. Tuyns AJ, Kaaks R, Haelterman M: Colorectal cancer and the consumption of foods: a case-control study in Belgium. Nutr Cancer 11(3):189–204, 1988.

87. van Duijnhoven FJ, Bueno-De-Mesquita HB, Ferrari P, et al: Fruit, vegetables, and colorectal cancer risk: the European Prospective Investigation into cancer and nutrition. Am J Clin Nutr 89(5):1441–1452, 2009.

88. Steinmetz KA, Potter JD: Food-group consumption and colon cancer in the Adelaide case-control study. I. Vegetables and fruit. Int J Cancer 53(5):711–719, 1993.

89. Steinmetz KA, Kushi LH, Bostick RM, et al: Vegetables, fruit, and colon cancer in the Iowa Women's Health Study. Am J Epidemiol 139(1):1–15, 1994.

90. Dorant E, van den Brandt PA, Goldbohm RA: A prospective cohort study on the relationship between onion and leek consumption, garlic supplement use and the risk of colorectal carcinoma in the Netherlands. Carcinogenesis 17(3):477–484, 1996.

91. Haenszel W, Berg JW, Segi M, et al: Large-bowel cancer in Hawaiian Japanese. J Natl Cancer Inst 51(6):1765–1779, 1973.

92. Haenszel W, Locke FB, Segi M: A case-control study of large bowel cancer in Japan. J Natl Cancer Inst 64(1):17–22, 1980.

93. Hu JF, Liu YY, Yu YK, et al: Diet and cancer of the colon and rectum: a case-control study in China. Int J Epidemiol 20(2):362–367, 1991.

94. Tajima K, Tominaga S: Dietary habits and gastro-intestinal cancers: a comparative case-control study of stomach and large intestinal cancers in Nagoya, Japan. Jpn J Cancer Res 76(8):705–716, 1985.

95. Tanaka S, Haruma K, Kunihiro M, et al: Effects of aged garlic extract (AGE) on colorectal adenomas: a double-blinded study. Hiroshima J Med Sci 53(3–4):39–45, 2004.

96. Tanaka S, Haruma K, Yoshihara M, et al: Aged garlic extract has potential suppressive effect on colorectal adenomas in humans. J Nutr 136(3 Suppl):821S–826S, 2006.

97. Fleischauer AT, Poole C, Arab L: Garlic consumption and cancer prevention: meta-analyses of colorectal and stomach cancers. Am J Clin Nutr 72(4):1047–1052, 2000.

98. Ngo SN, Williams DB, Cobiac L, Head RJ: Does garlic reduce risk of colorectal cancer? A systematic review. J Nutr 137(10):2264–2269, 2007.

99. Will JC, Galuska DA, Vinicor F, Calle EE: Colorectal cancer: another complication of diabetes mellitus? Am J Epidemiol 147(9):816–825, 1998.

100. Nilsen TI, Vatten LJ: Prospective study of colorectal cancer risk and physical activity, diabetes, blood glucose and BMI: exploring the hyperinsulinaemia hypothesis. Br J Cancer 84(3):417–422, 2001.

101. Giovannucci E: Insulin and colon cancer. Cancer Causes Control 6(2):164–179, 1995.

102. Hu FB, Manson JE, Liu S, et al: Prospective study of adult onset diabetes mellitus (type 2) and risk of colorectal cancer in women. J Natl Cancer Inst 91(6):542–547, 1999.

103. La Vecchia C, Negri E, Decarli A, Franceschi S: Diabetes mellitus and colorectal cancer risk. Cancer Epidemiol Biomarkers Prev 6(12):1007–1010, 1997.

104. Kono S, Honjo S, Todoroki I, et al: Glucose intolerance and adenomas of the sigmoid colon in Japanese men (Japan). Cancer Causes Control 9(4):441–446, 1998.

105. Boing H, Martinez L, Frentzel-Beyme R, Oltersdorf U: Regional nutritional pattern and cancer mortality in the Federal Republic of Germany. Nutr Cancer 7(3):121–130, 1985.

106. Bristol JB, Emmett PM, Heaton KW, Williamson RC: Sugar, fat, and the risk of colorectal cancer. Br Med J (Clin Res Ed) 291(6507):1467–1470, 1985.

107. Centonze S, Boeing H, Leoci C, et al: Dietary habits and colorectal cancer in a low-risk area. Results from a population-based case-control study in southern Italy. Nutr Cancer 21(3):233–246, 1994.

108. de Verdier MG, Longnecker MP: Eating frequency—a neglected risk factor for colon cancer? Cancer Causes Control 3(1):77–81, 1992.

109. La Vecchia C, Franceschi S, Dolara P, et al: Refined-sugar intake and the risk of colorectal cancer in humans. Int J Cancer 55(3):386–389, 1993.

110. Macquart-Moulin G, Riboli E, Cornee J, et al: Colorectal polyps and diet: a case-control study in Marseilles. Int J Cancer 40(2):179–188, 1987.

111. Peters RK, Garabrant DH, Yu MC, Mack TM: A case-control study of occupational and dietary factors in colorectal cancer in young men by subsite. Cancer Res 49(19):5459–5468, 1989.

112. Tuyns AJ, Haelterman M, Kaaks R: Colorectal cancer and the intake of nutrients: oligosaccharides are a risk factor, fats are not. A case-control study in Belgium. Nutr Cancer 10(4):181–196, 1987.

113. Benito E, Obrador A, Stiggelbout A, et al: A population-based case-control study of colorectal cancer in Majorca. I. Dietary factors. Int J Cancer 45(1):69–76, 1990.

114. Llopis A, Morales M, Rodriguez R: Digestive cancer in relation to diet in Spain. J Environ Pathol Toxicol Oncol 11(3):169–175, 1992.

115. Modan B, Barell V, Lubin F, et al: Low-fiber intake as an etiologic factor in cancer of the colon. J Natl Cancer Inst 55(1):15–18, 1975.

116. Pickle LW, Greene MH, Ziegler RG, et al: Colorectal cancer in rural Nebraska. Cancer Res 44(1):363–369, 1984.

117. Zaridze D, Filipchenko V, Kustov V, et al: Diet and colorectal cancer: results of two case-control studies in Russia. Eur J Cancer 29A(1):112–115, 1992.

118. Ma J, Giovannucci E, Pollak M, et al: A prospective study of plasma C-peptide and colorectal cancer risk in men. J Natl Cancer Inst 96(7):546–553, 2004.

119. Kaaks R, Toniolo P, Akhmedkhanov A, et al: Serum C-peptide, insulin-like growth factor (IGF)-I, IGF-binding proteins, and colorectal cancer risk in women. J Natl Cancer Inst 92(19):1592–1600, 2000.

120. Baron JA, Gerhardsson de Verdier M, Ekbom A: Coffee, tea, tobacco, and cancer of the large bowel. Cancer Epidemiol Biomarkers Prev 3(7):565–570, 1994.

121. Baron JA, Greenberg ER, Haile R, et al: Coffee and tea and the risk of recurrent colorectal adenomas. Cancer Epidemiol Biomarkers Prev 6(1):7–10, 1997.

122. Jacobsen BK, Bjelke E, Kvale G, Heuch I: Coffee drinking, mortality, and cancer incidence: results from a Norwegian prospective study. J Natl Cancer Inst 76(5):823–831, 1986.

123. La Vecchia C, Ferraroni M, Negri E, et al: Coffee consumption and digestive tract cancers. Cancer Res 49(4):1049–1051, 1989.

124. Rosenberg L: Coffee and tea consumption in relation to the risk of large bowel cancer: a review of epidemiologic studies. Cancer Lett 52(3):163–171, 1990.

125. Dales LG, Friedman GD, Ury HK, et al: A case-control study of relationships of diet and other traits to colorectal cancer in American blacks. Am J Epidemiol 109(2):132–144, 1979.

126. Graham S, Dayal H, Swanson M, et al: Diet in the epidemiology of cancer of the colon and rectum. J Natl Cancer Inst 61(3):709–714, 1978.

127. Hartman TJ, Tangrea JA, Pietinen P, et al: Tea and coffee consumption and risk of colon and rectal cancer in middle-aged Finnish men. Nutr Cancer 31(1):41–48, 1998.

128. Miller AB, Howe GR, Jain M, et al: Food items and food groups as risk factors in a case-control study of diet and colo-rectal cancer. Int J Cancer 32(2):155–161, 1983.

129. Nomura A, Heilbrun LK, Stemmermann GN: Prospective study of coffee consumption and the risk of cancer. J Natl Cancer Inst 76(4):587–590, 1986.

130. Phillips RL, Snowdon DA: Dietary relationships with fatal colorectal cancer among Seventh-Day Adventists. J Natl Cancer Inst 74(2):307–317, 1985.

131. Shannon J, White E, Shattuck AL, Potter JD: Relationship of food groups and water intake to colon cancer risk. Cancer Epidemiol Biomarkers Prev 5(7):495–502, 1996.

132. Ekbom A: Review: substantial coffee consumption was associated with a lower risk of colorectal cancer in the general population. Gut 44(5):597, 1999.
133. Goldbohm RA, Hertog MG, Brants HA, et al: Consumption of black tea and cancer risk: a prospective cohort study. J Natl Cancer Inst 88(2):93–100, 1996.
134. Kohlmeier L, Weterings KG, Steck S, Kok FJ: Tea and cancer prevention: an evaluation of the epidemiologic literature. Nutr Cancer 27(1):1–13, 1997.
135. Yang CS, Wang ZY: Tea and cancer. J Natl Cancer Inst 85(13):1038–1049, 1993.
136. Kumar N, Shibata D, Helm J, et al: Green tea polyphenols in the prevention of colon cancer. Front Biosci 12:2309–2315, 2007.
137. Bushman JL: Green tea and cancer in humans: a review of the literature. Nutr Cancer 31(3):151–159, 1998.
138. Ji BT, Chow WH, Hsing AW, et al: Green tea consumption and the risk of pancreatic and colorectal cancers. Int J Cancer 70(3):255–258, 1997.
139. Kono S, Shinchi K, Ikeda N, et al: Physical activity, dietary habits and adenomatous polyps of the sigmoid colon: a study of self-defense officials in Japan. J Clin Epidemiol 44(11):1255–1261, 1991.
140. Kato I, Tominaga S, Matsuura A, et al: A comparative case-control study of colorectal cancer and adenoma. Jpn J Cancer Res 81(11):1101–1108, 1990.
141. Pufulete M: Intake of dairy products and risk of colorectal neoplasia. Nutr Res Rev 21(1):56–67, 2008.
142. Wu AH, Paganini-Hill A, Ross RK, Henderson BE: Alcohol, physical activity and other risk factors for colorectal cancer: a prospective study. Br J Cancer 55(6):687–694, 1987.
143. Cho E, Smith-Warner SA, Spiegelman D, et al: Dairy foods, calcium, and colorectal cancer: a pooled analysis of 10 cohort studies. J Natl Cancer Inst 96(13):1015–1022, 2004.
144. Norat T, Riboli E: Dairy products and colorectal cancer. A review of possible mechanisms and epidemiological evidence. Eur J Clin Nutr 57(1):1–17, 2003.
145. Singh PN, Fraser GE: Dietary risk factors for colon cancer in a low-risk population. Am J Epidemiol 148(8):761–764, 1998.
146. Steinmetz KA, Potter JD: Food-group consumption and colon cancer in the Adelaide case-control study. II. Meat, poultry, seafood, dairy foods and eggs. Int J Cancer 53(5):720–727, 1993.
147. Hayatsu H, Hayatsu T: Suppressing effect of lactobacillus casei administration on the urinary mutagenicity arising from ingestion of fried ground beef in the human. Cancer Lett 73(2–3):173–179, 1993.
148. Biasco G, Paganelli GM, Brandi G, et al: Effect of lactobacillus acidophilus and bifidobacterium bifidum on rectal cell kinetics and fecal pH. Ital J Gastroenterol 23(3):142, 1991.
149. Boutron MC, Faivre J, Marteau P, et al: Calcium, phosphorus, vitamin D, dairy products and colorectal carcinogenesis: a French case-control study. Br J Cancer 74(1):145–151, 1996.
150. Kampman E, Giovannucci E, van 't Veer P, et al: Calcium, vitamin D, dairy foods, and the occurrence of colorectal adenomas among men and women in two prospective studies. Am J Epidemiol 139(1):16–29, 1994.
151. Kampman E, Goldbohm RA, van den Brandt PA, van 't Veer P: Fermented dairy products, calcium, and colorectal cancer in The Netherlands Cohort Study. Cancer Res 54(12):3186–3190, 1994.
152. Peters RK, Pike MC, Garabrant D, Mack TM: Diet and colon cancer in Los Angeles County, California. Cancer Causes Control 3(5):457–473, 1992.
153. Young TB, Wolf DA: Case-control study of proximal and distal colon cancer and diet in Wisconsin. Int J Cancer 42(2):167–175, 1988.
154. Buehring GC, Philpott SM, Choi KY: Humans have antibodies reactive with bovine leukemia virus. AIDS Res Hum Retroviruses 19(12):1105–1113, 2003.
155. Schwartz I, Levy D: Pathobiology of bovine leukemia virus. Vet Res 25(6):521–536, 1994.
156. Sellers TA, Vierkant RA, Djeu J, et al: Unpasteurized milk consumption and subsequent risk of cancer. Cancer Causes Control 19(8):805–811, 2008.
157. Newmark HL, Wargovich MJ, Bruce WR: Colon cancer and dietary fat, phosphate, and calcium: a hypothesis. J Natl Cancer Inst 72(6):1323–1325, 1984.
158. Lipkin M, Newmark H: Effect of added dietary calcium on colonic epithelial-cell proliferation in subjects at high risk for familial colonic cancer. N Engl J Med 313(22):1381–1384, 1985.
159. Martinez ME, Willett WC: Calcium, vitamin D, and colorectal cancer: a review of the epidemiologic evidence. Cancer Epidemiol Biomarkers Prev 7(2):163–168, 1998.
160. Wu K, Willett WC, Fuchs CS, et al: Calcium intake and risk of colon cancer in women and men. J Natl Cancer Inst 94(6):437–446, 2002.
161. Sellers TA, Bazyk AE, Bostick RM, et al: Diet and risk of colon cancer in a large prospective study of older women: an analysis stratified on family history (Iowa, United States). Cancer Causes Control 9(4):357–367, 1998.
162. Baron JA, Beach M, Mandel JS, et al: Calcium supplements for the prevention of colorectal adenomas. Calcium Polyp Prevention Study Group. N Engl J Med 340(2):101–107, 1999.
163. Hofstad B, Vatn MH, Andersen SN, et al: The relationship between faecal bile acid profile with or without supplementation with calcium and antioxidants on recurrence and growth of colorectal polyps. Eur J Cancer Prev 7(4):287–294, 1998.
164. Martinez ME, Marshall JR, Sampliner R, et al: Calcium, vitamin D, and risk of adenoma recurrence (United States). Cancer Causes Control 13(3):213–220, 2002.
165. Duris I, Hruby D, Pekarkova B, et al: Calcium chemoprevention in colorectal cancer. Hepato-gastroenterology 43(7):152–154, 1996.
166. Grau MV, Baron JA, Sandler RS, et al: Prolonged effect of calcium supplementation on risk of colorectal adenomas in a randomized trial. J Natl Cancer Inst 99(2):129–136, 2007.
167. Martinez ME, Jacobs ET: Calcium supplementation and prevention of colorectal neoplasia: lessons from clinical trials. J Natl Cancer Inst 99(2):99–100, 2007.
168. Research, W.C.R.F.A.I.f.C: Food, Nutrition, Physical Activity, and the Prevention of Cancer: a Global Perspective. Washington, DC: American Institute for Cancer Research, 2007.
169. Kushi LH, Byers T, Doyle T, et al: American Cancer Society Guidelines on Nutrition and Physical Activity for cancer prevention: reducing the risk of cancer with healthy food choices and physical activity. CA Cancer J Clin 56(5):254–281; quiz 313–314, 2006.
170. Garland CF, Garland FC: Do sunlight and vitamin D reduce the likelihood of colon cancer? Int J Epidemiol 9(3):227–231, 1980.
171. Shabahang M, Buras RR, Davoodi F, et al: 1,25-Dihydroxyvitamin D3 receptor as a marker of human colon carcinoma cell line differentiation and growth inhibition. Cancer Res 53(16):3712–3718, 1993.
172. Sheikh MS, Rochefort H, Garcia M: Overexpression of p21WAF1/CIP1 induces growth arrest, giant cell formation and apoptosis in human breast carcinoma cell lines. Oncogene 11(9):1899–1905, 1995.
173. Donohue MM, Demay MB: Rickets in VDR null mice is secondary to decreased apoptosis of hypertrophic chondrocytes. Endocrinology 143(9):3691–3694, 2002.
174. Garland C, Shekelle RB, Barrett-Connor E, et al: Dietary vitamin D and calcium and risk of colorectal cancer: a 19-year prospective study in men. Lancet 1(8424):307–309, 1985.
175. Bostick RM, Potter JD, Sellers TA, et al: Relation of calcium, vitamin D, and dairy food intake to incidence of colon cancer among older women. The Iowa Women's Health Study. Am J Epidemiol 137(12):1302–1317, 1993.
176. Kearney J, Giovannucci E, Rimm EB, et al: Calcium, vitamin D, and dairy foods and the occurrence of colon cancer in men. Am J Epidemiol 143(9):907–917, 1996.
177. Martinez ME, Giovannucci EL, Colditz GA, et al: Calcium, vitamin D, and the occurrence of colorectal cancer among women. J Natl Cancer Inst 88(19):1375–1382, 1996.
178. Mizoue T, Kimura Y, Toyomura K, et al: Calcium, dairy foods, vitamin D, and colorectal cancer risk: the Fukuoka Colorectal Cancer Study. Cancer Epidemiol Biomarkers Prev 17(10):2800–2807, 2008.
179. Ferraroni M, LaVecchia C, D'Vanzo B, et al: Selected micronutrient intake and the risk of colorectal cancer. Br J Cancer 70(6):1150–1155, 1994.
180. Wei MY, Garland CF, Gorham ED, et al: Vitamin D and prevention of colorectal adenoma: a meta-analysis. Cancer Epidemiol Biomarkers Prev 17(11):2958–2969, 2008.

181. Grau MV, Baron JA, Sandler RS, et al: Vitamin D, calcium supplementation, and colorectal adenomas: results of a randomized trial. J Natl Cancer Inst 95(23):1765–1771, 2003.
182. Blount BC, Mack MM, Wehr CM, et al: Folate deficiency causes uracil misincorporation into human DNA and chromosome breakage: implications for cancer and neuronal damage. Proc Natl Acad Sci U S A 94(7):3290–3295, 1997.
183. Tseng M, Murray SC, Kupper LL, Sandler RS: Micronutrients and the risk of colorectal adenomas. Am J Epidemiol 144(11):1005–1014, 1996.
184. Baron JA, Sandler RS, Haile RW, et al: Folate intake, alcohol consumption, cigarette smoking, and risk of colorectal adenomas. J Natl Cancer Inst 90(1):57–62, 1998.
185. Giovannucci E, Stampfer MJ, Colditz GA, et al: Multivitamin use, folate, and colon cancer in women in the Nurses' Health Study. Ann Intern Med 129(7):517–524, 1998.
186. Sanjoaquin MA, Allen N, Couto E, et al: Folate intake and colorectal cancer risk: a meta-analytical approach. Int J Cancer 113(5):825–828, 2005.
187. Cole BF, Baron JA, Sandler RS, et al: Folic acid for the prevention of colorectal adenomas: a randomized clinical trial. JAMA 297(21):2351–2359, 2007.
188. Luebeck EG, Moolgavkar SH, Liu AY, et al: Does folic acid supplementation prevent or promote colorectal cancer? Results from model-based predictions. Cancer Epidemiol Biomarkers Prev 17(6):1360–1367, 2008.
189. Kim YI: Role of folate in colon cancer development and progression. J Nutr 133(11 Suppl 1):3731S–3739S, 2003.
190. Ibrahim EM, Zekri JM: Folic acid supplementation for the prevention of recurrence of colorectal adenomas: metaanalysis of interventional trials. Med Oncol 2009 Sep 12. [Epub ahead of print.]
191. Frosst P, Blom HJ, Milos R, et al: A candidate genetic risk factor for vascular disease: a common mutation in methylenetetrahydrofolate reductase. Nat Genet 10(1):111–113, 1995.
192. Ma J, Stampfer MJ, Giovannucci E, et al: Methylenetetrahydrofolate reductase polymorphism, dietary interactions, and risk of colorectal cancer. Cancer Res 57(6):1098–1102, 1997.
193. Slattery ML, Potter JD, Samowitz W, et al: Methylenetetrahydrofolate reductase, diet, and risk of colon cancer. Cancer Epidemiol Biomarkers Prev 8(6):513–518, 1999.
194. Ulrich CM, Kampman E, Bigler J, et al: Colorectal adenomas and the C677T MTHFR polymorphism: evidence for gene-environment interaction? Cancer Epidemiol Biomarkers Prev 8(8):659–668, 1999.
195. Nelson RL: Dietary minerals and colon carcinogenesis (review). Anticancer Res 7(3 Pt A):259–269, 1987.
196. Clark LC, Hixson LJ, Combs GF Jr, et al: Plasma selenium concentration predicts the prevalence of colorectal adenomatous polyps. Cancer Epidemiol Biomarkers Prev 2(1):41–46, 1993.
197. Psathakis D, Wedemeyer N, Oevermann E, et al: Blood selenium and glutathione peroxidase status in patients with colorectal cancer. Dis Colon Rectum 41(3):328–335, 1998.
198. Clark LC, Combs GF Jr, Turnbull BW, et al: Effects of selenium supplementation for cancer prevention in patients with carcinoma of the skin. A randomized controlled trial. Nutritional Prevention of Cancer Study Group. JAMA 276(24):1957–1963, 1996.
199. Duffield-Lillico AJ, Reid ME, Turnbull BW, et al: Baseline characteristics and the effect of selenium supplementation on cancer incidence in a randomized clinical trial: a summary report of the Nutritional Prevention of Cancer Trial. Cancer Epidemiol Biomarkers Prev 11(7):630–639, 2002.
200. Greenberg ER, Baron JA, Tosteson TD, et al: A clinical trial of antioxidant vitamins to prevent colorectal adenoma. Polyp Prevention Study Group. N Engl J Med 331(3):141–147, 1994.
201. Giovannucci E: An updated review of the epidemiological evidence that cigarette smoking increases risk of colorectal cancer. Cancer Epidemiol Biomarkers Prev 10(7):725–731, 2001.
202. Doll R, Peto R: Mortality in relation to smoking: 20 years' observations on male British doctors. Br Med J 2(6051):1525–1536, 1976.
203. Rogot E, Murray JL: Smoking and causes of death among U.S. veterans: 16 years of observation. Public Health Rep 95(3):213–222, 1980.
204. Hammond EC: Smoking in relation to the death rates of one million men and women. Natl Cancer Inst Monogr 127–204, 1966.
205. Doll R, Gray R, Hafner B, Peto R: Mortality in relation to smoking: 22 years' observations on female British doctors. Br Med J 280(6219):967–971,1980.
206. Kono S, Ikeda N, Yanai F, et al: Alcoholic beverages and adenomatous polyps of the sigmoid colon: a study of male self-defence officials in Japan. Int J Epidemiol 19(4):848–852, 1990.
207. Higginson J: Etiological factors in gastrointestinal cancer in man. J Natl Cancer Inst 37(4):527–545, 1966.
208. Staszewski J: Smoking and cancer of the alimentary tract in Poland. Br J Cancer 23(2):247–253, 1969.
209. Williams RR, Horm JW: Association of cancer sites with tobacco and alcohol consumption and socioeconomic status of patients: interview study from the Third National Cancer Survey. J Natl Cancer Inst 58(3):525–547, 1977.
210. D'Avanzo B, La Vecchia C, Franceschi S, et al: Cigarette smoking and colorectal cancer: a study of 1,584 cases and 2,879 controls. Prev Med 24(6):571–579, 1995.
211. Nordlund LA, Carstensen JM, Pershagen G: Cancer incidence in female smokers: a 26-year follow-up. Int J Cancer 73(5):625–628, 1997.
212. Sharpe CR, Siemiatycki JA, Rachet BP: The effects of smoking on the risk of colorectal cancer. Dis Colon Rectum 45(8):1041–1050, 2002.
213. Giovannucci E, Colditz GA, Stampfer MJ, et al: A prospective study of cigarette smoking and risk of colorectal adenoma and colorectal cancer in U.S. women. J Natl Cancer Inst 86(3):192–199, 1994.
214. Cope GF, Wyatt JI, Pinder IF, et al: Alcohol consumption in patients with colorectal adenomatous polyps. Gut 32(1):70–72, 1991.
215. Kikendall JW, Bowen PE, Burgess MB, et al: Cigarettes and alcohol as independent risk factors for colonic adenomas. Gastroenterology 97(3):660–664, 1989.
216. Martinez ME, McPherson RS, Annegers JF, Levin B: Cigarette smoking and alcohol consumption as risk factors for colorectal adenomatous polyps. J Natl Cancer Inst 87(4):274–279, 1995.
217. Olsen J, Kronborg O: Coffee, tobacco and alcohol as risk factors for cancer and adenoma of the large intestine. Int J Epidemiol 22(3):398–402, 1993.
218. Honjo S, Kono S, Shinchi K, et al: Cigarette smoking, alcohol use and adenomatous polyps of the sigmoid colon. Jpn J Cancer Res 83(8):806–811, 1992.
219. Hoff G, Vatn MH, Larsen S: Relationship between tobacco smoking and colorectal polyps. Scand J Gastroenterol 22(1):13–16, 1987.
220. Zahm SH, Cocco P, Blair A: Tobacco smoking as a risk factor for colon polyps. Am J Public Health 81(7):846–849, 1991.
221. Monnet E, Allemand H, Farina H, Carayon P: Cigarette smoking and the risk of colorectal adenoma in men. Scand J Gastroenterol 26(7):758–762, 1991.
222. Nagata C, Shimizu H, Kametani M, et al: Cigarette smoking, alcohol use, and colorectal adenoma in Japanese men and women. Dis Colon Rectum 42(3):337–342, 1999.
223. Almendingen K, Hofstad B, Trygg K, et al: Smoking and colorectal adenomas: a case-control study. Eur J Cancer Prev 9(3):193–203, 2000.
224. Boutron MC, Faivre J, Dop MC, et al: Tobacco, alcohol, and colorectal tumors: a multistep process. Am J Epidemiol 141(11):1038–1046, 1995.
225. Breuer-Katschinski B, Nemes K, Marr A, et al: Alcohol and cigarette smoking and the risk of colorectal adenomas. Dig Dis Sci 45(3):487–493, 2000.
226. Demers RY, Neale AV, Demers P, et al: Serum cholesterol and colorectal polyps. J Clin Epidemiol 41(1):9–13, 1988.
227. Longnecker MP, Chen MJ, Probst-Hensch NM, et al: Alcohol and smoking in relation to the prevalence of adenomatous colorectal polyps detected at sigmoidoscopy. Epidemiology 7(3):275–280, 1996.
228. Potter JD, Bigler J, Fosdick L, et al: Colorectal adenomatous and hyperplastic polyps: smoking and N-acetyltransferase 2 polymorphisms. Cancer Epidemiol Biomarkers Prev 8(1):69–75, 1999.
229. Terry MB, Neugut AI: Cigarette smoking and the colorectal adenoma-carcinoma sequence: a hypothesis to explain the paradox. Am J Epidemiol 147(10):903–910, 1998.
230. Chao A, Thun MJ, Jacobs EJ, et al: Cigarette smoking and colorectal cancer mortality in the cancer prevention study II. J Natl Cancer Inst 92(23):1888–1896, 2000.

231. Chute CG, Willett WC, Colditz GA, et al: A prospective study of body mass, height, and smoking on the risk of colorectal cancer in women. Cancer Causes Control 2(2):117–124, 1991.

232. Chyou PH, Nomura AM, Stemmermann GN: A prospective study of colon and rectal cancer among Hawaii Japanese men. Ann Epidemiol 6(4):276–282, 1996.

233. Doll R, Peto R, Boreham J, Sutherland I: Mortality in relation to smoking: 50 years' observations on male British doctors. BMJ 328(7455):1519, 2004.

234. Doll R, Peto R, Wheatley K, et al: Mortality in relation to smoking: 40 years' observations on male British doctors. BMJ 309(6959):901–911, 1994.

235. Heineman EF, Zahm SH, McLaughlin JK, Vaught JB: Increased risk of colorectal cancer among smokers: results of a 26-year follow-up of US veterans and a review. Int J Cancer 59(6):728–738, 1994.

236. Hsing AW, McLaughlin JK, Chow WH, et al: Risk factors for colorectal cancer in a prospective study among U.S. white men. Int J Cancer 77(4):549–543, 1998.

237. Jarebinski M, Adanja B, Vlajinac H: Case-control study of relationship of some biosocial correlates to rectal cancer patients in Belgrade, Yugoslavia. Neoplasma 36(3):369–374, 1989.

238. Jarebinski M, Vlajinac H, Adanja B: Biosocial and other characteristics of the large bowel cancer patients in Belgrade (Yugoslavia). Arch Geschwulstforsch 58(6):411–417, 1988.

239. Klatsky AL, Armstrong MA, Friedman GD, Hiatt RA: The relations of alcoholic beverage use to colon and rectal cancer. Am J Epidemiol 128(5):1007–1015, 1988.

240. Knekt P, Hakama M, Jarvinen R, et al: Smoking and risk of colorectal cancer. Br J Cancer 78(1):136–139, 1998.

241. Le Marchand L, Wilkens LR, Kolonel LN, et al: Associations of sedentary lifestyle, obesity, smoking, alcohol use, and diabetes with the risk of colorectal cancer. Cancer Res 57(21):4787–4794, 1997.

242. Newcomb PA, Storer BE, Marcus PM: Cigarette smoking in relation to risk of large bowel cancer in women. Cancer Res 55(21):4906–4909, 1995.

243. Sandler RS, Sandler DP, Comstock GW, et al: Cigarette smoking and the risk of colorectal cancer in women. J Natl Cancer Inst 80(16):1329–1333, 1988.

244. Slattery ML, Potter JD, Friedman GD, et al: Tobacco use and colon cancer. Int J Cancer 70(3):259–264, 1997.

245. Slattery ML, West DW, Robison LM, et al: Tobacco, alcohol, coffee, and caffeine as risk factors for colon cancer in a low-risk population. Epidemiology 1(2):141–145, 1990.

246. Sturmer T, Glynn RJ, Lee IM, et al: Lifetime cigarette smoking and colorectal cancer incidence in the Physicians' Health Study I. J Natl Cancer Inst 92(14):1178–1181, 2000.

247. Tverdal A, Thelle D, Stensvold I, et al: Mortality in relation to smoking history: 13 years' follow-up of 68,000 Norwegian men and women 35–49 years. J Clin Epidemiol 46(5):475–487, 1993.

248. Welfare MR, Cooper J, Bassendine MF, Daly AK: Relationship between acetylator status, smoking, and diet and colorectal cancer risk in the north-east of England. Carcinogenesis 18(7):1351–1354, 1997.

249. Hinds MW, Kolonel LN, Lee J, Hirohata T: Associations between cancer incidence and alcohol/cigarette consumption among five ethnic groups in Hawaii. Br J Cancer 41(6):929–940, 1980.

250. Vobecky J, Caro J, Devroede G: A case-control study of risk factors for large bowel carcinoma. Cancer 51(10):1958–1963, 1983.

251. Breslow NE, Enstrom JE: Geographic correlations between cancer mortality rates and alcohol-tobacco consumption in the United States. J Natl Cancer Inst 53(3):631–639, 1974.

252. Choi SY, Kahyo H: Effect of cigarette smoking and alcohol consumption in the etiology of cancers of the digestive tract. Int J Cancer 49(3):381–386, 1991.

253. Enstrom JE: Colorectal cancer and beer drinking. Br J Cancer 35(5):674–683, 1977.

254. Freudenheim JL, Graham S, Marshall JR, et al: Lifetime alcohol intake and risk of rectal cancer in western New York. Nutr Cancer 13(1–2):101–109, 1990.

255. Knox EG: Foods and diseases. Br J Prev Soc Med 31(2):71–80, 1977.

256. Kune GA, Vitetta L: Alcohol consumption and the etiology of colorectal cancer: a review of the scientific evidence from 1957 to 1991. Nutr Cancer 18(2):97–111, 1992.

257. Kabat GC, Howson CP, Wynder EL: Beer consumption and rectal cancer. Int J Epidemiol 15(4):494–501, 1986.

258. Longnecker MP, Orza MJ, Adams ME, et al: A meta-analysis of alcoholic beverage consumption in relation to risk of colorectal cancer. Cancer Causes Control 1(1):59–68, 1990.

259. Potter JD, McMichael AJ, Hartshorne JM: Alcohol and beer consumption in relation to cancers of bowel and lung: an extended correlation analysis. J Chronic Dis 35(11):833–842, 1982.

260. Riboli E, Cornee J, Macquart-Moulin G, et al: Cancer and polyps of the colorectum and lifetime consumption of beer and other alcoholic beverages. Am J Epidemiol 134(2):157–166, 1991.

261. Tuyns AJ, Pequignot G, Gignoux M, Valla A: Cancers of the digestive tract, alcohol and tobacco. Int J Cancer 30(1):9–11, 1982.

262. Wynder EL, Shigematsu T: Environmental factors of cancer of the colon and rectum. Cancer 20(9):1520–1561, 1967.

263. Bagnardi V, Blangiardo M, La Vecchia C, Corrao G: A meta-analysis of alcohol drinking and cancer risk. Br J Cancer 85(11):1700–1705, 2001.

264. Meyer F, White E: Alcohol and nutrients in relation to colon cancer in middle-aged adults. Am J Epidemiol 138(4):225–236, 1993.

265. Baron JA, Sandler RS, Haile RW, et al: Folate intake, alcohol consumption, and risk of colorectal adenomas. J Natl Cancer Inst 90(1):57–62, 1998.

266. Wolin KY, Yan Y, Colditz GA, Lee IM: Physical activity and colon cancer prevention: a meta-analysis. Br J Cancer 100(4):611–616, 2009.

267. Renehan AG, Tyson M, Egger M, et al: Body-mass index and incidence of cancer: a systematic review and meta-analysis of prospective observational studies. Lancet 371(9612):569–578, 2008.

268. Larsson SC, Wolk A: Obesity and colon and rectal cancer risk: a meta-analysis of prospective studies. Am J Clin Nutr 86(3):556–565, 2007.

269. Harriss DJ, Atkinson G, George K, et al: Lifestyle factors and colorectal cancer risk (1): systematic review and meta-analysis of associations with body mass index. Colorectal Dis 11(6):547–563, 2009.

270. McMichael AJ, McCall MG, Hartshorne JM, Woodings TL: Patterns of gastro-intestinal cancer in European migrants to Australia: the role of dietary change. Int J Cancer 25(4):431–437, 1980.

271. Parkin DM: International variation. Oncogene 23(38):6329–6340, 2004.

272. Kolonel LN: Cancer incidence among Filipinos in Hawaii and the Philippines. Natl Cancer Inst Monogr 69:93–98, 1985.

273. King H, Haenszel W: Cancer mortality among foreign- and native-born Chinese in the United States. J Chronic Dis 26(10):623–646, 1973.

274. Lee J, Demissie K, Lu SE, Rhoads GG: Cancer incidence among Korean-American immigrants in the United States and native Koreans in South Korea. Cancer Control 14(1):78–85, 2007.

275. Petrakis NL: Some preliminary observations on the influence of genetic admixture on cancer incidence in American Negroes. Int J Cancer 7(2):256–258, 1971.

276. Young JL Jr, Devesa SS, Cutler SJ: Incidence of cancer in United States blacks. Cancer Res 35(11 Pt. 2):3523–3536, 1975.

277. McCredie M, Williams S, Coates M: Cancer mortality in migrants from the British Isles and continental Europe to New South Wales, Australia, 1975–1995. Int J Cancer 83(2):179–185, 1999.

278. Bouchardy C, Khlat M, Mirra AP, Parkin D: Cancer risks among European migrants in Sao Paulo, Brazil. Eur J Cancer 29A(10):1418–1423, 1993.

6

Chemoprevention of Colorectal Cancer

Melissa A. Munsell and Francis M. Giardiello

KEY POINTS

- The chemopreventive effect of nonsteroidal anti-inflammatory drugs (NSAIDs) is supported by in vitro experiments, animal models, epidemiologic studies, and clinical trials.
- Currently, the American Cancer Society and the U.S. Preventive Services Task Force do not recommend aspirin and NSAIDs for colorectal cancer prevention in the average-risk person.
- Additional studies are needed to elucidate the effect of estrogen and medroxyprogesterone acetate on colorectal cancer prevention.
- Certain diets and some vitamins, minerals, and antioxidants appear to protect against colorectal cancer.

Introduction

Colorectal cancer is a leading cause of cancer-related deaths in the United States. Currently, the goal of screening programs is early detection of a preinvasive lesion or early cancer. An alternative or conjunctive approach is chemoprevention of colon cancer. Chemoprevention involves using drugs or natural compounds to inhibit or reverse carcinogenesis. Nonsteroidal anti-inflammatory drugs (NSAIDs), vitamins, hormones, and dietary factors have been implicated in primary prevention of colon cancer (Box 6-1).

Nonsteroidal Anti-inflammatory Drugs

NSAIDs, cyclooxygenase-2 (COX-2) inhibitors, and aspirin all have been studied in the prevention of colon cancer. Strong support for a chemopreventive effect of NSAIDs is provided by in vitro experiments, animal models, epidemiologic studies, and clinical trials.[1] The mechanism of action of NSAIDs is inhibition of cyclooxy-genase, which is a key enzyme in the conversion of arachidonic acid to prostaglandins, prostacyclin, and thromboxanes. Prostaglandins affect cell proliferation and tumor growth through activation of second messengers in signal transduction pathways, and prostaglandin levels are increased in many cancers including colorectal adenomas and adenocarcinomas.[2] COX-1 is present in most tissues, whereas COX-2 is expressed in response to growth factors, cytokines, mitogens, and tumor promoters.[3] COX-2 inhibition also has anti-angiogenic[4] and apoptotic effects.[5] COX-2 independent targets have been suggested as well, including β-catenin, transcription factor NF-κB, and transforming growth factor-β (TGF-β).[6–8]

Much of the initial data on NSAIDs and chemoprevention of colon cancer in humans came from literature on familial adenomatous polyposis (FAP), which is an autosomal dominant disorder characterized by innumerable colorectal adenomas and eventual carcinoma. Giardiello and colleagues[9] conducted the first randomized controlled trial evaluating sulindac in patients with FAP who had not undergone colectomy. Twenty-two patients with FAP received either sulindac 300 mg daily for 9 months or placebo, and the number and size of polyps were evaluated every 3 months for 1 year. The group treated with sulindac had a statistically significant reduction in both the number and size of polyps when compared with the placebo group. Many studies have evaluated sulindac in FAP, and all report either complete or partial regression of adenomas after 3 to 6 months of treatment with sulindac at doses of 300 to 400 mg per day.[10]

NSAIDs such as sulindac have gastrointestinal toxicity that may limit use for prevention in

---

Box 6-1. Potential Chemopreventive Agents

NSAIDs
  Sulindac
  Celecoxib
  Aspirin
Ursodeoxycholic Acid
Hormones
  Estrogen
  Medroxyprogesterone acetate
Calcium
Folate
Selenium
Curcumin

---

colorectal cancer. This has led to studies on COX-2 inhibitors. COX-2 is expressed in inflammatory states, premalignant lesions, and colorectal cancer. Thus, COX-2 inhibitors were speculated to have a role in the chemoprevention of colon cancer. Again, using patients with FAP, Steinbach and colleagues[11] randomized patients to celecoxib at 100 mg or 400 mg twice daily or placebo for 6 months. Endoscopy done at the beginning and end of the 6 months demonstrated a significant reduction in the mean number of polyps and the polyp burden in the group receiving high-dose celecoxib (Fig. 6-1).

The finding that NSAIDs lead to polyp regression in patients with FAP led to investigation of NSAIDs in sporadic adenomas and colorectal neoplasia (see Box 6-1). Epidemiologic studies have shown a reduction in colorectal cancer in individuals taking NSAIDs.[1,12] A series of case-control studies revealed a 40% to 50% reduction in the risk of colonic adenomas or colorectal cancer among patients taking aspirin.[1] Thun and colleagues[13] reported results of a large observational study on aspirin and colon cancer showing that aspirin reduced the relative risk of cancer mortality by 40% when consumed more than 16 times per month for at least 1 year. Giovannucci and associates[14] measured cancer incidence in a cohort of women and found that regular aspirin use at doses similar to those recommended for cardiovascular disease prevention reduced the risk of colorectal cancer; however, this effect may require more than a decade of use to occur (Fig. 6-2). A controlled trial with the primary endpoint of cardiovascular events involved 22,071 male physicians randomized to aspirin 325 mg or placebo every other day for 5 years found no difference between the two groups in the incidence of colorectal cancer. These findings may be accounted for by the short treatment period.[15]

Two large randomized trials have evaluated the role of aspirin in colorectal adenoma recurrence. Baron and colleagues[16] randomized 1121 patients (with removed polyps) to aspirin 81 mg or 325 mg daily or placebo. Ninety-seven percent of patients had a follow-up colonoscopy at least 1 year after randomization, and the incidence of adenomas was 38% in the low-dose aspirin group

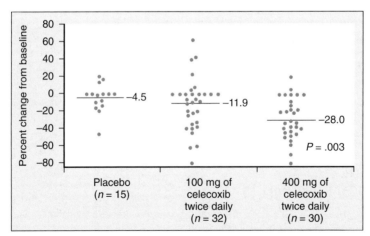

Figure 6-1. Percent change from baseline in the number of colorectal polyps in 77 patients with familial adenomatous polyposis who were treated with placebo or celecoxib (100 mg or 400 mg twice daily) for 6 months.   A decrease from baseline represents disease regression; an increase represents disease progression. The horizontal lines show the mean changes. *P* value is for comparison with the placebo group. (From Steinbach G, Lynch PM, Phillips RK, et al: The effect of celecoxib, a cyclooxygenase-2 inhibitor, in familial adenomatous polyposis. N Engl J Med 342:1946–1952, 2000, Fig. 1.)

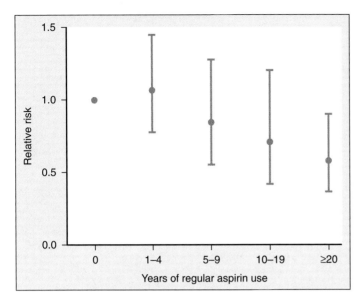

Figure 6-2. Age-adjusted relative risks of colorectal cancer and 95% confidence intervals according to the number of consecutive years of regular aspirin use among users compared with nonusers of aspirin.   *P* value for trend over time is .008. Regular aspirin use was defined as the consumption of two or more tablets per week. (From Giovannucci E, Egan KM, Hunter DJ, et al: Aspirin and the risk of colorectal cancer in women. N Engl J Med 333:609–614, 1995, Fig. 2.)

compared with 47% in the placebo group and 45% in the high-dose aspirin group. These investigations concluded that low-dose aspirin prevents recurrence of adenomas in the colon. Of note, a higher but not statistically significant incidence of stroke was found in the aspirin group. Also, the reason why higher-dose aspirin did not have the same effect as low-dose aspirin is unclear.

A second study randomized 635 patients with previous colorectal cancer to either aspirin 325 mg daily or placebo and found that the aspirin group had fewer adenomas and a longer time to detection of a first adenoma (Fig. 6-3).[17] This study concluded that daily aspirin can significantly reduce the incidence of colorectal adenomas in patients with previous colorectal cancer. In a smaller randomized control trial, Benamouzig and colleagues[18] showed that daily soluble aspirin was associated with a reduction in the risk of recurrent adenomas found at colonoscopy 1 year after beginning treatment (Table 6-1).

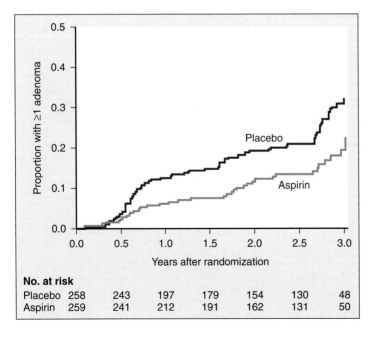

Figure 6-3. Kaplan-Meier estimates of the time to a first adenoma. (From Sandler RS, Halabi S, Baron JA, et al: A randomized trial of aspirin to prevent colorectal adenomas in patients with previous colorectal cancer. N Engl J Med 348:883–890, 2003, Fig. 1.)

Table 6-1. Major Trials of Chemoprevention in Colorectal Cancer with Aspirin

First Author	Reference	Study Design	Patients	Effect
Thun	13	Prospective cohort	662,424 patients providing information on frequency and duration of aspirin use	Regular aspirin use associated with reduced risk of colorectal cancer
Giovannucci	14	Prospective cohort	89,446 women reporting number of consecutive years of aspirin use	Regular, long-term aspirin use associated with reduced risk of colorectal cancer
Sturmer	15	Prospective cohort, following randomized placebo controlled	22,071 male physicians randomly assigned aspirin use	No association of aspirin use with colorectal cancer protection
Baron	16	Randomized, placebo controlled	1,121 patients with sporadic adenomas randomized to aspirin or placebo	Low-dose aspirin prevents recurrence of adenomas
Sandler	17	Randomized, placebo controlled	635 patients with previous colorectal cancer with curative resection randomized to aspirin or placebo	Daily aspirin use associated with reduction of adenomas in patients with previous colorectal cancer

Ursodeoxycholic Acid

Another drug that may show benefits in chemoprevention is ursodeoxycholic acid (UDCA), also called ursodiol, a synthetic bile acid. Preclinical studies demonstrate that UDCA has chemopreventive effects. In a cross-sectional study on patients with ulcerative colitis and primary sclerosing cholangitis, the use of UDCA was associated with lower incidence of colonic dysplasia. The hypothesized mechanism of action is that UDCA reduces levels of the secondary bile acid deoxycholic acid, which is cytotoxic to colonic epithelial cells and induces hyperproliferation.[19] Pardi and colleagues[20] studied UDCA in a similar population and found that those taking the drug had a relative risk of 0.26 (95% confidence interval [CI], 0.06–0.92) for developing colorectal dysplasia or cancer (Fig. 6-4). A phase III, double-blind, placebo-controlled trial of UDCA was conducted to evaluate its ability to prevent colorectal adenoma recurrence. This trial found a nonstatistically significant reduction in total adenoma recurrence but did have a 39%

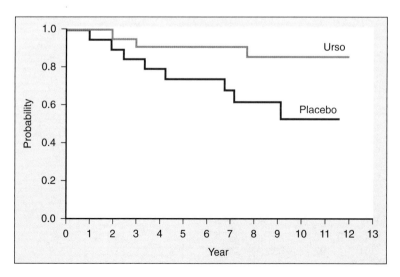

Figure 6-4. Kaplan-Meier estimates of the proportion of patients free of dysplasia or cancer according to initial treatment assignment. (From Pardi DS, Loftus EV Jr, Kremers WK, et al: Ursodeoxycholic acid as a chemopreventive agent in patients with ulcerative colitis and primary sclerosing cholangitis. Gastroenterology 124:889–893, 2003, Fig. 1.)

reduction in recurrence of adenomas with high-grade dysplasia.[21] Further investigation is needed to evaluate the role of UDCA in chemoprevention of high-grade dysplasia.

Hormones

Over the last 20 years, mortality from colon cancer has decreased slightly in both sexes but more prominently in women.[22] From 1982 to 1992, there was a 2.3-fold increase in the use of oral menopausal estrogens and a 4.9-fold increase in oral medroxyprogesterone use.[23] This increase in hormonal therapy led to the postulation that hormones may reduce the risk of colon cancer. Biologic evidence includes findings that estrogens decrease the production of secondary bile acids, which can promote malignant change in colonic epithelium. Also, estrogens decrease the production of insulin-like growth factor I, an important mitogen, which may exert a direct effect on colorectal epithelium.[22] Epidemiologic studies of postmenopausal hormone replacement therapy (HRT) showed a 20% reduction (relative risk [RR] 0.80, 95% CI, 0.74–0.86) in risk of colon cancer in postmenopausal women

who had ever taken HRT compared with women who had never used hormones.[24]

The Women's Health Initiative (WHI) evaluated 16,608 postmenopausal women in a randomized controlled trial. Participants were given either estrogen .625 mg daily plus medroxyprogesterone acetate 2.5 mg daily or placebo. The primary outcomes of this study were coronary heart disease and adverse outcome of invasive breast cancer. A global index summarized the risks and benefits of HRT, including colorectal cancer. The study did show a hazard ratio for colorectal cancer of 0.63 (0.43–0.93), indicating a reduction in colorectal cancer in the HRT group. However, the study was stopped after 5.2 years of follow-up because of an increased risk of breast cancer, stroke, coronary disease, and venous thromboembolism.[25] Using the data from the WHI, Chlebowski and colleagues[26] showed a statistically significant decrease in colorectal cancer among users of HRT. However, patients who were diagnosed with colorectal cancer were more likely to have a more advanced stage of cancer than women taking placebo (Fig. 6-5). These findings were not easily explainable. Again using the WHI data, a randomized con-

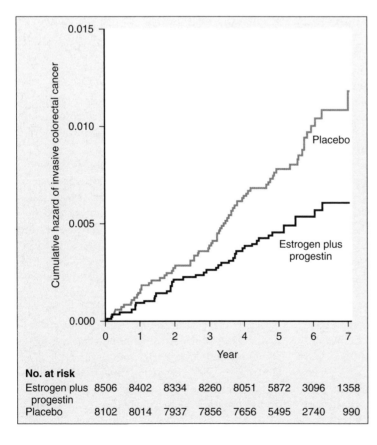

Figure 6-5. Kaplan-Meier plots of the cumulative hazard of invasive colorectal cancer, according to treatment group. The hazard ratio for colorectal cancer in the group who received estrogen plus progestin, compared with the group who received placebo, was 0.56 (95% confidence interval, 0.38–0.81). The data shown do not include two carcinoid tumors among women in the estrogen-plus-progestin group and one squamous cell carcinoma in a woman in the placebo group. (From Chlebowski RT, Wactawski-Wende J, Ritenbaugh C, et al: Estrogen plus progestin and colorectal cancer in postmenopausal women. N Engl J Med 350:991–1004, 2004, Fig. 1.)

trolled trial evaluated use of estrogen alone in postmenopausal women with hysterectomy and found no significant differences in rates of colorectal cancer when compared with those with placebo.[27] This study and others[28] may suggest that progesterone, rather than estrogen, is the chemopreventive agent.

Minerals and Vitamins

Vitamins such as calcium, folate, and selenium have also been implicated in chemoprevention of colon cancer. The first suggestion of a protective effect of dietary calcium for colorectal cancer was by Newmark and colleagues[29] in 1984. These investigators hypothesized that dietary calcium could neutralize fatty acids and free bile acids, which have an irritative effect on the colonic epithelium. Numerous murine studies have shown that calcium decreases colonic mucosal hyperproliferation, decreases markers of colorectal mucosal proliferation, and inhibits colonic tumor development.[30] Although two early meta-analyses showed little or no protection against colorectal cancer with calcium,[31,32] numerous subsequent prospective cohort studies have reported a modest decrease of colorectal cancer in high-intake calcium groups compared with that in low-intake groups.[33-36] Baron and associates[37] conducted a randomized control trial of 930 subjects on the effect of calcium carbonate supplementation on the recurrence of colorectal adenomas. Patients received either 3 g of calcium carbonate (1200 mg of elemental calcium) daily or placebo, with colonoscopies at 1 and 4 years after the qualifying examination. Results showed a significant reduction in the risk of colorectal adenomas in the calcium group. Finally, a meta-analysis of three randomized controlled trials suggested that calcium prevents recurrent colorectal adenomas, with an overall relative risk of 0.80 (95% CI, 0.68–0.93).[38] Vitamin D has also been found to be inversely associated with risk of colorectal cancer.[32]

Several cohort and case-control studies have suggested a reduced risk of colorectal cancer with a higher consumption of vegetables and fruits.[22] Folate is a B vitamin found in leafy green vegetables, citrus fruits, and dried beans and peas. Folic acid is involved in DNA synthesis and repair, DNA methylation, and modulation of cell proliferation shown in both in vitro and animal studies.[39,40] Murine models of colorectal cancer report that folate administration is associated with decreased risk of colonic neoplasm,[41,42] and epidemiologic studies show an inverse relationship between dietary folate and colorectal cancer incidence.[22] Also, two large prospective cohort studies show an association between folate intake and reduced incidence of colorectal cancer.[43,44] In the Nurses' Health Study, 88,756 women provided diet assessments including multivitamin use. This investigation found that long-term use of folate at doses higher than 400 mcg daily was associated with a substantial decreased risk of colon cancer.[43] In the National Health and Nutrition Epidemiologic Follow-up Study, subjects were followed up for 20 years, and an inverse relationship of folate intake and colon cancer was found for men (RR 0.40; 95% CI, 0.18–0.88).[44]

Selenium is an essential trace element in the human diet and is incorporated into proteins. Selenoproteins are involved in the neutralization of reactive oxygen species and are important for the antioxidative defense of cells.[45] Selenium is found in plant foods, and the concentration of selenium in food correlates with the content of the soil where plants are grown. In ecologic studies, selenium intake has an inverse relationship to colon cancer risk.[46] In colon cancer cell lines, selenomethionine inhibits growth and decreases levels of cyclooxygenase proteins in the cells,[47] and animal studies have consistently shown that selenium has activity against colorectal cancer.[48]

Although in vitro and animal studies show activity of selenium against colorectal cancer, epidemiologic studies have been inconsistent. In a case-control analysis by Nomura and colleagues,[49] low selenium levels were associated with an increase in relative risk of colon cancer, although the results were not statistically significant. Similarly, prospective cohort studies have not consistently shown that patients with colorectal cancer are selenium-deficient.[50,51] However, several investigations reveal a protective relationship of selenium and colorectal adenomas and cancer.[52-54] A randomized, placebo-controlled trial in 1996 evaluated selenium supplementation for prevention of skin cancer in 1312 patients with a history of skin carci-

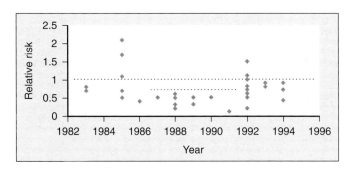

HO
CH₃O
OH
OCH₃
O O

Curcumin

Figure 6-6. Chemical structure of curcumin [1,7-bis-(4-hydroxy-3-methoxyphenyl)-1,6-heptadiene-3,5-dione]. (From Kawamori T, Lubet R, Steele VE, et al: Chemopreventive effect of curcumin, a naturally occurring anti-inflammatory agent, during the promotion/progression stages of colon cancer. Cancer Res 59:597–601, 1999, Fig. 1.)

noma. The primary endpoint of skin carcinoma was not affected by selenium supplementation. However, the selenium group did have decreased total cancer mortality, with a lower incidence of colorectal cancer (RR 0.58; 95% CI, 0.18–0.95).[55] More recently, a pooled analysis of three randomized trials of 1763 subjects found an inverse association between higher blood selenium concentration and adenoma risk.[56] Other vitamins have been studied as well. In a prospective, randomized trial, beta carotene and vitamins C and E failed to prevent colorectal adenomas.[57]

Curcumin

Curcumin, a diferuloylmethane derived from the plant *Curcuma longa*, is a potent antioxidant with anti-inflammatory and antitumor activities[58] (Fig. 6-6). It is commonly consumed as turmeric spice. Both in vitro studies and animal models have demonstrated a chemopreventive effect of curcumin.[59,60] Curcumin inhibits COX-2 expression, inhibits growth in human colon cancer cell models, and suppresses nuclear factor κB, a transcription factor that controls expression of cytokines.[59,61,62] In patients with advanced colorectal cancer refractory to standard chemotherapy, 5 of 15 individuals given daily oral curcumin had stable disease after 2 to 4 months of treatment.[63] In a phase I clinical trial, treatment with oral curcumin for 3 months showed docu-

mented histologic improvement of precancerous lesions in 1 of 2 patients with resected bladder cancer, 2 of 7 patients with oral leukoplakia, 1 of 6 patients with gastric intestinal metaplasia, and 1 of 4 patients with cervical intraepithelial neoplasm.[64] Furthermore, a recent study of 5 FAP patients with prior colectomy treated with oral curcumin and quercetin (flavonoid found in green tea, onions, and red wine) had a reduction in number and size of ileal and rectal adenomas after 6 months of treatment.[65]

Diet and Exercise

Diet has also been implicated in colon cancer, including meats, vegetables, fruit, and fiber. Prospective cohort studies have demonstrated an increase in risk of colorectal cancer in patients who consume red meat frequently.[66,67] However, when vegetarians were compared with matched controls, there was no difference in mortality from colorectal cancer.[68] There does appear to be convincing evidence, however, for a correlation between high vegetable and fruit intake and low colorectal neoplasia. Most published case-control and cohort studies show a relative risk of less than 0.8 for colorectal neoplasia in subjects with the highest intake of fruits and vegetables[69] (Fig. 6-7). Fiber has a less clear role in the risk of colorectal cancer. About 60% of epidemiologic studies have linked high-fiber diets with a decreased risk of colorectal adenomas

Figure 6-7. Summary of a series of case-control and cohort studies examining the relation between dietary intake of fruits and vegetables and the relative risk of colorectal cancer. Each study is plotted in the year that the data were published. The dotted line reflects a relative risk of 1. (From Gatof D, Ahnen D: Primary prevention of colorectal cancer: diet and drugs. Gastroenterol Clin North Am 31:587–623, 2002.)

and cancer, and a large European prospective study showed similar results.[70] On the contrary, two large prospective, randomized, controlled studies showed that adopting a diet low in fat and high in fiber, fruits, and vegetables did not influence the risk of recurrence of colorectal adenomas.[71,72]

Along with diet, body habitus and physical activity have been studied in relation to colon cancer. Overall, case-control and cohort studies have demonstrated a positive association between obesity and cancer risk, whereas the majority of studies have shown an inverse relationship between physical activity and colorectal cancer risk.[69]

Summary

More studies are needed to elucidate effective agents for chemoprevention of colorectal cancer. Of course, any protective benefit of a chemopreventive agent must be weighed against its potential adverse effects, such as gastrointestinal irritation with NSAIDs. The American Cancer Society and the U.S. Preventive Services Task Force currently do not recommend the routine use of aspirin and NSAIDS to prevent colorectal cancer in the average-risk person, given the potential adverse effects.[73] Aspirin may be added in selected patients who may gain additional benefit. Patients should be recommended to follow a well-balanced diet high in fruits, vegetables, and fiber and to consider calcium supplementation.

References

1. DuBois RN, Giardiello FM, Smalley WE: Nonsteroidal anti-inflammatory drugs, eicosanoids, and colorectal cancer prevention. Gastroenterol Clin North Am 25:773–791, 1996.
2. Giardiello FM, Offerhaus GJ, DuBois RN: The role of nonsteroidal anti-inflammatory drugs in colorectal cancer prevention. Eur J Cancer 31A:1071–1076, 1995.
3. Vane JR, Botting RM: The mechanism of action of aspirin. Thromb Res 110:255–258, 2003.
4. Boon EM, Keller JJ, Wormhoudt TA, et al: Sulindac targets nuclear beta-catenin accumulation and Wnt signalling in adenomas of patients with familial adenomatous polyposis and in human colorectal cancer cell lines. Br J Cancer 90:224–229, 2004.
5. Sheng H, Shao J, Morrow JD, et al: Modulation of apoptosis and Bcl-2 expression by prostaglandin E2 in human colon cancer cells. Cancer Res 58:362–366, 1998.
6. Smith ML, Hawcroft G, Hull MA: The effect of non-steroidal anti-inflammatory drugs on human colorectal cancer cells: evidence of different mechanisms of action. Eur J Cancer 36:664–674, 2000.
7. Stark LA, Reid K, Sansom OJ, et al: Aspirin activates the NF-κB signalling pathway and induces apoptosis in intestinal neoplasia in two in vivo models of human colorectal cancer. Carcinogenesis 28:968–976, 2007. Epub 2006 Nov 28.
8. Baek SJ, Kim KS, Nixon JB, et al: Cyclooxygenase inhibitors regulate the expression of a TGF-beta superfamily member that has proapoptotic and antitumorigenic activities. Mol Pharmacol 59:901–908, 2001.
9. Giardiello FM, Hamilton SR, Krush AJ, et al: Treatment of colonic and rectal adenomas with sulindac in familial adenomatous polyposis. N Engl J Med 328:1313–1316, 1993.
10. Keller JJ, Giardiello FM: Chemoprevention strategies using NSAIDs and COX-2 inhibitors. Cancer Biol Ther 2:S140–S149, 2003.
11. Steinbach G, Lynch PM, Phillips RK, et al: The effect of celecoxib, a cyclooxygenase-2 inhibitor, in familial adenomatous polyposis. N Engl J Med 342:1946–1952, 2000.
12. Serrano D, Lazzeroni M, Decensi A: Chemoprevention of colorectal cancer: an update. Tech Coloproctol 8:S248–S252, 2004.
13. Thun MJ, Namboodiri MM, Heath CW: Aspirin use and reduced risk of fatal colon cancer. N Engl J Med 325:1593–1596, 1991.
14. Giovannucci E, Egan KM, Hunter DJ, et al: Aspirin and the risk of colorectal cancer in women. N Engl J Med 333:609–614, 1995.
15. Sturmer T, Glynn RJ, Lee IM, et al: Aspirin use and colorectal cancer: post-trial follow-up data from the Physicians' Health Study. Ann Intern Med 128:713–720, 1983.
16. Baron JA, Cole BF, Sandler RS, et al: A randomized trial of aspirin to prevent colorectal adenomas. N Engl J Med 348:891–899, 2003.
17. Sandler RS, Halabi S, Baron JA, et al: A randomized trial of aspirin to prevent colorectal adenomas in patients with previous colorectal cancer. N Engl J Med 348:883–890, 2003.
18. Benamouzig R, Deyra J, Martin A, et al: Daily soluble aspirin and prevention of colorectal adenoma recurrence: one-year results of the APACC trial. Gastroenterology 125:328–336, 2003.
19. Tung BY, Emond MJ, Haggitt RC, et al: Ursodiol use is associated with lower prevalence of colonic neoplasia in patients with ulcerative colitis and primary sclerosing cholangitis. Ann Intern Med 134:89–95, 2001.
20. Pardi DS, Loftus EV Jr, Kremers WK, et al: Ursodeoxycholic acid as a chemopreventive agent in patients with ulcerative colitis and primary sclerosing cholangitis. Gastroenterology 124:889–893, 2003.
21. Alberts DS, Martinez ME, Hess LM, et al: Phase III trial of ursodeoxycholic acid to prevent colorectal adenoma recurrence. J Natl Cancer Inst 97:846–853, 2005.
22. Janne PA, Mayer RJ: Chemoprevention of colorectal cancer. N Engl J Med 342:1960–1968, 2000.
23. Wysowski DK, Golden L, Burke L: Use of menopausal estrogens and medroxyprogesterone in the United States, 1982–1992. Obstet Gynecol 85:6–10, 1995.
24. Grodstein F, Newcomb PA, Stampfer MJ: Postmenopausal hormone therapy and the risk of colorectal cancer: a review and meta-analysis. Am J Med 106:574–582, 1999.
25. Rossouw JE, Anderson GL, Prentice RL, et al: Risks and benefits of estrogen plus progestin in healthy postmenopausal women: principal results from the Women's Health Initiative randomized controlled trial. JAMA 288:321–333, 2002.
26. Chlebowski RT, Wactawski-Wende J, Ritenbaugh C, et al: Estrogen plus progestin and colorectal cancer in postmenopausal women. N Engl J Med 350:991–1004, 2004.
27. Anderson GL, Limacher M, Assaf AR, et al: Effects of conjugated equine estrogen in postmenopausal women with hysterectomy: the Women's Health Initiative randomized controlled trial. JAMA 291:1701–1712, 2004.
28. Giardiello FM, Hylind LM, Trimbath JD, et al: Oral contraceptives and polyp regression in familial adenomatous polyposis. Gastroenterology 128:1077–1080, 2005.
29. Newmark HL, Wargovich MJ, Bruce WR: Colon cancer and dietary fat, phosphate, and calcium: a hypothesis. J Natl Cancer Inst 72:1323–1325, 1984.
30. Lipkin M: Update on preclinical and human studies of calcium and colon cancer prevention. W J Gastroenterol 5:461–464, 1999.
31. Bergsma-Kadijk JA, van't Veer P, Kampman E, Burema J: Calcium does not protect against colorectal neoplasia. Epidemiology 7:590–597, 1996.
32. Martinez ME, Willett WC: Calcium, vitamin D, and colorectal cancer: a review of the epidemiologic evidence. Cancer Epidemiol Biomarkers Prev 7:163–168, 1998.

33. McCullough ML, Robertson AS, Rodriguez C, et al: Calcium, vitamin D, dairy products, and risk of colorectal cancer in the Cancer Prevention Study II Nutrition Cohort (United States). Cancer Causes Control 14:1–12, 2003.
34. Wu K, Willett WC, Fuchs CS, et al: Calcium intake and risk of colon cancer in women and men. J Natl Cancer Inst 94:437–446, 2002.
35. Sellers TA, Bazyk AE, Bostick RM, et al: Diet and risk of colon cancer in a large prospective study of older women: an analysis stratified on family history (Iowa, United States). Cancer Causes Control 9:357–367, 1998.
36. Flood A, Peters U, Chatterjee N, et al: Calcium from diet and supplements is associated with reduced risk of colorectal cancer in a prospective cohort of women. Cancer Epidemiol Biomarkers Prev 14:126–132, 2005.
37. Baron JA, Beach M, Mandel JS, et al: Calcium supplements for the prevention of colorectal adenomas. Calcium Polyp Prevention Study Group. N Engl J Med 340:101–107, 1999.
38. Shaukat A, Scouras N, Schunemann HJ: Role of supplemental calcium in the recurrence of colorectal adenomas: a metaanalysis of randomized controlled trials. Am J Gastroenterol 100:390–394, 2005.
39. Turini ME, DuBois RN: Primary prevention: phytoprevention and chemoprevention of colorectal cancer. Hematol Oncol Clin North Am 16:811–840, 2002.
40. Choi SW, Mason JB: Folate status: effects on pathways of colorectal carcinogenesis. J Nutr 132:2413S–2418S, 2002.
41. Cravo ML, Mason JB, Dayal Y, et al: Folate deficiency enhances the development of colonic neoplasia in dimethylhydrazine-treated rats. Cancer Res 52:5002–5006, 1992.
42. Kim YI, Salomon RN, Graeme-Cook F, et al: Dietary folate protects against the development of macroscopic colonic neoplasia in a dose responsive manner in rats. Gut 39:732–740, 1996.
43. Giovannucci E, Stampfer MJ, Colditz GA, et al: Multivitamin use, folate, and colon cancer in women in the Nurses' Health Study. Ann Intern Med 129:517–524, 1998.
44. Su LJ, Arab L: Nutritional status of folate and colon cancer risk: evidence from NHANES I epidemiologic follow-up study. Ann Epidemiol 11:65–72, 2001.
45. Al-Taie OH, Seufert J, Karvar S, et al: Selenium supplementation enhances low selenium levels and stimulates glutathione peroxidase activity in peripheral blood and distal colon mucosa in past and present carriers of colon adenomas. Nutr Cancer 46:125–130, 2003.
46. Shamberger RJ, Tytko SA, Willis CE: Antioxidants and cancer. Part VI. Selenium and age-adjusted human cancer mortality. Arch Environ Health 31:231–235, 1976.
47. Baines A, Taylor-Parker M, Goulet AC, et al: Selenomethionine inhibits growth and suppresses cyclooxygenase-2 (COX-2) protein expression in human colon cancer cell lines. Cancer Biol Ther 1:370–374, 2002.
48. Duffield-Lillico AJ, Shureiqi I, Lippman SM: Can selenium prevent colorectal cancer? A signpost from epidemiology. J Natl Cancer Inst 96:1645–1647, 2004.
49. Nomura A, Yamakawa H, Ishidate T, et al: Intestinal metaplasia in Japan: association with diet. J Natl Cancer Inst 68:401–405, 1982.
50. Early DS, Hill K, Burk R, et al: Selenoprotein levels in patients with colorectal adenomas and cancer. Am J Gastroenterol 97:745–748, 2002.
51. van den Brandt PA, Goldbohm RA, van't Veer P, et al: A prospective cohort study on toenail selenium levels and risk of gastrointestinal cancer. J Natl Cancer Inst 85:224–229, 1993.
52. Willett WC, Polk BF, Morris JS, et al: Prediagnostic serum selenium and risk of cancer. Lancet 2:130–134, 1983.
53. Clark LC, Hixson LJ, Combs GF Jr, et al: Plasma selenium concentration predicts the prevalence of colorectal adenomatous polyps. Cancer Epidemiol Biomarkers Prev 2:41–46, 1993.
54. Fernandez-Banares F, Cabre E, Esteve M, et al: Serum selenium and risk of large size colorectal adenomas in a geographical area with a low selenium status. Am J Gastroenterol 97:2103–2108, 2002.
55. Clark LC, Combs GF Jr, Turnbull BW, et al: Effects of selenium supplementation for cancer prevention in patients with carcinoma of the skin. A randomized controlled trial. Nutritional Prevention of Cancer Study Group. JAMA 276:1957–1963, 1996.
56. Jacobs ET, Jiang R, Alberts DS, et al: Selenium and colorectal adenoma: results of a pooled analysis. J Natl Cancer Inst 96:1669–1675, 2004.
57. Greenberg ER, Baron JA, Tosteson TD, et al: A clinical trial of antioxidant vitamins to prevent colorectal adenoma. Polyp Prevention Study Group. N Engl J Med 331:141–147, 1994.
58. Lev-Ari S, Strier L, Kazanov D, et al: Celecoxib and curcumin synergistically inhibit the growth of colorectal cancer cells. Clin Cancer Res 11:6738–6744, 2005.
59. Li L, Aggarwal BB, Shishodia S, et al: Nuclear factor-kappaB and IkappaB kinase are constitutively active in human pancreatic cells, and their down-regulation by curcumin (diferuloylmethane) is associated with the suppression of proliferation and the induction of apoptosis. Cancer 101:2351–2362, 2004.
60. Kawamori T, Lubet R, Steele VE, et al: Chemopreventive effect of curcumin, a naturally occurring anti-inflammatory agent, during the promotion/progression stages of colon cancer. Cancer Res 59:597–601, 1999.
61. Goel A, Boland CR, Chauhan DP: Specific inhibition of cyclooxygenase-2 (COX-2) expression by dietary curcumin in HT-29 human colon cancer cells. Cancer Lett 172:111–118, 2001.
62. Singh S, Aggarwal BB: Activation of transcription factor NF-kappa B is suppressed by curcumin (diferuloylmethane). J Biol Chem 270:24995–25000, 1995.
63. Sharma RA, McLelland HR, Hill KA, et al: Pharmacodynamic and pharmacokinetic study of oral Curcuma extract in patients with colorectal cancer. Clin Cancer Res 7:1894–1900, 2001.
64. Cheng AL, Hsu CH, Lin JK, et al: Phase I clinical trial of curcumin, a chemopreventive agent, in patients with high-risk or pre-malignant lesions. Anticancer Res 21:2895–2900, 2001.
65. Cruz-Correa M, Shoskes DA, Sanchez P, et al: Combination treatment with curcumin and quercetin of adenomas in familial adenomatous polyposis. Clin Gastroenterol Hepatol 4:1035–1038, 2006.
66. Willett WC, Stampfer MJ, Colditz GA, et al: Relation of meat, fat, and fiber intake to the risk of colon cancer in a prospective study among women. N Engl J Med 323:1664–1672, 1990.
67. Giovannucci E, Rimm EB, Stampfer MJ, et al: Intake of fat, meat, and fiber in relation to risk of colon cancer in men. Cancer Res 54:2390–2397, 1994.
68. Norat T, Lukanova A, Ferrari P, et al: Meat consumption and colorectal cancer risk: dose-response meta-analysis of epidemiological studies. Int J Cancer 98:241–256, 2002.
69. Gatof D, Ahnen D: Primary prevention of colorectal cancer: diet and drugs. Gastroenterol Clin North Am 31:587–623, 2002.
70. Bingham SA, Day NE, Luben R, et al: Dietary fibre in food and protection against colorectal cancer in the European Prospective Investigation into Cancer and Nutrition (EPIC): an observational study. Lancet 361:1496–1501, 2003.
71. Alberts DS, Martinez ME, Roe DJ, et al: Lack of effect of a high-fiber cereal supplement on the recurrence of colorectal adenomas. N Engl J Med 342:1156–1162, 2000.
72. Schatzkin A, Lanza E, Corle D, et al: Lack of effect of a low-fat, high-fiber diet on the recurrence of colorectal adenomas. N Engl J Med 342:1149–1155, 2000.
73. Routine aspirin or nonsteroidal anti-inflammatory drugs for the primary prevention of colorectal cancer: U.S. Preventive Services Task Force recommendation statement. Ann Intern Med 146:361–364, 2007.

7

Fecal Occult Blood Test

Michel I. Kafrouni and John H. Kwon

KEY POINTS

- Screening with the fecal occult blood test (FOBT) is less useful in the prevention of cancer compared with the invasive tests available.
- Colorectal cancer screening with FOBT should be performed annually at home on two samples from each of three consecutive bowel movements.
- All positive FOBTs should be followed by a colonoscopy for direct visualization.
- Two forms of FOBTs are available: the guaiac-based FOBT (g-FOBT) and the fecal immunochemical-based test (FIT).
- The g-FOBT is less expensive than FIT but requires dietary restrictions.
- The FIT is more sensitive than the g-FOBT and is also more specific for lower gastrointestinal bleeding sources.

Introduction

Stool tests for screening are known as fecal occult blood tests (FOBTs) because they are designed to detect the presence of blood in the stool. Since colorectal cancer (CRC) or large polyps (larger than 1 to 2 cm) tend to bleed, these tests are designed to detect these types of lesions. Smaller adenomas do not tend to bleed and are not generally detected with FOBT technique. Therefore, stool tests are considered useful for the detection of CRC and advanced neoplasia and are considered less beneficial in CRC prevention. Since the goal of ultrasound screening programs is colorectal cancer prevention, routine use of FOBT over invasive testing is discouraged.[1] Presently, FOBT is the second most commonly used screening modality for CRC in the United States, with lower endoscopic examinations being the most common.[2]

The use of FOBT is on the decline and has decreased from 21.8% in 2002 to 18.7% in 2004 in favor of lower endoscopic examinations, which increased from 45.2% in 2002 to 50.6% in 2004.[2] Although the FOBT cannot localize the source of gastrointestinal (GI) bleeding (Table 7-1) and although polyps and cancers may exhibit only intermittent bleeding, the efficacy of the FOBT as a CRC screening modality for people of *average risk* has been confirmed in multiple studies.[3-6] In this chapter, current recommendations regarding the use of the FOBT for CRC screening and the relative advantages and disadvantages of specific FOBTs are addressed.

Types of Fecal Occult Blood Tests

The most commonly used FOBT is the guaiac-based test (g-FOBT). Guaiac is a natural resin extracted from the wood of the *Guaiacum officinale* plant. The basis of the test depends on the presence of the heme moiety from the hemoglobin that helps hydrogen peroxide (the main component of the developer) oxidize the paper-embedded guaiac into a blue-colored quinone product (Fig. 7-1A). Examples of commercially available FOBTs are shown in Figure 7-2A and B. The most commonly used g-FOBTs used in the United States are the Hemoccult II (Beckman Coulter, Brea, California) and the more sensitive Hemoccult II SENSA *elite* (Beckman Coulter), used by 72.4% and 13.1% of physicians surveyed, respectively.[7] The U.S. Preventive Services Task Force (USPSTF) and the Gastrointestinal (GI) Consortium recommend the annual use of guaiac-based test cards prepared at home by patients with two samples from each of three consecutive stool samples[8,9]

Table 7-1. Common Gastrointestinal Sources of Occult Blood

Bleeding Source	Most Common Lesions
Oral	Bleeding gums, dental work
Esophageal	Adenocarcinoma, hemorrhagic erosions
Gastric	Hemorrhagic erosions, hemorrhagic ulcer, vascular ectasia
Small intestinal	Hemorrhagic polyps, hemorrhagic ulcer, vascular ectasia, adenocarcinoma
Colonic	Vascular ectasia, diverticular bleeding, adenocarcinoma, polyps
Rectal	Hemorrhoids, anal fissures

(Table 7-2). A single stool specimen obtained during digital rectal examination is not recommended as an adequate screening strategy for CRC.[9]

The fecal immunochemical test (FIT) that was approved by the United States Food and Drug Administration in 2001 has been added to recent American Cancer Society (ACS) and GI Consortium guidelines for colorectal cancer screening[9,10] (see Table 7-2). FIT is based on antibody detection of partial sequences of specific antigenic sites on the globin portion of human hemoglobin (see Fig. 7-1B). Currently, several FITs are commercially available; examples include the Hemoccult ICT (Fig. 7-2C; Beckman Coulter), the HemeSelect (Smith-

Kline Diagnostics, Palo Alto, California), and the InSure (Enterix Inc., Edison, New Jersey) tests. As with the g-FOBT, the ACS also recommends the annual use of multiple stool samples (three consecutive bowel movements) for FIT CRC screening. FIT is processed only in a clinical laboratory, whereas g-FOBT can be processed in a physician's office.

General Advantages and Disadvantages of Fecal Occult Blood Tests

The primary advantage of the FOBT is that evidence demonstrates a reduction in CRC mortality rate, with an annual g-FOBT decreasing the 13-year CRC mortality by 33%.[3] Similarly, the biennial g-FOBT was shown to decrease the 10-year CRC mortality rate by 14% to 18%.[4-6,11] Mandel and associates[4] in a randomized controlled trial (RCT) described a reduced incidence of CRC with either annual or biennial FOBT after 18 years of follow-up. However, the extensive follow-up and subsequent removal of precancerous lesions were thought to have contributed to the reduced CRC-associated mortality. Another randomized controlled trial by Kronborg and associates[5] confirmed the CRC mortality reduction at 18% after 10 years (Table 7-3). Additional studies from Nottingham, UK, and Burgundy, France, reported comparable results with a 15% and 16% reduction of CRC mortality, respectively.[6,11] These studies were pooled in two meta-analyses that concluded that

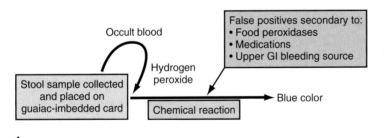

Figure 7-1. Schematic of the g-FOBT (**A**) and i-FOBT (**B**) blood detection reactions. g-FOBT, guaiac-based fecal occult blood test; i-FOBT, immunochemical fecal occult blood test.

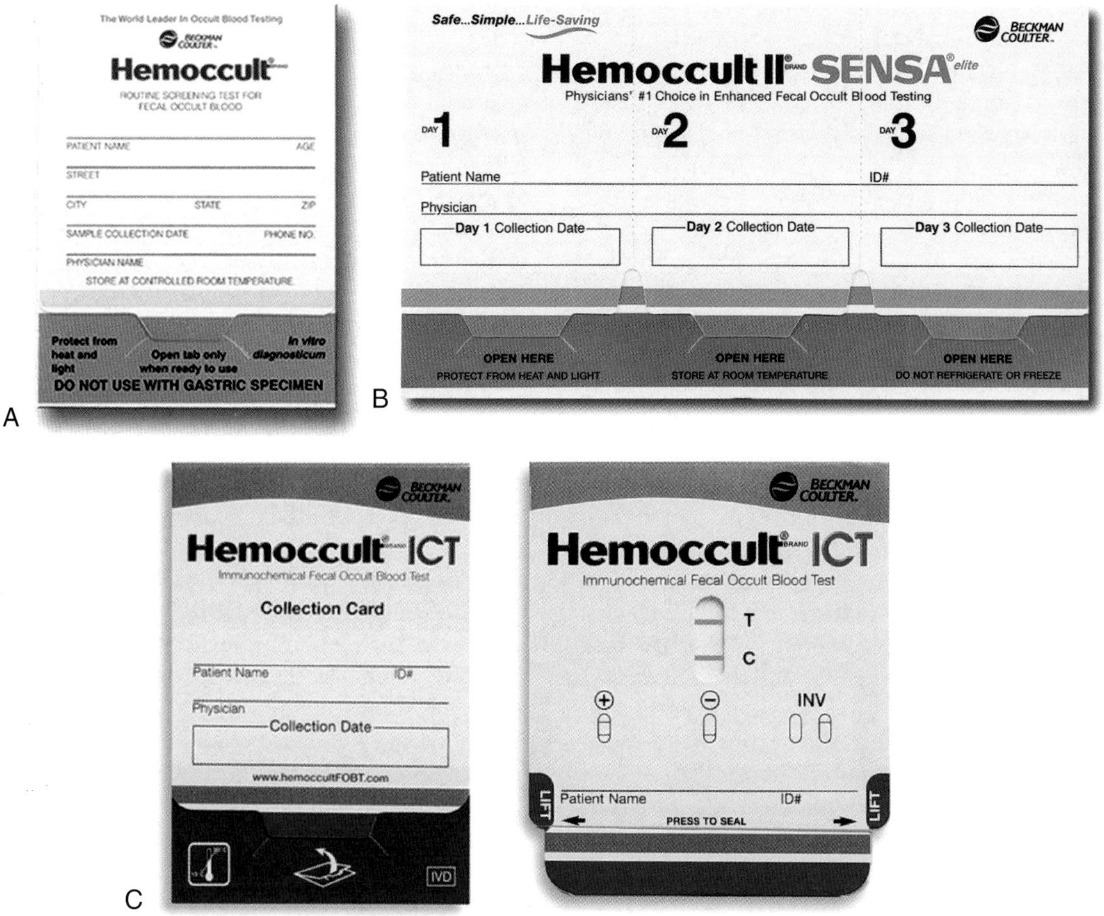

Figure 7-2. Fecal occult blood tests. The Hemoccult FOBT (**A**), the Hemoccult II Sensa Elite FOBT (**B**), and the Hemoccult ICT (**C**). (Photographs provided courtesy of Beckman Coulter, Brea, California.)

Table 7-2. Recommendations Regarding the Use of FOBT for Colorectal Cancer Screening

	American Cancer Society	Gastrointestinal Consortium	Preventive Services Task Force
Year of recommendation	2007[10]	2003[9]	2002[8]
g-FOBT	Yearly*	Yearly*	Yearly*
i-FOBT	Yearly*	Yearly*	n/a

*Either g-FOBT or i-FOBT and preferably in combination with sigmoidoscopy every 5 years.
g-FOBT, guaiac-based fecal occult blood test; i-FOBT, immunochemical fecal occult blood test; n/a, not applicable.

biennial FOBT decreased CRC mortality by 14%[12] and 15%[13] over the first 10 years. There was no evidence-based improvement in CRC mortality if FOBT was performed over longer periods.[12] Of note, although most studies report a reduction in CRC mortality, a recent systematic review of biennial g-FOBT screening for CRC did not demonstrate a reduced effect on total mortality rate.[14]

The second advantage of the FOBT as a CRC screening modality, compared with all other tests, includes its ease of administration. Both the g-FOBT and the FIT are noninvasive tests administered from the patient's home.[15] Frazier and associates[16] showed that the g-FOBT compares favorably with other CRC screening modalities with cost-per-year of life saved ($17,805). Sonnenberg and associates,[8,17] using

18% as percentage of mortality reduction, calculated an incremental cost effectiveness ratio of $10,463 per year of life saved. The results from the above studies and three others were summarized by Pignone and colleagues.[8] The findings were consistent with the cost-effectiveness of other modalities used to screen CRC and other cancers.

Because of its ease of administration and low cost (for the g-FOBT), the FOBT may be of particular benefit as a CRC screening modality in poor countries, where facilities and resources for more invasive tests, including sigmoidoscopies and colonoscopies, are not widely available. For example, in China, with its aging population and lack of a widely subsidized health care system, the FOBT has been proposed as the most compelling method for CRC screening because of its cost-effectiveness and ease of implementation.[18]

The major disadvantage of the FOBT has been improper implementation. Despite published guidelines by the ACS and the USPSTF,[8,10] 32.5% of primary care physicians performed office-based FOBTs rather than home-based FOBTs.[7] The randomized controlled studies demonstrating a reduction in CRC mortality required the analysis of two stool samples in three consecutively obtained bowel movements.[4-6] Collins and associates[19] demonstrated that a single g-FOBT on a stool obtained by digital rectal examination in an in-office setting resulted in a sensitivity of only 4.9% for cancer or large polyps compared with 24% using the home-based g-FOBT protocol. Similarly, a single FIT also demonstrated a low sensitivity in detecting both advanced (27.1%) and nonad-

vanced neoplasms (10.4%) of the colon, especially if the lesions were in the proximal colon.[20] Furthermore, a single FIT was unable to detect one third of the invasive cancers.[20] The propensity for intermittent bleeding of polyps and CRCs likely contributes to the poor sensitivity of a single FOBT. In addition, the intermittent bleeding likely contributes to the necessity for testing on sequential stool samples and the increased sensitivity of annual FOBTs, compared with biennial screening protocols. Mandel and colleagues[3] demonstrated a 33% reduction in CRC mortality rate with annual testing compared with a 21% reduction with biennial testing for 10 years (Table 7-3).

FOBT as a CRC screening modality has seen poor compliance. A CDC survey performed in 1999 reported that only 40.3% of eligible, average-risk subjects for CRC ever had an FOBT and 20.6% received an FOBT within 1 year before the survey.[21] Compliance and adherence to CRC screening guidelines were improved with the implementation of a postage-paid return kit and follow-up telephone reminders.[22] In addition, education of both patients and physicians regarding FOBTs was recommended after a study of a low-income, average-risk African-American population in Harlem, New York, demonstrated a greater adherence if the patients had more knowledge regarding the FOBT or received relevant recommendations from their physician.[23] The use of multifaceted, culturally appropriate patient education materials nearly doubled the rate of FOBT screening in a group of low-income minority patients over a 6-month period.[24]

Table 7-3. Major Studies Using FOBT for Colorectal Cancer Screening

	Location	Study Type	Frequency	Length of Follow-up	CRC Mortality Relative Risk Reduction
Mandel et al (1993)[3]	Minnesota, USA	RCT	Yearly FOBT	13 yr	33%
Mandel et al (2000)[4]	Minnesota, USA	RCT	Biennial FOBT	18 yr	21%
Kronborg et al (1996)[5]	Funen, Denmark	RCT	Biennial FOBT	10 yr	18%
Hardcastle et al (1996)[6]	Nottingham, UK	RCT	Biennial FOBT	10 yr	15%
Faivre et al (2004)[11]	Burgundy, France	RCT	Biennial FOBT	11 yr	16%
Heresbach et al (2006)[12]	n/a	Meta-analysis	Biennial FOBT	10 yr	14%
			Biennial FOBT	>10 yr	No significant reduction
Hewitson et al (2007)[13]	n/a	Meta-analysis	Biennial FOBT	10 yr	15%
			At least 1 FOBT	10 yr	25%

FOBT, fecal occult blood test; n/a, not applicable; RCT, randomized controlled study.

Of note, an inappropriate reliance on a repeat FOBT for a positive FOBT has been documented, with one study demonstrating 29.7% of primary care physicians recommending repeat FOBT rather than endoscopic diagnostic testing for positive FOBTs.[7] Baig and associates[25] reported that 46% of primary care providers relied on a negative repeat FOBT and failed to refer their patients for colonoscopy, or referred them for barium enemas or sigmoidoscopies. Similarly, in a Veterans Administration–based study, follow-up colonoscopy was performed in only 59% of patients with a positive FOBT.[26] A colonoscopy should be performed on all patients with a positive FOBT.[27]

Specific Characteristics of the g-FOBT and FIT

In addition to general FOBT considerations, the g-FOBT and FIT have distinct characteristics that influence the utilization and accuracy of the tests as CRC screening modalities (Box 7-1). The differences between the g-FOBT and FIT include factors that contribute to false-positive and false-negative results, their relative specificities and sensitivities for CRC diagnosis, and their relative costs.

The first major benefit to using the g-FOBT is that significantly more evidence has been accumulated demonstrating that annual CRC screening with home-based g-FOBT protocols reduces CRC mortality (see Table 7-3). The first study demonstrating a reduction in CRC

mortality using the g-FOBT was published in 1993.[3] Since then, many studies that used biennial testing[5,6,11–13] confirmed that screening with g-FOBT showed a statistically significant reduction in CRC mortality. Although no studies have demonstrated a decrease in mortality associated with the use of FIT over g-FOBT, Allison and associates[28] recently demonstrated an increased sensitivity of FIT (82% versus 64%) for the detection of left-sided CRC of FIT over sensitive g-FOBT tests. It is believed that this finding will correlate with a decrease in CRC mortality. More important is that this study evaluated a highly sensitive g-FOBT and demonstrated that the sensitivity varies greatly among test types such that some g-FOBT products can be listed as low sensitivity and others as highly sensitive.

The second advantage to using the g-FOBT over FIT is the relative cost per screen. Based on Medicare schedules, the base costs for each cycle of g-FOBT and FIT were estimated at $15 and $22, respectively.[29] Although an early study by Castiglione and associates[30] suggested that screening with FIT can be more cost-effective than with g-FOBT, no further studies are available to confirm the cost-effectiveness of FIT over g-FOBT. Although FIT has been recommended by the GI Consortium and ACS as an alternative to g-FOBT,[10,31] its benefit over g-FOBT is uncertain.[1]

One disadvantage of the g-FOBT is that its sensitivity and specificity are affected by rehydration of stool sample cards before analysis. Rehydration of stool samples increased the sensitivity of the g-FOBT from 2.4% to 9.8%; however, it increased the rate of false positives as the specificity decreased from 97.7% to 90.4%.[4] Thus, to avoid the increased false positives and subsequent overutilization of follow-up colonoscopies, the USPSTF has recommended not rehydrating samples.[31]

Many factors may contribute to false-positives and false-negatives of the g-FOBT (Box 7-2). False-positive results have been attributed to many foods and drugs that contain either blood or oxidizing agents. Specific drugs that may lead to false positives include aspirin, iron, steroids, and colchicine. Specific foods that may lead to false positives include red meats and vegetables containing peroxidases, such as radishes, turnips, and broccoli. Delaying the development of the g-FOBT for more than 48 hours

Box 7-1. Advantages and Disadvantages of g-FOBT and i-FOBT

Advantages
Ease of administration
Low cost
Noninvasiveness
Can be implemented on large-scale basis
Proved to reduce CRC mortality*
Cost effective*

Disadvantages and Limitations
Poor sensitivity*
Inadequate follow-up
Poor compliance
Dietary restrictions*

*Applies to g-FOBT but not i-FOBT.
CRC, colorectal cancer; g-FOBT, guaiac-based fecal occult blood test; i-FOBT, immunochemical fecal occult blood test.

Box 7-2. Factors Contributing to False-positive and False-negative g-FOBT Results

False Positives

Other sources of bleeding (see Table 7-1)
Anticoagulants and blood thinners like aspirin
Medications: steroids, iron, colchicine
Oxidizing drugs such as iodine and boric acid
Consumption of red meat within three days of the test
Consumption of fish
Consumption of broccoli, turnips, and horseradish

False Negatives

Vitamin C consumption
Intermittent bleeding of polyps and cancers

---

decreased the false positives caused by plant peroxidases. However, rehydrating stool samples recapitulated the false positives caused by plant peroxidases.[32] Specific foods may lead to false-negative results, including large doses of vitamin C. Therefore, dietary restrictions are required for an adequate g-FOBT. Before the g-FOBT, individuals should avoid nonsteroidal anti-inflammatory drugs (NSAIDs) and 325 mg of aspirin for 7 days prior to testing. Furthermore, red meat and vitamin C supplements of more than 250 mg should be avoided for 3 days before the test. The decreased dietary restrictions associated with the FIT have been cited as a reason for increased compliance using the FIT compared with the g-FOBT.[33] However, a recent study demonstrated a similar compliance to the FIT compared with the g-FOBT.[34]

A clear disadvantage of g-FOBT is its poor sensitivity. Upper GI sources of bleeding are responsible for a large number of false positives in CRC screening. In a study by Rockey and colleagues,[35] 71 out of 248 subjects referred for occult bleeding detected by positive g-FOBT were found to have an upper GI bleeding source, whereas only 54 had a lower GI bleeding source. FIT has a clear advantage over g-FOBT in distinguishing lower GI bleeding, with its sensitivity for lesions in the lower GI tract being 91% compared with 19% for upper GI sources.[36] The globin protein from sources in the upper GI tract gets degraded by GI enzymes, making FIT a poor test to screen for upper GI sources of bleeding and a more specific test for bleeds originating in the lower GI tract.[36,37]

Other cited advantages of FIT over g-FOBT include recent evidence that FIT is more sensi-

tive in detecting high-risk adenomas.[15] Also, automated FIT reading technology has been developed, allowing for adjustments in the reading threshold to optimize its sensitivity and specificity and eliminate user/reader variability.[15,38] The utilization of a brush-sampling FIT (InSure FOBT) compared with g-FOBT was also associated with an increased compliance, attributed to increased ease of use.[39]

Conclusions

Both guaiac-based and immunochemical-based FOBTs are recommended by the ACS and the GI Consortium as screening modalities for CRC. In general, the FOBT is a cost-effective CRC screening method for people of average risk and should not be used as a screening method for people with an increased risk for CRC. FOBT should be implemented yearly, either solely or in combination with flexible sigmoidoscopy every 5 years. g-FOBTs are the most frequently used test. However, utilization of FIT is increasing. Although FIT is more expensive, it has been associated with improved compliance and decreased false-positive results. Regardless of which test is used, educating both patients and physicians about administering the test improves compliance. FOBT as a CRC screening tool is decreasing in the United States, but it remains a viable option for CRC screening in the United States as much as in societies with limited resources and access to endoscopic facilities.

References

1. Levin B, Lieberman DA, McFarland B, et al: Screening and surveillance for the early detection of colorectal cancer and adenomatous polyps, 2008: a joint guideline from the American Cancer Society, the US Multi-Society Task Force on Colorectal Cancer, and the American College of Radiology. Gastroenterology 134:1570–1595, 2008.
2. Ouyang DL, Chen JJ, Getzenberg RH, et al: Noninvasive testing for colorectal cancer: a review. Am J Gastroenterol 100: 1393–1403, 2005.
3. Mandel JS, Bond JH, Church TR, et al: Reducing mortality from colorectal cancer by screening for fecal occult blood. Minnesota Colon Cancer Control Study. N Engl J Med 328:1365–1371, 1993.
4. Mandel JS, Church TR, Bond JH, et al: The effect of fecal occult-blood screening on the incidence of colorectal cancer. N Engl J Med 343:1603–1607, 2000.
5. Kronborg O, Fenger C, Olsen J, et al: Randomised study of screening for colorectal cancer with faecal-occult-blood test. Lancet 348:1467–1471, 1996.
6. Hardcastle JD, Chamberlain JO, Robinson MH, et al: Randomised controlled trial of faecal-occult-blood screening for colorectal cancer. Lancet 348:1472–1477, 1996.
7. Nadel MR, Shapiro JA, Klabunde CN, et al: A national survey of primary care physicians' methods for screening for fecal occult blood. Ann Intern Med 142:86–94, 2005.

8. Pignone M, Saha S, Hoerger T, et al: Cost-effectiveness analyses of colorectal cancer screening: a systematic review for the U.S. Preventive Services Task Force. Ann Intern Med 137:96–104, 2002.

9. Winawer S, Fletcher R, Rex D, et al: Gastrointestinal Consortium Panel. Colorectal cancer screening and surveillance: clinical guidelines and rationale—update based on new evidence. Gastroenterology 124:544–560, 2003.

10. American Cancer Society: Guidelines for the Early Detection of Cancer. 2007.

11. Faivre J, Dancourt V, Lejeune C, et al: Reduction in colorectal cancer mortality by fecal occult blood screening in a French controlled study. Gastroenterology 126:1674–1680, 2004.

12. Heresbach D, Manfredi S, D'halluin PN, et al: Review in depth and meta-analysis of controlled trials on colorectal cancer screening by faecal occult blood test. Eur J Gastroenterol Hepatol 18:427–433, 2006.

13. Hewitson P, Glasziou P, Irwig L, et al: Screening for colorectal cancer using the faecal occult blood test, Hemoccult. Cochrane Database Syst Rev 2007;(1):CD001216.

14. Moayyedi P, Achkar E: Does fecal occult blood testing really reduce mortality? A reanalysis of systematic review data. Am J Gastroenterol 101:380–384, 2006.

15. Guittet L, Bouvier V, Mariotte N, et al: Comparison of a guaiac based and an immunochemical faecal occult blood test in screening for colorectal cancer in a general average risk population. Gut 56:210–214, 2007.

16. Frazier AL, Colditz GA, Fuchs CS, et al: Cost-effectiveness of screening for colorectal cancer in the general population. JAMA 284:1954–1961, 2000.

17. Sonnenberg A, Delco F, Inadomi JM: Cost-effectiveness of colonoscopy in screening for colorectal cancer. Ann Intern Med 133:573–584, 2000.

18. Sung J: Does fecal occult blood test have a place for colorectal cancer screening in China in 2006? Am J Gastroenterol 101:213–215, 2006.

19. Collins JF, Lieberman DA, Durbin TE, et al: Veterans Affairs Cooperative Study #380 Group. Accuracy of screening for fecal occult blood on a single stool sample obtained by digital rectal examination: a comparison with recommended sampling practice. Ann Intern Med 142:81–85, 2005.

20. Morikawa T, Kato J, Yamaji Y, et al: A comparison of the immunochemical fecal occult blood test and total colonoscopy in the asymptomatic population. Gastroenterology 129:422–428, 2005.

21. Centers for Disease Control and Prevention (CDC). Trends in screening for colorectal cancer: United States, 1997 and 1999. MMWR Morb Mortal Wkly Rep 50:162–166, 2001.

22. Church TR, Yeazel MW, Jones RM, et al: A randomized trial of direct mailing of fecal occult blood tests to increase colorectal cancer screening. J Natl Cancer Inst 96:770–780, 2004.

23. Lawsin C, DuHamel K, Weiss A, et al: Colorectal cancer screening among low-income African Americans in East Harlem: a theoretical approach to understanding barriers and promoters to screening. J Urban Health 84:32–44, 2007.

24. Tu SP, Taylor V, Yasui Y, et al: Promoting culturally appropriate colorectal cancer screening through a health educator: a randomized controlled trial. Cancer 107:959–966, 2006.

25. Baig N, Myers RE, Turner BJ, et al: Physician-reported reasons for limited follow-up of patients with a positive fecal occult blood test screening result. Am J Gastroenterol 98:2078–2081, 2003.

26. Etzioni DA, Yano EM, Rubenstein LV, et al: Measuring the quality of colorectal cancer screening: the importance of follow-up. Dis Colon Rectum 49:1002–1010, 2006.

27. Ransohoff DF, Lang CA: Screening for colorectal cancer with the fecal occult blood test: a background paper. American College of Physicians. Ann Intern Med 126:811–822, 1997.

28. Allison JE, Sakoda LC, Levin TR, et al: Screening for colorectal neoplasms with new fecal occult blood tests: update on performance characteristics. J Natl Cancer Inst 99:1462–1470, 2000.

29. Parekh M, Fendrick AM, Ladabaum U: As tests evolve and costs of cancer care rise: reappraising stool-based screening for colorectal neoplasia. Aliment Pharmacol Ther 27(8):697–712, 2008.

30. Castiglione G, Zappa M, Grazzini G, et al: Cost analysis in a population based screening programme for colorectal cancer: comparison of immunochemical and guaiac faecal occult blood testing. J Med Screen 4:142–146, 1997.

31. Pignone M, Rich M, Teutsch SM, et al: Screening for colorectal cancer in adults at average risk: a summary of the evidence for the U.S. Preventive Services Task Force. Ann Intern Med 137:132–141, 2002.

32. Sinatra MA, Young GP, St John DJ, et al: A study of laboratory based faecal occult blood testing in Melbourne, Australia. The Faecal Occult Blood Testing Study Group. J Gastroenterol Hepatol 13:396–400, 1998.

33. Smith A, Young GP, Cole SR, et al: Comparison of a brush-sampling fecal immunochemical test for hemoglobin with a sensitive guaiac-based fecal occult blood test in detection of colorectal neoplasia. Cancer 107:2152–2159, 2006.

34. Ko CW, Dominitz JA, Nguyen TD: Fecal occult blood testing in a general medical clinic: comparison between guaiac-based and immunochemical-based tests. Am J Med 115:111–114, 2003.

35. Rockey DC, Koch J, Cello JP, et al: Relative frequency of upper gastrointestinal and colonic lesions in patients with positive fecal occult-blood tests. N Engl J Med 339:153–159, 1998.

36. Nakama H, Kamijo N, Fattah AS, et al: Immunologic detection of fecal occult blood from upper digestive tract diseases. Hepatogastroenterology 45:752–754, 1998.

37. Nakama H, Zhang B: Immunochemical fecal occult blood test is inadequate for screening test of stomach cancer. Dig Dis Sci 45:2195–2198, 2000.

38. Vilkin A, Rozen P, Levi Z, et al: Performance characteristics and evaluation of an automated-developed and quantitative, immunochemical, fecal occult blood screening test. Am J Gastroenterol 100:2519–2525, 2005.

39. Cole SR, Young GP, Esterman A, et al: A randomised trial of the impact of new faecal haemoglobin test technologies on population participation in screening for colorectal cancer. J Med Screen 10:117–122, 2003.

8 Colonoscopy and Flexible Sigmoidoscopy in Colorectal Cancer Screening and Surveillance

Michelle N. Zikusoka and John H. Kwon

KEY POINTS

- Persons with average risk for colorectal cancer should undergo flexible sigmoidoscopy every 5 years or colonoscopy every 10 years after the age of 50.
- Those with a positive family history should start screening as early as 40 years old.
- Special consideration with regard to screening should be given to patients with a positive family history, history of polypectomy or surgical resection, as well as those with hereditary syndromes or inflammatory bowel disease.

Introduction

With increasing recognition of the prevalence of colorectal cancer (CRC) and the effect it has on the health of Americans, the medical community has gradually adopted screening and surveillance guidelines. The current modalities for screening and surveillance include fecal occult blood testing, flexible sigmoidoscopy, colonoscopy, and radiographic studies, including double-contrast barium enema and virtual colonoscopy. This discussion focuses on flexible sigmoidoscopy and colonoscopy.

The earliest known tool for luminal evaluation of the gastrointestinal tract was the *Lichtleiter*, or light conductor. Invented by Philipp Bozzini in Frankfurt, Germany, in 1806, this instrument used a candle as the source of illumination for rectoscopy[1] (Fig. 8-1). Almost a century later, in 1894, Howard Kelly[2] of Johns Hopkins University introduced the first rigid rectosigmoidoscopes, which allowed visualization to a depth of 30 cm. Over the next 5 decades, poor illumination, limited depth, and patient discomfort continued to present challenges to the clinician. Not until the 1950s did a true revolution in endoscopy occur. During this period, Narinder Singh Kapany[3] invented flexible optical fibers. Using this newfound technology, Basil Hirschowitz[4] of the University of Michigan created the first fiber optic endoscope. As the earliest tool to overcome the seemingly inherent obstacles associated with prior techniques, this modality of luminal gastrointestinal investigation soon came into common practice. The incorporation of new technologies such as the snare device for polypectomy in the late 1960s[5] augmented not only the diagnostic but also the therapeutic potential of colonoscopy and flexible sigmoidoscopy.[6]

Indications for Screening

The goal of a CRC screening program is to detect precancerous and cancerous lesions early so that interventions will lead to improved outcome while appropriately making use of available resources. CRC or the precursor lesion, adenomatous polyps, may affect diverse patient populations, including asymptomatic persons, those who have had a polypectomy, and those who have had a CRC surgical resection, and special populations such as those with inflammatory bowel disease (IBD) or with hereditary/genetic predispositions. The creation of a viable screening and surveillance program needs to be diverse enough to incorporate all those at risk for CRC. To that end, risk stratification is of paramount importance to ensure appropriate implementation of screening and surveillance guidelines. However, this task is fraught with challenges, such as resource limitations, the economic burden of covering expenses, and clinician aptitude. Also vital to the success of a CRC

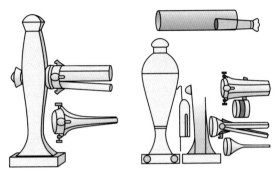

Figure 8-1. Lichtleiter or light conductor for luminal evaluation of the rectum.

Table 8-1. Percentage of Adults Aged ≥50 Years Who Reported Receiving a Fecal Occult Blood Test (FOBT) Within 12 Months Preceding Survey and/or Lower Endoscopy Within 5 and 10 Years Preceding Survey, by Test Type

Test	%	(95% CI)
FOBT within 12 mo	23.5	(±0.5)
Lower endoscopy within 5 yr	38.7	(±0.5)
Lower endoscopy within 10 yr	43.4	(±0.6)
FOBT within 12 mo and/or lower endoscopy within 10 yr	59.1	(±0.6)

*Age-adjusted to the 2001 BRFSS population.
CI, confidence interval.
From Behavioral Risk Factor Surveillance Systems (BRFSS), United States, 2001; Colorectal cancer test use among persons aged >50 years, United States, 2001. MMWR Morbidity and Mortality Weekly Rep 52:193–196, 2003, Fig. 1.

screening program are patient compliance and willingness to participate, sensitivity and specificity of screening modalities, accessibility, and overall benefit with minimized risk.

According to the Behavior Risk Factor Surveillance System (BRFSS), only 30% to 50% of individuals for whom screening is recommended are currently being screened in the United States. Moreover, the percentage of those undergoing screening varies widely by region within the United States (Fig. 8-2, Table 8-1). Furthermore, according to the Centers for Disease Control and Prevention, there are approximately 41 million average-risk persons older than 50 years who are eligible for screening.[7] Only an estimated 2.8 million flexible sigmoidoscopies and 14.2 million colonoscopies were performed in 2002. To meet the demands

if all individuals were to be screened, at least 18 million more colonoscopies would have to be performed annually. To provide more resources, one solution is to increase the number of persons trained in endoscopy. However, ensuring that quality control measures are in place is an important aspect of a screening program. Recent reports in the literature have demonstrated that adenoma detection rates may vary greatly with endoscopist experience such that endoscopists who have performed more than 400 endoscopies were better at detecting adenomas than those who had not[8] (Fig. 8-3). If appropriately

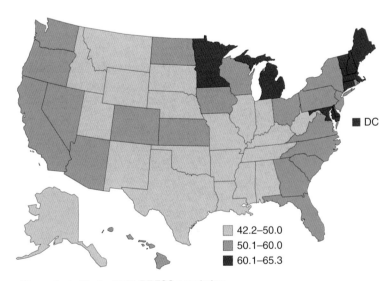

■ DC

42.2–50.0
50.1–60.0
60.1–65.3

*Age-adjusted to the 2001 BRFSS population

Figure 8-2. Percentage of adults age ≥50 who reported receiving a fecal occult blood test (FOBT) within 12 months preceding survey and/or lower endoscopy within 5 and 10 years preceding survey, by state. Figures are age-adjusted to the 2001 BRFSS population. (From Behavioral Risk Factor Surveillance Systems [BRFSS], United States, 2001: Colorectal cancer test use among persons aged >50 years, United States, 2001. MMWR Morb Mortal Wkly Rep 52:193–196, 2003, Fig. 1.)

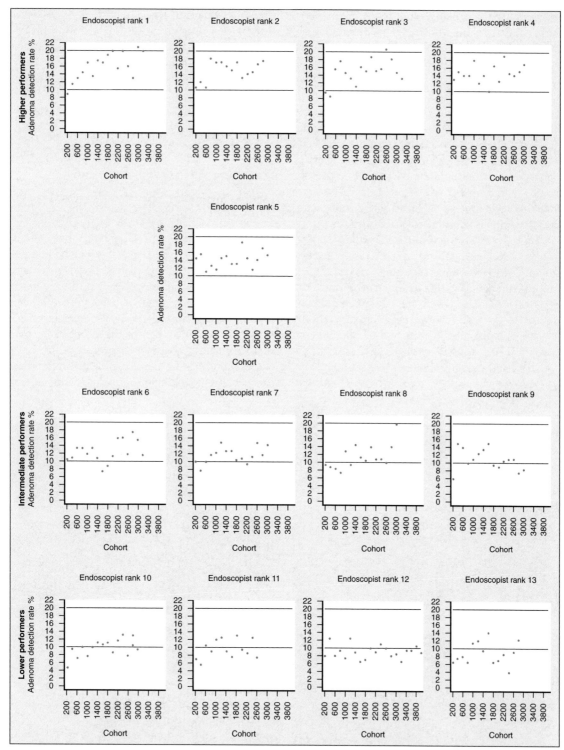

Figure 8-3. Endoscopist experience and performance affect detection rates in flexible sigmoidoscopy. The investigators demonstrated that average adenoma detection rate (ADR) increased with screening experience (up to 400 cases). There was also a wide variation in ADRs among endoscopists. Eleven more adenomas were detected per 100 people screened by the highest-ranking endoscopist compared with the lowest-ranking endoscopist (21.7 versus 10.4), which is equivalent to a 50% miss rate of adenomas. (From Atkin W, Rogers P, Cardwell C, et al: Wide variation in adenoma detection rates at screening flexible sigmoidoscopy. Gastroenterology 126:1247–1256, 2004, Fig. 2.)

implemented, regular colonoscopic screening and adherence to screening guidelines may prevent 76% to 90% of colon cancers.[9]

Findings on Endoscopic Evaluation

Lesions found on endoscopic examination can be broadly categorized as polyps and nonpolypoid lesions (Fig. 8-4). Polyps are characterized as neoplastic or non-neoplastic. Non-neoplastic polyps are further subdivided into hyperplastic polyps, hamartomas, lymphoid aggregrates, and inflammatory polyps. Those with malignant potential include tubular, tubulovillous, and villous polyps. Serrated and microtubular adenomas as well as invasive carcinoma may also be found.[10] Histologically, features indicating a more favorable prognosis include the absence of poor differentiation and the absence of lymphatic or vascular involvement.[11] Nonpolypoid lesions have been more difficult to detect, yet make up 30% to 40% of all CRC lesions.[12–14] Today's endoscopic techniques are beginning to incorporate staining and microscopy techniques

that further aid in the detection and classification of such lesions. Regarding anatomic distribution, about 50% of polyps are found in the proximal colon, whereas 20% are found distally. Synchronous polyps are found in about 30% of cases. Adenomas and carcinomas, however, have a right-sided predominance that increases with age.[15]

Screening and Surveillance Tools

Flexible Sigmoidoscopy

The flexible sigmoidoscope is an endoscopic tool that allows visualization of the large bowel to the depth of about 70 cm (Fig. 8-5). The benefits of flexible sigmoidoscopy include lower cost, lack of necessity for full bowel preparation, and no sedation. The preparation for this procedure can usually be accomplished with enemas given no more than 3 hours before the procedure. This modality is often used in conjunction with fecal occult blood testing. This screening combination has been reported to have a detection rate of

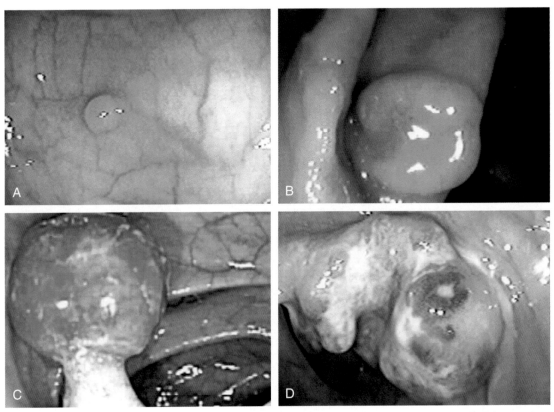

Figure 8-4. Colonoscopy findings.   A, Hyperplastic polyp. **B,** Sessile polyp. **C,** Pedunculated polyp. **D,** Adenocarcinomatous mass.

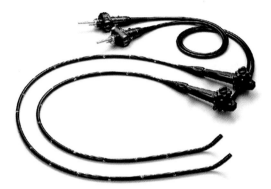

Figure 8-5. Colonoscope and flexible sigmoidoscope.
(Courtesy of Olympus America, Inc.)

76% in contrast to 70% with flexible sigmoidoscopy alone.[16]

Flexible sigmoidoscopy, although limited in extent of colonic visualization, is associated with decreased morbidity and mortality.[17] A large Veterans' Administration population study by Muller and Sonnenberg[18] revealed a 50% reduction in risk of developing CRC (odds ratio 0.55) through endoscopic procedures. This protective influence lasted about 6 years. Others have noted protection sustainable for as long as 16 years.[19] Current guidelines set by the U.S. Preventive Services Task Force, the American Cancer Society (ACS), and the American College of Radiology recommend examination by flexible sigmoidoscopy every 5 years for average-risk persons[20] (Table 8-2).

The obvious limitation of performing flexible sigmoidoscopy is the depth of visualization, limited mainly to the left colon and part of the transverse colon. In an effort to overcome the inherent hindrance, multiple studies have attempted to predict the potential presence of proximal lesions otherwise missed by this imaging modality by examining distal findings. Advanced proximal adenomas may occur in patients, regardless of the presence of advanced lesions in the distal colon. Advanced distal lesions, however, are indicative of a higher risk of advanced proximal lesions. Imperiale and colleagues[21] reported a 2.6 relative risk of advanced proximal neoplasia for patients with distal hyperplastic polyps, whereas patients with distal tubular adenomas or advanced distal polyps had a relative risk ratio of 4.0 or 6.7, respectively, compared with patients with no distal polyps. Furthermore, age greater than 65 years, family history of CRC, villous histology in distal adenomas, adenomas larger than or equal to 1 cm, and multiplicity of distal adenomas are associated with increased risk of advanced proximal lesions.[22] In such populations, it may be prudent to proceed directly to total colonic examination through colonoscopy. Despite the potential pitfalls associated with limited visualization, flexible sigmoidoscopy remains a frequently used screening option.

Colonoscopy

Colonoscopy allows complete visualization of the large intestine. This examination technique requires adequate preparation, including a clear liquid diet as well as an oral cathartic regimen (i.e., sodium phosphate, magnesium citrate, polyethylene glycol). The preparation is often the least tolerated step in the procedure. Unlike the flexible sigmoidoscopy, intravenous sedation is necessary for examination. Aside from the risks associated with sedation, colonoscopic examination itself bears some degree of morbidity and mortality. Compared with sigmoidoscopy, colonoscopy has a higher rate of perforation (1 per 1000 procedures overall compared with an estimated rate of 1 per 10,000 for sigmoidoscopic procedures).[23]

Table 8-2. A Comparison of Flexible Sigmoidoscopy and Colonoscopy in Colorectal Cancer Screening in the Average-Risk, Asymptomatic Person

	Flexible Sigmoidoscopy	Colonoscopy
Screening interval in the asymptomatic individual	5 years	10 years
Age for average-risk screening initiation	50 years	50 years
Depth of visualization	Distal transverse colon	Entire colon
Preparation	Enema, laxative	Liquid cathartic
Sedation	None	Light, intravenous
Perforation risk	1 per 10,000	1 per 1000

Colonoscopy offers the benefit of complete examination of the large bowel. A prospective study of 116 proximal CRC patients noted that 65% of patients lacked distal findings.[24] If flexible sigmoidoscopy was the only means of colonic examination, the proximal neoplasms could have potentially gone undetected. The sensitivity of colonoscopy for adenomas is 87.5% to 90% for polyps 1 cm or larger and 75% to 91.5% for polyps smaller than 1 cm.[25,26] In combination with polypectomy, colonoscopy leads to a lower-than-expected incidence of CRC. With polypectomy, the incidence of CRC decreases by 76% to 90%.[9]

Recently, quality measures have been defined by the U.S. Multi-Society Task Force (USMSTF) on CRC (consisting of the American College of Gastroenterology, American College of Physicians/American Society of Internal Medicine, American Gastroenterological Association, and the American Society for Gastrointestinal Endoscopy). The task force defines a high-quality colonoscopy as one that reaches the cecum, has little fecal residue, and has a minimum time of withdrawal from the cecum of 6 to 10 minutes.[27] These recommendations are based on findings that lower rates of adenoma detection have been seen in patients undergoing colonoscopy in which the time of withdrawal is less than 6 minutes.[28]

Despite the benefit of complete evaluation of the entire colon, colonoscopy remains one of the less popular options for CRC screening among patients. Barriers to successful implementation of a CRC screening program through colonoscopy include the patient's concerns regarding procedure risk, the preparation, and the fear of pain and discomfort. This, combined with the impact of cost, insurance access, long waiting periods, absence from work, need for transportation to and from the procedure, and scheduling conflicts have also proved to be hindrances to the application of a successful screening campaign.

Current Recommendations

Official guidelines for the use of flexible sigmoidoscopy and colonoscopy in the screening and surveillance of CRC were first published in 1997 by a consortium of gastroenterologic societies, including the American Gastroenterological Association.[29] The current and revised edition, published in 2003, expands on familial, hereditary syndrome, as well as high-risk cases.[30] More recently, new guidelines addressed postpolypectomy and postsurgical resection populations.[31] In 2008, similar updates summarizing screening and surveillance guidelines for the average-risk person have been published that begin to look more closely at the economic burden of the disease and quality measures to improve screening results.[20] The recommendations gleaned from these published guidelines are summarized in the text that follows.

Asymptomatic, Average-Risk Persons

The USMSTF and ACS recommendations for colonoscopy and sigmoidoscopy in asymptomatic, average-risk persons are summarized in Table 8-2. The lifetime risk for development of nonhereditary CRC is 6%.[32] Average-risk persons are defined as those with no family history of CRC or a history of conditions, such as IBD, which may predispose them to CRC. About 75% of new CRC cases are found in individuals of average risk. The recommendation from the USMSTF on CRC and the American Cancer Society is for colonoscopic examination every 10 years, beginning at age 50. If sigmoidoscopy is chosen as a means of screening, it should be performed every 5 years.

Familial Risk

One of the earliest studies supporting CRC screening of persons with familial risk reported a higher risk of colonic adenoma in patients with a history of CRC in first-degree relatives compared with that of controls. This risk increased substantially in those with two or more afflicted relatives. First-degree relatives are defined as parents, siblings, and children; second-degree relatives include aunts, uncles, and grandparents. Relatives such as great-grandparents and cousins are considered third-degree relatives.

Current recommendations from the USMSTF and the ACS include early initiation of colonoscopic screening in persons with (1) one first-degree relative with CRC or adenomatous polyps diagnosed before age 60 or (2) two or more first-degree relatives diagnosed at any age. Screening should begin at age 40, or 10 years younger than the person with earliest familial diagnosis. Subsequent examinations should

---

Box 8-1. Colorectal Cancer Screening Guidelines in Persons with Familial Risk

- For individuals with (a) a first-degree relative diagnosed with colorectal cancer (CRC) or adenomatous polyps *before* the age of 60 or (b) two or more first-degree relatives diagnosed with CRC at any age, screening should be initiated at age 40, or 10 years younger than the earliest familial diagnosis. Subsequent examinations should occur at 5-year intervals.
- For individuals with (a) a first-degree relative diagnosed *after* age 60 or (b) two or more second-degree relatives with CRC, screening should begin at age 40. Subsequent examinations should occur every 10 years.
- For individuals with one second-degree or third-degree relative with CRC, screening should follow recommendations for average-risk individuals.

Adapted from Levin B, Lieberman DA, McFarland B, et al: Screening and surveillance for the early detection of colorectal cancer and adenomatous polyps, 2008: a joint guideline from the American Cancer Society, the US Multi-Society Task Force on Colorectal Cancer, and the American College of Radiology. Gastroenterology 134:1570–1595, 2008.

Box 8-2. Colorectal Cancer Surveillance Guidelines for the Postpolypectomy Patient

Patients should be subdivided according to risk.
- Lower-risk patients include those with 1 or 2 small (<1 cm) tubular adenomas with no high-grade dysplasia. Follow-up should occur in 5–10 years.
- Increased-risk patients include those with 3–10 adenomas, high-grade dysplasia, villous features, or an adenoma ≥1 cm or larger; colonoscopic examination should occur every 3 years.
- If subsequent examination is normal or shows only 1 or 2 small tubular adenomas with low-grade dysplasia, the subsequent examination should be in 5 years.
- If follow-up examination reveals ≥10 adenomas, the next colonoscopy should occur within less than 3 years.

Adapted from Levin B, Lieberman DA, McFarland B, et al: Screening and surveillance for the early detection of colorectal cancer and adenomatous polyps, 2008: a joint guideline from the American Cancer Society, the US Multi-Society Task Force on Colorectal Cancer, and the American College of Radiology. Gastroenterology 134:1570–1595, 2008.

---

occur at 5-year intervals. Persons with (1) a first-degree relative diagnosed after age 60 or (2) two second-degree relatives with CRC should initiate screening at age 40, but subsequent examinations should occur every 10 years. Those with one second-degree or third-degree relative with CRC should undergo screening as average-risk individuals (Box 8-1).

Postpolypectomy

For patients with significant findings on initial screening colonoscopy, follow-up is warranted. Again, risk stratification is used in this patient population. According to the USMSTF and the ACS, patients who have 3 to 10 adenomas, high-grade dysplasia, villous features, or an adenoma 1 cm or larger on initial screening colonoscopy are in the "increased risk" category. These individuals should undergo the next colonoscopic examination in 3 years. If this examination is normal or shows only one or two small tubular adenomas with low-grade dysplasia, the subsequent examination should be 5 years later. For those with 10 or more adenomas on follow-up evaluation, the next colonoscopy should occur in less than 3 years.

Patients are categorized as lower risk when one or two small (less than 1 cm) tubular adeno-

mas with no high-grade dysplasia are found on initial screening colonoscopy. These patients should follow up in 5 to 10 years. If only hyperplastic lesions are found, colonoscopy should occur within the same time interval as that of average-risk persons at 10 years[20] (Box 8-2).

Postsurgical Resection

The USMSTF and the ACS recommend that patients with stage I, II, III, or IV CRC who have undergone surgical resection with intent to cure should undergo colonoscopy either 1 year after the preoperative colonoscopy for detection of synchronous disease or 1 year after resection. If the initial colonoscopy could not be performed as a result of an obstructing lesion, either a virtual colonoscopy should be performed before resection or a colonoscopy 3 to 6 months after resection. If the examination is normal, subsequent examinations should be in 3 years, then again in 5 years. For surveillance after resection for rectal cancer, endoscopic evaluation of the rectum for local recurrence every 3 to 6 months for the first 2 to 3 years is recommended. The endoscopist should tailor follow-up intervals according to subsequent findings, potentially shortening surveillance intervals (Box 8-3).

Box 8-3. Colorectal Cancer Surveillance Guidelines for the Postsurgical Resection Patient

Surveillance recommendations for colorectal cancer are:

- Colonoscopy should be performed 1 year after resection or 1 year after the colonoscopy that was performed in the preoperative period to clear the colon of synchronous disease.
- If the examination is normal, subsequent examinations should be carried out in 3 years, then again in 5 years.
- For surveillance for local recurrence after surgery for rectal cancer, endoscopic evaluation of the rectum every 3–6 months for the first 2–3 years is recommended.

Adapted from Levin B, Lieberman DA, McFarland B, et al: Screening and surveillance for the early detection of colorectal cancer and adenomatous polyps, 2008: a joint guideline from the American Cancer Society, the US Multi-Society Task Force on Colorectal Cancer, and the American College of Radiology. Gastroenterology 134:1570–1595, 2008.

Special Populations

Inflammatory Bowel Disease

Ulcerative colitis and Crohn's disease account for 1% to 2% of CRC cases. To facilitate early detection and intervention, surveillance colonoscopy in patients with inflammatory bowel disease (IBD) has been shown to decrease mortality.[33-35] Risk factors for the development of CRC in the IBD population include disease duration and extent.[36] Particularly among ulcerative colitis patients, there is a noted increased risk of CRC in those who develop primary sclerosing cholangitis (PSC). In a study of 132 ulcerative colitis patients with primary sclerosing cholangitis, 25% developed CRC compared with 5.6% of controls.[37] These patients are more likely to develop advanced-stage proximal CRC.

For dysplasia screening in the IBD patient population, colonoscopies are generally performed every 1 to 2 years either after 8 years of disease in patients with pancolitis or after 15 years in those with left-sided colitis. During surveillance, biopsies should be taken every 10 cm in all four quadrants and in areas of stricture.[38]

Hereditary Colon Cancers

Hereditary colon cancers represent 20% of all CRC. Persons included in this category include those with familial adenomatous polyposis, hereditary nonpolyposis colorectal cancer (HNPCC)/ Lynch syndrome, and Peutz-Jeghers syndrome. CRC detection and incidence are discussed in Chapter 3.

New Directions

Endoscopic examination of the gastrointestinal tract has undergone a tremendous evolution through the centuries. Accelerated by the introduction of fiber optics, endoscopy is now a vital component to everyday health care.

As with any technology, the pursuit of advancement and refinement remains. The future of endoscopic evaluation of the colon lies within the incorporation of chromoendoscopy and the use of magnification/microscopy to further increase lesion detection rates. Chromoendoscopy involves spraying a biocompatible dye, such as 0.2% indigo carmine, to the epithelial surface of the gastrointestinal tract. This enables the endoscopist to view the fine details of the mucosa as well as a more defined shape and border of a potential lesion. Further enhancement occurs when combined with microscopy to magnification ×100. Chromoendoscopy may become increasingly important with the findings by Soetikno and associates[39] of a 6% to 15% incidence of nonpolypoid colorectal neoplasms in asymptomatic adults. These neoplasms are difficult to detect on routine colonoscopy; however, they are associated with a higher likelihood to contain cancer (odds ratio 9.78).

A study comparing conventional colonoscopy, chromoendoscopy, and chromoendoscopy with magnification has been conducted. This study included 122 patients with 206 lesions (10 mm or less; 22% non-neoplastic, 78% neoplastic by histology). Conventional colonoscopy detected 84% of these lesions, whereas chromoendoscopy and chromoendoscopy with magnification detected 89.3% and 95.6% of lesions, respectively.[40]

Originally devised by Kudo and associates,[41] the pit pattern classification system serves as a means of interpreting findings on chromoendoscopic/microscopic examination. This system has five major subtypes: (I) normal round pit, (II) cross- or star-shaped pit, (III) tubular pit, (IV) branched or gyrus-like pit, and (V) irregular pit. Subtypes I and II are typically nonneoplastic whereas subtypes III, IV, and V are associated with neoplasia.[42,43]

The chromoendoscopic technique, in combination with microscopy, is noted to be especially helpful in patients with ulcerative colitis.[44] Since current surveillance guidelines for patients with IBD require multiple random biopsies, staining and microscopy may allow streamlining of current techniques while potentially improving the detection of lesions. Although of obvious benefit, the incorporation of these two techniques may meet obstacles, mainly because of the labor-intensive nature of this form of examination and because of the additional costs. These challenges are in the setting of an already high endoscopic demand.

Conclusion

As one of the leading health threats to American lives, CRC has garnered much attention within the realm of public health. Similar to other screening programs, such as those for breast and cervical cancer, CRC screening and surveillance have great potential for decreasing morbidity and mortality. Impediments to program success include the invasive nature of endoscopic studies, lack of knowledge of appropriate screening guidelines, and limited manpower and resources to ensure full public participation. Through the proactivity of physicians and patients, great strides can be made in the early detection and treatment of CRC. Flexible sigmoidoscopy and colonoscopy are two major tools that can facilitate this process. The continual refinement of current techniques, as well as the incorporation of new technologies, will ultimately lead to further evolution of guidelines and recommendations.

References

1. Engel RM: Philipp Bozzini—The father of endoscopy. J Endourol 17(10):859–862, 2003.
2. Kelly HA: A new method of examination and treatment of disease of the rectum and sigmoid flexure. Ann Surg 21: 468–478, 1895.
3. Kapany N: Fiber Optics. Principles and Applications. New York: Academic Press, 1967.
4. Hirschowitz BI, Curtiss LE, Peters CW, Pollard HM: Demonstration of a new gastroscope, the "fiberscope." Gastroenterology 35:50–53, 1958.
5. Wolff WI, Shinya H: Polypectomy via the fiberoptic colonoscope. N Engl J Med 288:329–332, 1973.
6. Edmonson JM: Focus on ... fiberoptic colonoscope. Gastrointest Endosc 52(3):17A–20A, 2000.
7. Seeff LC, Richards TB, Shapiro JA, et al: How many endoscopies are performed for colorectal cancer screening? Results from CDC's survey of endoscopic capacity. Gastroenterology 127(6): 1670–1677, 2004.
8. Atkin W, Rogers P, Cardwell C, et al: Wide variation in adenoma detection rates at screening flexible sigmoidoscopy. Gastroenterology 126:1247–1256, 2004.
9. Winawer SJ, Zauber AG, Ho MN, et al: Prevention of colorectal cancer by colonoscopic polypectomy. The National Polyp Study Workgroup. N Engl J Med 329(27):1977–1981, 1993.
10. Rubio CA, Jaramillo E, Lindblom A, Fogt F: Classification of colorectal polyps: guidelines for the endoscopist. Endoscopy 34(3):226–236, 2002.
11. Colucci PM, Yale SH, Rall CJ: Colorectal polyps. Clin Med Res 1(3):261–262, 2003.
12. Saitoh Y, Waxman I, West AB, et al: Prevalence and distinctive biologic features of flat colorectal adenomas in a North American population. Gastroenterology 120(7):1657–1665, 2001.
13. Hurlstone DP, Fujii T, Lobo AJ: Early detection of colorectal cancer using high-magnification chromoscopic colonoscopy. Br J Surg 89(3):272–282, 2002.
14. Rembacken BJ, Fujii T, Cairns A, et al: Flat and depressed colonic neoplasms: a prospective study of 1000 colonoscopies in the UK. Lancet 355(9211):1211–1214, 2000.
15. Patel K, Hoffman NE: The anatomical distribution of colorectal polyps at colonoscopy. J Clin Gastroenterol 33(3):222–225, 2001.
16. Lieberman DA, Weiss DG; Veterans Affairs Cooperative Study Group 380: One-time screening for colorectal cancer with combined fecal occult-blood testing and examination of the distal colon. N Engl J Med 345(8):555–560, 2001.
17. Selby JV, Friedman GD, Quesenberry CP Jr, Weiss NS: A case-control study of screening sigmoidoscopy and mortality from colorectal cancer. N Engl J Med 326(10):653–657, 1992.
18. Muller AD, Sonnenberg A: Prevention of colorectal cancer by flexible endoscopy and polypectomy. A case-control study of 32,702 veterans. Ann Intern Med 123(12):904–910, 1995.
19. Newcomb PA, Storer BE, Morimoto LM, et al: Long-term efficacy of sigmoidoscopy in the reduction of colorectal cancer incidence. J Natl Cancer Inst 95(8):622–625, 2003.
20. Levin B, Lieberman DA, McFarland B, et al: Screening and surveillance for the early detection of colorectal cancer and adenomatous polyps, 2008: a joint guideline from the American Cancer Society, the US Multi-Society Task Force on Colorectal Cancer, and the American College of Radiology. Gastroenterology 134:1570–1595, 2008.
21. Imperiale TF, Wagner DR, Lin CY, et al: Risk of advanced proximal neoplasms in asymptomatic adults according to the distal colorectal findings. N Engl J Med 343(3):169–174, 2000.
22. Rubio CA, Jaramillo E, Lindblom A, Fogt F: Classification of colorectal polyps: guidelines for the endoscopist. Endoscopy 34(3):226–236, 2002.
23. Pignone M, Rich M, Teutsch S, et al: Screening for colorectal cancer in adults at average risk: a summary of the evidence for the U.S. Preventive Services Task Force. Ann Intern Med 137:132–141, 2002.
24. Rex DK, Chak A, Vasudeva R, et al: Prospective determination of distal colon findings in average-risk patients with proximal colon cancer. Gastrointest Endosc 49(6):727–730, 1999.
25. Rex DK, Cutler CS, Lemmel GT, et al: Colonoscopic miss rates of adenomas determined by back-to-back colonoscopies. Gastroenterology 112(1):24–28, 1997.
26. Pickhardt PJ, Choi JR, Hwang I, et al: Computed tomographic virtual colonoscopy to screen for colorectal neoplasia in asymptomatic adults. N Engl J Med 349(23):2191–2200, 2003.
27. Rex DK, Bond JH, Winawer S, et al; U.S. Multi-Society Task Force on Colorectal Cancer: Quality in the technical performance of colonoscopy and the continuous quality improvement process for colonoscopy: recommendations of the U.S. Multi-Society Task Force on Colorectal Cancer. Am J Gastroenterol 97(6):1296–1308, 2002.
28. Barclay RL, Vicari JJ, Doughty AS, et al: Colonoscopic withdrawal times and adenoma detection during screening colonoscopy. N Engl J Med 355(24):2533–2541, 2006.
29. Winawer SJ, Fletcher RH, Miller L, et al: Colorectal cancer screening: clinical guidelines and rationale. Gastroenterology 112(2):594–642, 1997.
30. Winawer S, Fletcher R, Rex D, et al; Gastrointestinal Consortium Panel: Colorectal cancer screening and surveillance: clinical guidelines and rationale—update based on new evidence. Gastroenterology 124(2):544–560, 2003.

31. Winawer SJ, Zauber AG, Fletcher RH, et al: Guidelines for colonoscopy surveillance after polypectomy: a consensus update by the US Multi-Society Task Force on Colorectal Cancer and the American Cancer Society. CA Cancer J Clin 56(3):143–159, 2006.
32. Jemal A, Thomas A, Murray T, Thun M: Cancer statistics 2002. CA Cancer J Clin 52:32–47, 2002.
33. Choi PM, Nugent FW, Schoetz DJ Jr, et al: Colonoscopic surveillance reduces mortality from colorectal cancer in ulcerative colitis. Gastroenterology 105(2):418–424, 1993.
34. Provenzale D, Onken J: Surveillance issues in inflammatory bowel disease: ulcerative colitis. J Clin Gastroenterol 32(2): 99–105, 2001.
35. Collins PD, Mpofu C, Watson AJ, Rhodes JM: Strategies for detecting colon cancer and/or dysplasia in patients with inflammatory bowel disease. Cochrane Database Syst Rev 19(2), 2006, CD000279.
36. Bansal P, Sonnenberg A: Risk factors for colorectal cancer in inflammatory bowel disease. Am J Gastroenterol 91:44–48, 1996.
37. Shetty K, Rybicki L, Brzezinski A, et al: The risk for cancer or dysplasia in ulcerative colitis patients with primary sclerosing cholangitis. Am J Gastroenterol 94(6):1643–1649, 1999.
38. Rubin DT, Kavitt RT: Surveillance for cancer and dysplasia in inflammatory bowel disease. Gastroenterol Clin North Am 35(3):581–604, 2006.
39. Soetikno R, Kaltenbach T, Rouse R, et al: Prevalence of nonpolypoid (flat and depressed) colorectal neoplasms in asymptomatic and symptomatic adults. JAMA 299:1027–1035, 2008.
40. Fu KI, Sano Y, Kato S, et al: Chromoendoscopy using indigo carmine dye spraying with magnifying observation is the most reliable method for differential diagnosis between non-neoplastic and neoplastic colorectal lesions: a prospective study. Endoscopy 36(12):1089–1093, 2004.
41. Kudo S, Hirota S, Nakajima T, et al: Colorectal tumours and pit pattern. J Clin Pathol 47(10):880–885, 1994.
42. Kudo S, Tamura S, Nakajima T, et al: Diagnosis of colorectal tumorous lesions by magnifying endoscopy. Gastrointest Endosc 44(1):8–14, 1996.
43. Kudo S, Rubio CA, Teixeira CR, et al: Pit pattern in colorectal neoplasia: endoscopic magnifying view. Endoscopy 33(4): 367–373, 2001.
44. Kiesslich R, Goetz M, Lammersdorf K, et al: Chromoscopy-guided endomicroscopy increases the diagnostic yield of intraepithelial neoplasia in ulcerative colitis. Gastroenterology 132(3):874–882, 2007.

9 Stool and Blood Sampling for Early Detection of Colorectal Cancer

Jason K. Sicklick and Nita Ahuja

KEY POINTS

- Screening methods have been applied for the detection of premalignant colonic polyps and the early diagnosis of colorectal tumors.
- Current recommendation for the screening of sporadic colorectal cancer consists of noninvasive and invasive measures that should begin at age 50 years.
- The majority of colorectal tumors result from sporadic genetic mutations, but 10% to 25% of tumors are considered hereditary.
- Sporadic colorectal cancers contain a multitude of genetic abnormalities acquired during the progression of normal mucosa to adenocarcinoma.
- There is little evidence, at present, to suggest that blood genetic markers may be used for screening for sporadic colorectal cancers or premalignant lesions, whereas there is clear evidence for their usefulness in patients with hereditary nonpolyposis colorectal cancer (HNPCC) and familial adenomatous polyposis (FAP).
- Stool screening is based on the evaluation of stool specimens for the presence of exfoliated DNA from tumors.
- Fecal DNA testing for genetic mutations and epigenetic alterations may provide the potential to improve colorectal cancer screening in a noninvasive manner.
- Currently, genetic screening methods are expensive and labor-intensive and require the corroboration of additional larger studies.

Introduction

Colorectal cancer is the third most common malignancy in the United States and the third leading cause of cancer deaths amongst all men and women.[1] Overall, colorectal cancer has an incidence of 61.3 in 100,000 men and 44.9 in 100,000 women. The lifetime risk for an individual to develop colorectal cancer in the United States is approximately 6%. In an attempt to decrease the incidence of cancer diagnoses and its complications and cancer-related deaths, new methods of genetic screening are being investigated for the detection of premalignant colonic lesions as well as for earlier diagnosis of colorectal tumors.

The current recommendation for the screening of sporadic colorectal cancer consists of noninvasive and invasive measures that should begin at age 50. Screening options are outlined in Box 9-1.[2] In general, annual fecal occult blood test (FOBT) in combination with sigmoidoscopy every 5 years is the most common method for screening. In addition, to assess the entire length of colon and rectum, colonoscopic evaluation should be performed every 10 years. Despite evidence that annual FOBT screening has resulted in a reduction of cancer-related deaths from colorectal cancer over a decade, no studies have proved a concurrent reduction in the incidence of cancer. This is primarily due to the lack of sensitivity of these tests for detecting many dysplastic adenomas and early-stage tumors.[3-5]

Most recently, consensus guidelines were released by the American Cancer Society, the American College of Radiology, and the U.S. Multi-Society Task Force on Colorectal Cancer (a group made up of representatives from the American College of Gastroenterology, the American Gastroenterological Association, and the American Society for Gastrointestinal Endoscopy). Computed tomography (CT) colonography is now included as one of several options for colorectal cancer screening every 5 years in average-risk adults, beginning at age 50.[6] Moreover, the consensus group now recommends fecal immunochemical testing (FIT) and stool DNA testing (sDNA) as tests that

---

Box 9-1. Current Adenomatous Polyp and Colorectal Cancer Screening Options Beginning at Age 50

Adenomatous Polyp and Colorectal Cancer Screening Options

Flexible sigmoidoscopy every 5 years

or

Double-contrast barium enema every 5 years

or

CT colonography (CTC, also known as virtual colonoscopy), every 5 years

or

Colonoscopy every 10 years (should also be performed if any of the above tests are positive)

Colorectal Cancer Detection Options

Fecal occult blood test (FOBT) every year

Fecal immunochemical test (FIT) every year

Stool DNA test (sDNA), interval uncertain

Data from Smith RA, Cokkinides V, Eyre HJ: American Cancer Society guidelines for the early detection of cancer, 2006. CA Cancer J Clin. 56(1):11–25; quiz 49–50, 2006; and Levin B, Lieberman DA, McFarland B, et al: Screening and surveillance for the early detection of colorectal cancer and adenomatous polyps, 2008: a joint guideline from the American Cancer Society, the US Multi-Society Task Force on Colorectal Cancer, and the American College of Radiology. Gastroenterology 134(5):1570–1595, 2008.

---

primarily detect cancer.[6] In addition to the aforementioned modalities, genetic screening has been applied to patients with a strong history of colorectal cancer.

Over the past two decades, numerous advances have been made in our understanding of the genetic and epigenetic events that lead to colorectal cancers. Although most colorectal tumors (65% to 85%) result from sporadic genetic mutations, 10% to 25% of tumors are considered hereditary. The latter includes about 1% to 3% of patients with hereditary nonpolyposis colon cancer (HNPCC, or Lynch syndrome) and 0.5% with familial adenomatous polyposis (FAP). HNPCC primarily results from germline autosomal dominant gene mutations, truncations, and frameshifts in the DNA mismatch repair genes, *MLH1* and *MSH2*. After the discovery of these two genes, mutations in *MSH6* and *PMS2* were also linked to HNPCC.[7] According to the current InSiGHT (International Society for Gastrointestinal Hereditary Tumors) database maintained by the International Collaborative Group on Hereditary Nonpolyposis Colorectal Cancer (ICG-HNPCC), approximately 500 unique HNPCC-associated mismatch repair gene mutations have been iden-

tified. Of these, approximately 50% involve *MLH1*, approximately 40% involve *MSH2*, and approximately 10% involve *MSH6*. In addition, *PMS2* mutations are associated with diverse clinical features of HNPCC, including those of Turcot syndrome.

FAP results from germline autosomal dominant mutations in the adenomatous polyposis colic (*APC*) gene, a tumor suppressor gene, in the Wnt signaling pathway. Inheritance of one or more than 400 known *APC* mutations carries a 100% lifetime risk of colorectal cancer. In the case of these two hereditary syndromes, as well as with patients with first-degree relative who had colorectal cancer, screening with sigmoidoscopy or colonoscopy as frequently as every 1 to 2 years is a medical necessity. Although these forms of screening have the potential to detect colorectal cancers at early stages, their sensitivity and specificity are not 100%, and there are clearly risks (colonic perforation and hemorrhage) from these invasive procedures. Moreover, compliance with screening is at most 50%.[8] Better and noninvasive assays may improve the accuracy, safety, affordability, and patient compliance rates of screening for colorectal cancers.

Numerous advances also have been made in identifying genetic factors that are responsible for the progression of sporadic colon cancers. This process is thought to be caused by the accumulation of alterations in DNA, resulting in changes to gene function (i.e., apoptosis resistance, aberrant cellular proliferation, and chromosomal or microsatellite instability), gene mutation or loss of heterozygosity, epigenetic alterations such as DNA methylation and histone changes, as well as over- and underexpression of oncogenes and tumor suppressor genes, respectively.[9-11] These genetic and epigenetic alterations lead to the gradual progression of colorectal cancer starting from normal colonic mucosa to metastatic disease through the stages of hyperplastic epithelium, low-grade dysplastic adenomas, high-grade dysplastic adenomas, adenocarcinoma in situ, and invasive adenocarcinoma.[12,13] Numerous genes have been identified in this process, and many of the key genes are listed in Table 9-1.

In recent years, researchers have not only used this knowledge to develop new chemotherapeutic agents to treat cancers but also have started to evaluate the usefulness of studying

Table 9-1. Genes Involved in the Progression of Colorectal Cancer

Gene	Name	Function	Alteration	From	To	References
					Epithelium	
APC	Adenomatous polyposis coli		Mutation, LOH DNA methylation	Normal	Hyperproliferative	38
Bat-26			Microsatellite instability	Normal	Hyperproliferative	19, 39–43
BRCA1	Breast cancer type 1, early onset		Mutation, LOH, DNA methylation	Normal	Hyperproliferative	44, 45
CDKN2A(p16) INK4, Mts1	Cyclin dependent kinase 2		DNA methylation	Normal	Hyperproliferative	23, 34, 46–48
Survivin		Inhibitor of apoptosis	Overexpression	Normal	Hyperproliferative	49–51
Bcl-2	B-cell lymphoma protein 2		Overexpression	Normal	Hyperproliferative	50, 52, 53
Nos-2	Nitric oxide synthase 2		Overexpression	Normal	Hyperproliferative	54, 55
Nf-κB	Nuclear factor kappa B		Overexpression	Normal	Hyperproliferative	56–58
Thioredoxin		Antioxidants	Overexpression	Normal	Hyperproliferative	59
C-Myc	MC29 avian myelocytomatosis virus	Proto-oncogene	Overexpression	Normal	Hyperproliferative	60–63
Terminal GalNAc	N-acetyl galactosamine		Underexpression	Normal	Hyperproliferative	
ER, Esr1	Estrogen receptor alpha 1		DNA methylation	Normal	Hyperproliferative	31, 64, 65
HIC1	Hypermethylated in cancer 1	Candidate tumor suppressor gene	DNA methylation	Normal	Hyperproliferative	29, 66
HPP1, Tenb2, Tpef	Hyperplastic polyposis protein 1, tomoregulin, transmembrane protein with epidermal growth factor-like and two follistatin-like domains 2		DNA methylation	Normal	Adenoma	67, 68

Continued

Table 9-1. Genes Involved in the Progression of Colorectal Cancer—cont'd

				Epithelium		
Gene	Name	Function	Alteration	From	To	References
K-Ras	GTPase Kras, Ki-ras		Mutation, LOH	Normal	Adenoma	42, 54, 69–74
Amacr	Alpha-methylacyl-CoA racemase		Overexpression	Normal	Adenoma	75–78
MLH1	MLH1 DNA mismatch repair protein		DNA methylation, mutations, truncations, frameshifts	Normal	Adenoma	12, 25, 79–82
SFRPs	Secreted frizzled-related proteins		DNA methylation, Underexpression	Normal	Adenocarcinoma	26, 27, 30, 83–85
Dcc	Deleted in colon cancer		Underexpression	Low-grade adenoma	High-grade adenoma	86–88
Telomerase	Telomerase		Overexpression	Low-grade adenoma	High-grade adenoma	12, 89, 90
p53	Tumor protein 53	Tumor suppressor gene	Mutation, LOH	High-grade adenoma	Adenocarcinoma	91–96
Src, c-src	pp60^c-src	Proto-oncogene	Overexpression	High-grade adenoma	Adenocarcinoma	97, 98
Ki-67	Antigen Ki-67		Overexpression	High-grade adenoma	Adenocarcinoma	52, 99, 100
MSH2	MSH2 DNA mismatch repair protein		Mutations, truncations, frameshifts			81, 101–103
MSH6	MSH6 DNA mismatch repair protein		Mutations			7, 104–106
PMS22	PMS2 DNA mismatch repair protein		Mutations			7, 107–109
MGMT	O-6-methylguanine-DNA methyltransferase		DNA methylation			24, 34, 110–112
MCC	Mutated in colorectal cancer	Cell differentiation	Mutation			13, 113, 114

LOH, loss of heterozygosity.

Box 9-2. Advantages and Disadvantages of Blood/Stool Screening for Colorectal Cancer Gene Mutations

Advantages	Disadvantages
Biologic rationale	New technology with only preliminary evidence to support
Potentially higher detection sensitivity for earlier-stage disease	Assays are labor-intensive
Less reliance on endoscopist experience and subjectivity	Currently expensive and therefore not cost-effective
No requirement for bowel preparations	Assays must be more streamlined for large-scale application
Potential application to screening for other cancers	

Data from Ahlquist DA: Molecular stool screening for colorectal cancer. Using DNA markers may be beneficial, but large scale evaluation is needed. Br Med J 321(7256):254–255, 2000.

---

these genes as markers of colorectal tumors with the aim of improving screening outcomes. Many current blood tumor markers, such as carcinoembryonic antigen (CEA), rely on the release of specific proteins into plasma, but these markers have not proved to be useful screening tools but rather are markers for disease recurrence or progression.[14]

Screening for genetic mutations via stool or blood specimens appears to have several advantages over current FOBT and endoscopic screening methods, as outlined in Box 9-2. The most obvious advantages include a clearer biologic rationale, potentially higher sensitivities for detecting disease at earlier stages, and less reliance on endoscopist experience/subjectivity for evaluating colorectal lesions. Alternatively, these screening methods are expensive and labor-intensive and require additional studies to confirm their validity. In the following sections, we detail some of the research in this growing field.

Screening Blood

According to the World Health Organization, more than 940,000 new cases of colorectal cancer are reported annually throughout the world. Of these, 10% to 25% (i.e., 94,000–235,000 cases) are considered hereditary, including FAP and HNPCC, in which there are clear links between hereditable gene mutations and disease. In these two heritable diseases, mutational screening has clear validity. However, for sporadic colorectal cancers and premalignant lesions, mutational screening of blood has not been well studied. This is because these mutations occur in the bowel and are not passed through the germline.

To begin developing a potential blood-screening method for sporadic colorectal cancers, one group has studied frequent APC and p53 gene mutations in the plasma of 240 colonoscopy patients with colorectal cancer or adenomas.[15] In their study, three plasma p53 mutations were identified. Two patients in the study had adenomas at biopsy, whereas one had a hyperplastic polyp. Despite identifying p53 mutations in the plasma, only one (33%) of the adenomas/polyps was positive for the mutation. In the study, only eight tumor specimens were analyzed for concordance with plasma results. One of eight (12.5%) tumors had a 5-base-pair APC gene deletion in the cancer, which was also detectable in that patient's plasma. Based on this small study, APC gene mutations were detectable in the plasma of a colorectal cancer patient, whereas p53 mutations were detectable in the plasma of adenoma patients. Despite these facts, at present limited data suggest that mutational screening of blood is reliable enough for widespread screening.

Proteomics and nuclear matrix proteins in the blood have also been explored. These limited studies require significantly more evaluation before potential clinical application can be considered.[8] Based on a lack of clear evidence, the 2006 American Society of Clinical Oncology recommendation for the use of blood tumor marker tests in the screening and surveillance of colorectal cancers states that data are insufficient to recommend the routine analysis of p53, K-ras, microsatellite instability, deleted in colon cancer (DCC), or other genes in the management of patients with colorectal cancer.[14] Current recommendations stipulate only that CEA be ordered preoperatively if it is to assist in staging and surgical planning, whereas postoperative CEA levels should be monitored every 3 months for at least 3 years for patients with stages II and III disease. The CEA blood marker may be used as a marker for monitoring the disease response, but there is no evidence from large study populations to suggest that malignant and premalignant DNA alterations in the colon are identifiable in the blood and may be used for the management of patients.[16]

Screening Stool

Unlike screening blood for inherited genetic mutations that predispose or lead to cancer, screening stool does not rely on heritability. Instead, it is based on the evaluation of stool specimens for exfoliated DNA from tumors. Because most colorectal cancers are sporadic, they may contain a multitude of genetic and epigenetic abnormalities acquired during the progression of normal mucosa to adenocarcinoma. Since these genetic, as well as epigenetic, alterations to the tumor DNA may not be found in the germline DNA of these patients, screening stool for such alterations appears compelling for identifying cancers. Table 9-2 outlines the biologic rationale for stool screening for colorectal cancer gene mutations and epigenetic alterations.

Despite the logic of this approach, targeting genetic alterations such as mutations for widespread screening is not sensitive enough for detecting cancer because no universal mutation and/or epigenetic alteration is common to all colorectal tumors. Rather, they are genetically heterogeneous, as seen in Table 9-1. For example, mutant *K-ras* is detected in less than 50% of colorectal neoplasms.[17,18] Thus, multiple DNA alterations must be selected as targets to obtain a high rate of detection. Furthermore, each marker within the assay must be specific enough to the neoplasm to prevent false-positive results.

Data from pilot projects suggest that the diagnostic yield improves when a stool assay with multiple targets is directed at a spectrum of DNA alterations commonly expressed by cancers.[19–21] In a blinded pilot study by Ahlquist and colleagues[19] published in 2000, they investigated 15 mutational "hot spots" on genes, including *K-ras*, *p53*, *APC*, and *Bat-26*.[19] DNA alterations were detected in 91% of patients ($n = 22$) with colorectal cancers, 82% of patients ($n = 11$) with adenomas larger than 1 cm, and 7% of controls ($n = 28$) who had had normal colonoscopies. (See Table 9-3 for selected series.).

A subsequent study by Dong and colleagues[21] in 2001 evaluated stool DNA isolated from 51

Table 9-2. Biologic Rationale for Stool Screening for Colorectal Cancer Gene Mutations and Epigenetic Alterations

Rationale	Note
Tumor DNA is continuously released into the fecal stream via exfoliation	As opposed to intermittent bleeding detected by FOBT, this could enhance screening sensitivity, obviating the need for multiple FOBT during each screening
DNA is derived directly from the neoplasm	May improve specificity
Colonic cell exfoliation from cancers is quantitatively higher than from normal mucosa[116,117]	
Genetic alterations in colorectal neoplasia are targets for assay development[118]	See Table 9-1.
DNA is stable during fecal transit and storage	In contrast, RNA is unstable and easily degradable which limits the ability to study the dysregulation of gene expression
Bowel preparation and its associated complications, including noncompliance and dehydration, would probably be unnecessary	
Sensitive techniques including polymerase chain reaction require only minute quantities of DNA for detection of mutations	

FOBT, fecal occult blood test.
Data from references 115 through 118.

Table 9-3. Sensitivity and Specificity of Selected Studies Using Stool DNA for Screening of Colorectal Adenomas and Cancers

Study	Number of Patients	Markers Used	Sensitivity (%)	Specificity (%)
Ahlquist et al (2000)[116]	33 adenomas/cancers 28 controls	Exact multitarget assay (K-Ras, p53, APC, Bat-26, L-DNA)	88	93
Dong et al (2001)[21]	51 cancers 0 controls	K-ras, p53, Bat-26	71	NR
Rengucci et al (2001)[119]	46 cancers 18 controls	K-ras, p53, microsatellite instability (MSI)	26	100
Tagore et al (2003)[120]	80 adenomas/cancers 212 controls	Exact multitarget assay (K-ras, p53, APC, Bat-26, L-DNA)	62	96
Calistri et al (2003)[121]	53 cancers 38 controls	K-ras, p53, APC, L-DNA, MSI	62	97
Imperiale et al (2004)[20]	2507 patients 31 cancers	Exact multitarget assay (K-ras, p53, APC, Bat-26, L-DNA)	52	95*
Syngal et al (2007)[122]	91 adenomas/cancers 0 controls	Exact multitarget assay (K-ras, p53, APC, Bat-26, L-DNA)	54	NR
Muller et al (2004)[30]	23 cancers 26 controls	Sfrp2 methylation	83	77
Lenhard et al (2005)[29]	39 adenomas/cancers 50 controls	HIC1 methylation	38	100
Itzkowitz et al (2007)[32]	40 cancers 122 controls	Exact multitarget assay (K-ras, p53, APC, Bat-26, L-DNA), and vimentin and Htlf methylation	87.5	82*

NR, not reported.
*Multicenter prospective trial.

patients with confirmed colorectal tumors. Three of the target genes previously evaluated were studied. These included *K-ras, p53,* and *Bat-26.* In this study, *p53* gene mutations were detected in the tumor DNA of 59% of patients. Tumors from 5.9% of patients had noninherited deletions at the *Bat-26* locus. The same alterations were also found in the respective patients' stool samples. Thirty-seven percent of the tumors had *K-ras* mutations in their tissue. Among the patients with *K-ras* mutations, 42% (8 of 19) had the identical mutation seen in the paired-stool DNA. Attesting to the specificity of the assays, no stool specimens contained DNA mutations not found in the primary tumors. Together, these markers detected 71% (36 of 51; 95% confidence interval [CI]: 56% to 83%) of all patients with colorectal cancers. In addition, the markers identified 36 of all 39 patients who had one of the genetic alterations with an overall sensitivity of 92% (95% CI: 79% to 98%). Both of these studies focused on evaluating patients with known disease. Given that the specificity of assays for detecting colorectal neoplasia in asymptomatic patients is unknown and

the true prevalence of the mutations is uncertain, there is clearly a need for more studies to evaluate the usefulness of these tests in the general population.

In 2004, Imperiale and colleagues[20] studied fecal DNA analysis compared with FOBT for colorectal cancer screening in the average-risk population over 50 years of age. In this study of 5486 subjects, stool specimens were obtained for DNA analysis, and patients underwent both FOBT and colonoscopy. Ultimately, 4404 subjects completed the study, and a subgroup of 2507 subjects was analyzed. This subgroup included all patients diagnosed with a colorectal tumor or advanced adenoma in addition to randomly selected subjects with minor polyps or without evidence of disease. The fecal DNA panel evaluated specimens for 21 mutations. In this study, the expanded fecal DNA panel detected 51.6% of 31 invasive cancers, whereas FOBT identified 12.9% (P = .003). The DNA panel also detected 40.8% of 71 invasive cancers plus adenomas with high-grade dysplasia, whereas FOBT identified 14.1% (P < .001). Among the 418 subjects with advanced neoplasia, which the authors defined as a tubular adenoma at least 1 cm in diameter, a polyp with a villous histologic appearance, a polyp with high-grade dysplasia, or invasive cancer, the DNA panel was positive in 18.2% of cases, whereas FOBT was positive in 10.8%. The authors concluded that the multi-target analysis of fecal DNA detected a greater proportion of important colorectal neoplasia than did FOBT without compromising specificity. (See Fig. 9-1 for an example.)

In addition to genetic alterations such as direct gene mutations, epigenetic alterations such as DNA hypermethylation are widespread in colon and rectal cancers.[22] DNA methylation of promoter-associated CpG islands is an alternate mechanism to mutation in silencing gene function and affects tumor suppressor genes, as well as growth and differentiation controlling genes. Multiple genes have now been identified that are silenced in colorectal cancer, including CDKN2A(p16),[23] MGMT,[24] and MLH1.[25] More specifically, the hypermethylation of the 5′ CpG island of MLH1 is found in most sporadic primary colorectal cancers with microsatellite instability. This methylation was often (but not invariably) associated with loss of MLH1 protein expression. Therefore, microsatellite instability in sporadic colorectal cancer often results from epigenetic inactivation of MLH1 in association with DNA methylation.

Epigenetic inactivation of secreted frizzled-related protein (SFRP) genes allows constitutive Wnt signaling in colorectal cancer and is found in the majority of colorectal cancers.[26,27] Some of these DNA methylation changes begin in the normal colonic epithelium as a function of age and may lead to a field defect that predisposes to cancer. In fact, age-related methylation may involve at least 50% of the genes that are hypermethylated in colon cancer and thus may serve as a useful screening marker.[22,28]

The detection of methylation alterations in tumor-derived DNA within stool is a novel, but less studied, approach to screening for colon and rectal cancers. However, since epigenetic alterations may be more common, screening for epigenetic alterations rather than genetic mutations in stool is a promising emerging target. In one of the few studies to analyze this approach, Lenhard and colleagues[29] investigated the single epigenetic marker, hypermethylated in cancer 1 (HIC1) promoter, compared with FOBT for distinguishing the patients with cancers and adenomas from those without disease. In a blinded fashion, stool samples were obtained from 26 patients with cancers, 13 patients with adenomas greater than or equal to 1 cm, 9 patients with hyperplastic

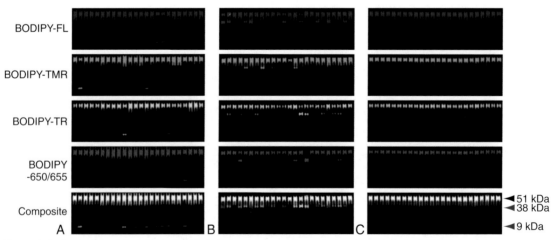

Figure 9-1. Examples of the multicolor digital protein truncation test conducted on fecal DNA samples.
A, Sample from a patient with an early-stage cancer. **B,** Sample from a patient with an adenoma. **C,** Sample from an individual free of colorectal neoplasia. The top four panels represent the individual signals for each fluorophore: BODIPY-FL, BODIPY-TMR, BODIPY-TR, and BODIPY-650/655. The bottom panel represents the composite of the four individual scans. A *black arrowhead* marks the full-length APC polypeptide, and *red arrowheads* mark the truncated mutant products. All the gels were scanned on a Typhoon 9410 instrument and the images analyzed using the ImageQuant software (both from Amersham Biosciences). (From Traverso G, Diehl F, Hurst R, et al: Multicolor in vitro translation. Nat Biotechnol 21[9]:1093–1037, 2003.)

polyps, 9 patients with inflammatory bowel disease, and 32 patients with endoscopically normal colons. Analysis of their samples demonstrated that 97% of the stool samples had amplifiable DNA. Of the patients analyzed, 42% of the samples from patients with tumors and 31% of the samples from patients with adenomas were positive for *HIC1* promoter methylation. None of the patients with endoscopically normal colons or hyperplastic polyps had aberrant *HIC1* promoter methylation.

In 2004, a study published in *Lancet* evaluated fecal DNA from patients with colorectal cancer compared with controls without cancer in order to determine the feasibility, sensitivity, and specificity of this approach.[30] The authors identified *SFRP2* methylation as a sensitive single DNA-based marker for the identification of colorectal cancer in stool samples. The sensitivity was 90% and specificity was 77% in a training set ($n = 23$). In follow-up independent testing, the sensitivity was 77% and specificity was 77% ($n = 26$). In another study, colorectal biopsies and fecal samples were obtained from 32 patients with adenomatous polyps or colorectal cancer, or no evidence disease.[31] An additional 18 fecal samples were obtained from healthy volunteers without bowel symptoms. Analysis was performed for CpG island methylation of *ER*, *HPP1*, *p16INK4a*, *APC*, *MLH1*, and *MGMT*. In this study, the levels of methylation at two CpG sites within *ER* significantly correlated with methylation in DNA from colorectal mucosa.

Most recently, Itzkowitz and colleagues[32] published the results of a prospective, multicenter trial that expands on earlier studies[33–35] by the same group. The latest study was conducted to determine the sensitivity and specificity of a second-generation assay (version 2) that used improved DNA stabilization/isolation techniques and evaluated a new promoter methylation marker.[35] In this study, 40 patients with colorectal cancer and 122 controls with normal colonoscopies provided stool samples to which DNA preservation buffer was added immediately. DNA was purified and analyzed for the original panel of 22 mutations, DNA integrity assay (DIA), which measures the susceptibility of DNA to denaturation in situ, and two promoter methylation markers, including *vimentin*. By using DNA that was optimally preserved and purified from stool, the sensitivity of the prototype version 1 assay increased from 52% to 72.5% because of enhanced DNA handling. The combination of *vimentin* gene methylation plus a DNA integrity assay resulted in 87.5% sensitivity and 82% specificity (Fig. 9-2). Moreover, cancers were detected regardless of the stage. Compared with the earlier version, this study demonstrated an improved fecal DNA test that incorporates two new markers and results in a higher sensitivity for colorectal cancers (see Imperiale and colleagues[20] for results of version 1 mentioned above).

In general, genetic mutations have a low sensitivity but high specificity. Thus, if a mutation is identified in a patient, it is likely to be

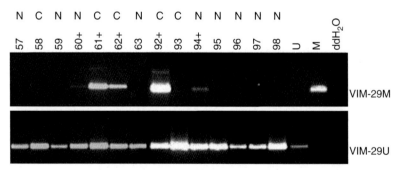

Figure 9-2. Fecal DNA test for colorectal cancer detection.   Detection of methylation of vimentin in fecal DNA from 9 normal (N) and 5 colon cancer (C) patients. The upper panel (VIM-29M) shows vimentin gene methylation, and the lower panel (VIM-29U) shows control wild-type amplification of unmethylated vimentin sequences derived from normal cells in all samples. Samples that have vimentin methylation are designated with a positive (+) sign next to patient sample number (60, 61, 62, 92, and 94). Assay controls include unmethylated (u) and methylated (m) DNA samples, and negative water blank (deionized water). (From Itzkowitz SH, Jandorf L, Brand R, et al: Improved fecal DNA test for colorectal cancer screening. Clin Gastroenterol Hepatol 5[1]:111–117, 2007.)

identified in the DNA. This suggests that the combination of more genetic and epigenetic markers might enhance the performance of these assays. However, mutational analysis is expensive. On the other hand, DNA methylation assays are easier to perform and are less expensive. However, all suffer from DNA degradation problems in the stool. Therefore, the solution may be a combination of genetic and epigenetic marks once optimal methods have been identified for collecting, storing, and transporting stool specimens. In addition, reliance on one stool sample may improve patient compliance, since FOBT requires multiple samples to improve the sensitivity of the assay.

Conclusion

Despite the low costs of FOBT, this test is well recognized to have high false-positive and false-negative rates, which lead to high-cost workups and missed colorectal cancer diagnoses when compared with endoscopic techniques. There is a need to develop reliable, specific molecular genetic tests for the noninvasive detection of premalignant colon lesions and colorectal cancers.[36,37]

Although the evidence for widespread screening for genetic mutations in sporadic tumors in the blood does not seem promising, fecal DNA testing for genetic mutations and epigenetic alterations appears to provide the potential to improve colorectal cancer screening in a noninvasive manner. Because of the heterogeneity of tumors, usually multiple markers distributed throughout the human genome need to be analyzed. This labor-intensive method does not allow for high-throughput screening. Therefore, markers with high sensitivity and good specificity are needed. Although many small trials of multiple target genetic assays demonstrate sensitivity for colorectal cancer of 62% to 91% and sensitivity for adenomas of 26% to 77%, the specificity of these assays is high, ranging from 93% to 100%. Thus, fecal DNA testing has shown greater sensitivity than guaiac-based occult blood tests for noninvasive colorectal cancer screening. Hypermethylation of cytosine residues in the CpG islands of tumor suppressor genes is also a key mechanism of colorectal carcinogenesis. Detection and quantification of CpG island methylation in human DNA isolated from stools may provide a novel strategy for the detection and investigation of colorectal neoplasia. Whether a combination of genetic and epigenetic markers will identify colorectal cancer at an early stage remains to be shown. However, early data also suggest that these results may be improved by additional analyses of gene promoter hypermethylation.[38]

The American Cancer Society, the American College of Radiology, and the U.S. Multi-Society Task Force on Colorectal Cancer now include the application of annual fecal immunohistochemical testing (FIT) and stool DNA testing (sDNA) of uncertain interval as adjuncts for detecting colorectal cancers given their high sensitivities for detecting malignancies. These may be performed in lieu of FOBT according to the recent recommendations, as shown in Box 9-1.[2,6] For FIT, the assay should be performed in a similar fashion to that of FOBT as a take-home multiple sample method. Like FOBT, the FIT assay looks for blood in the stool and should be followed up with additional investigations if positive. FIT and sDNA may offer improved sensitivity and specificity, but at an increased cost.[8]

In the meantime, the ACS Advisory Group has concluded that DNA stool testing remains an emerging technology. The best combination of markers remains unknown, and the results of studies in populations with an average risk of colorectal cancer are required before DNA stool testing can be recommended as a test for average-risk populations. Other groups have suggested using stool markers for screening of colorectal cancers to high-risk groups initially.[37] Another possibility is to use these stool screening tests for interval screening between colonoscopies; that is, if a colonoscopy is negative, then a repeat colonoscopy would be done in 10 years and such patients could get a stool DNA test at 5 years. Despite these facts, the major barrier to these assays is the cost. It remains unclear whether the added sensitivity merits the additional cost incurred from these sophisticated tests. Clearly, larger studies are needed to corroborate these early outcomes, including screening studies of larger cohorts of asymptomatic patients to reach conclusions regarding the future of these novel forms of colorectal cancer screening.

References

1. U.S. Cancer Statistics Working Group: United States Cancer Statistics: 2002 Incidence and Mortality. Atlanta: U.S. Depart-

ment of Health and Human Services, Centers for Disease Control and Prevention and National Cancer Institute, 2005.

2. Smith RA, Cokkinides V, Eyre HJ: American Cancer Society guidelines for the early detection of cancer, 2006. CA Cancer J Clin 56(1):11–25; quiz 49–50, 2006.

3. Mandel JS, Bond JH, Church TR, et al: Reducing mortality from colorectal cancer by screening for fecal occult blood. Minnesota Colon Cancer Control Study. N Engl J Med 328(19):1365–1371, 1993.

4. Hardcastle JD, Chamberlain JO, Robinson MH, et al: Randomised controlled trial of faecal-occult-blood screening for colorectal cancer. Lancet 348(9040):1472–1477, 1996.

5. Kronborg O, Fenger C, Olsen J, et al: Randomised study of screening for colorectal cancer with faecal-occult-blood test. Lancet 348(9040):1467–1471, 1996.

6. Levin B, Lieberman DA, McFarland B, et al: Screening and surveillance for the early detection of colorectal cancer and adenomatous polyps, 2008: a joint guideline from the American Cancer Society, the US Multi-Society Task Force on Colorectal Cancer, and the American College of Radiology. Gastroenterology 134(5):1570–1595, 2008.

7. Peltomaki P: Lynch syndrome genes. Fam Cancer 4(3):227–232, 2005.

8. Ouyang DL, Chen JJ, Getzenberg RH, Schoen RE: Noninvasive testing for colorectal cancer: a review. Am J Gastroenterol 100(6):1393–1403, 2005.

9. Papadopoulos N, Kinzler KW, Vogelstein B: The role of companion diagnostics in the development and use of mutation-targeted cancer therapies. Nat Biotechnol 24(8):985–995, 2006.

10. Vogelstein B, Kinzler KW: Cancer genes and the pathways they control. Nat Med 10(8):789–799, 2004.

11. Herman JG, Baylin SB: Gene silencing in cancer in association with promoter hypermethylation. N Engl J Med 349(21):2042–2054, 2003.

12. Gryfe R, Swallow C, Bapat B, et al: Molecular biology of colorectal cancer. Curr Probl Cancer 21(5):233–300, 1997.

13. Allen JI: Molecular biology of colon polyps and colon cancer. Semin Surg Oncol 11(6):399–405, 1995.

14. Locker GY, Hamilton S, Harris J, et al: ASCO 2006 update of recommendations for the use of tumor markers in gastrointestinal cancer. J Clin Oncol 24(33):5313–5327, 2006.

15. Gocke CD, Benko FA, Kopreski MS, McGarrity TJ: p53 and APC mutations are detectable in the plasma and serum of patients with colorectal cancer (CRC) or adenomas. Ann N Y Acad Sci 906:44–50, 2000.

16. Herman JG: Circulating methylated DNA. Ann N Y Acad Sci 1022:33–39, 2004.

17. Sidransky D, Tokino T, Hamilton SR, et al: Identification of ras oncogene mutations in the stool of patients with curable colorectal tumors. Science 256(5053):102–105, 1992.

18. Villa E, Dugani A, Rebecchi AM, et al: Identification of subjects at risk for colorectal carcinoma through a test based on K-ras determination in the stool. Gastroenterology 110(5):1346–1353, 1996.

19. Ahlquist DA, Skoletsky JE, Boynton KA, et al: Colorectal cancer screening by detection of altered human DNA in stool: feasibility of a multitarget assay panel. Gastroenterology 119(5):1219–1227, 2000.

20. Imperiale TF, Ransohoff DF, Itzkowitz SH, et al: Fecal DNA versus fecal occult blood for colorectal-cancer screening in an average-risk population. N Engl J Med 351(26):2704–2714, 2004.

21. Dong SM, Traverso G, Johnson C, et al: Detecting colorectal cancer in stool with the use of multiple genetic targets. J Natl Cancer Inst 93(11):858–865, 2001.

22. Schuebel KE, Chen W, Cope L, Glockner SC, et al: Comparing the DNA hypermethylome with gene mutations in human colorectal cancer. PLoS Genet 3(9):1709–1723, 2007.

23. Herman JG, Merlo A, Mao L, et al: Inactivation of the CDKN2/p16/MTS1 gene is frequently associated with aberrant DNA methylation in all common human cancers. Cancer Res 55(20):4525–4530, 1995.

24. Esteller M, Hamilton SR, Burger PC, et al: Inactivation of the DNA repair gene O6-methylguanine-DNA methyltransferase by promoter hypermethylation is a common event in primary human neoplasia. Cancer Res 59(4):793–797, 1999.

25. Herman JG, Umar A, Polyak K, et al: Incidence and functional consequences of hMLH1 promoter hypermethylation in

colorectal carcinoma. Proc Natl Acad Sci U S A 95(12):6870–6875, 1998.

26. Suzuki H, Watkins DN, Jair KW, et al: Epigenetic inactivation of SFRP genes allows constitutive WNT signaling in colorectal cancer. Nat Genet 36(4):417–422, 2004.

27. Taketo MM: Shutting down Wnt signal-activated cancer. Nat Genet 36(4):320–322, 2004.

28. Toyota M, Ahuja N, Ohe-Toyota M, et al: CpG island methylator phenotype in colorectal cancer. Proc Natl Acad Sci U S A 96(15):8681–8686, 1999.

29. Lenhard K, Bommer GT, Asutay S, et al: Analysis of promoter methylation in stool: a novel method for the detection of colorectal cancer. Clin Gastroenterol Hepatol 3(2):142–149, 2005.

30. Muller HM, Oberwalder M, Fiegl H, et al: Methylation changes in faecal DNA: a marker for colorectal cancer screening? Lancet 363(9417):1283–1285, 2004.

31. Belshaw NJ, Elliott GO, Williams EA, et al: Use of DNA from human stools to detect aberrant CpG island methylation of genes implicated in colorectal cancer. Cancer Epidemiol Biomarkers Prev 13(9):1495–1501, 2004.

32. Itzkowitz SH, Jandorf L, Brand R, et al: Improved fecal DNA test for colorectal cancer screening. Clin Gastroenterol Hepatol 5(1):111–117, 2007.

33. Traverso G, Shuber A, Olsson L, et al: Detection of proximal colorectal cancers through analysis of faecal DNA. Lancet 359(9304):403–404, 2002.

34. Petko Z, Ghiassi M, Shuber A, et al: Aberrantly methylated CDKN2A, MGMT, and MLH1 in colon polyps and in fecal DNA from patients with colorectal polyps. Clin Cancer Res 11(3):1203–1209, 2005.

35. Chen WD, Han ZJ, Skoletsky J, et al: Detection in fecal DNA of colon cancer-specific methylation of the nonexpressed vimentin gene. J Natl Cancer Inst 97(15):1124–1132, 2005.

36. Tagore KS, Levin TR, Lawson MJ: The evolution to stool DNA testing for colorectal cancer. Aliment Pharmacol Ther 19(12):1225–1233, 2004.

37. Moshkowitz M, Arber N. Emerging technologies in colorectal cancer screening. Surg Oncol Clin N Am 14(4):723–746, 2005.

38. Agrawal J, Syngal S: Colon cancer screening strategies. Curr Opin Gastroenterol 21(1):59–63, 2005.

39. Chialina SG, Fornes C, Landi C, et al: Microsatellite instability analysis in hereditary non-polyposis colon cancer using the Bethesda consensus panel of microsatellite markers in the absence of proband normal tissue. BMC Med Genet 7:5, 2006.

40. Chai SM, Zeps N, Shearwood AM, et al: Screening for defective DNA mismatch repair in stage II and III colorectal cancer patients. Clin Gastroenterol Hepatol 2(11):1017–1025, 2004.

41. Jover R, Paya A, Alenda C, et al: Defective mismatch-repair colorectal cancer: clinicopathologic characteristics and usefulness of immunohistochemical analysis for diagnosis. Am J Clin Pathol 122(3):389–394, 2004.

42. Berger BM, Vucson BM, Diteberg JS: Gene mutations in advanced colonic polyps: potential marker selection for stool-based mutated human DNA assays for colon cancer screening. Clin Colorectal Cancer 3(3):180–185, 2003.

43. Berger BM, Robison L, Glickman J: Colon cancer-associated DNA mutations: marker selection for the detection of proximal colon cancer. Diagn Mol Pathol 12(4):187–192, 2003.

44. Le Corre L, Vissac-Sabatier C, et al: Quantitative analysis of BRCA1, BRCA2 and Hmsh2 mRNA expression in colorectal Lieberkuhnien adenocarcinomas and matched normal mucosa: relationship with cellular proliferation. Anticancer Res 25(3B):2009–2016, 2005.

45. Peelen T, de Leeuw W, van Lent K, et al: Genetic analysis of a breast-ovarian cancer family, with 7 cases of colorectal cancer linked to BRCA1, fails to support a role for BRCA1 in colorectal tumorigenesis. Int J Cancer 88(5):778–782, 2000.

46. Samowitz WS, Albertsen H, Herrick J, et al: Evaluation of a large, population-based sample supports a CpG island methylator phenotype in colon cancer. Gastroenterology 129(3):837–845, 2005.

47. Lind GE, Thorstensen L, Løvig T, et al: A CpG island hypermethylation profile of primary colorectal carcinomas and colon cancer cell lines. Mol Cancer 3:28, 2004.

48. Trzeciak L, Hennig E, Kolodziejski J, et al: Mutations, methylation and expression of CDKN2a/p16 gene in colorectal cancer

and normal colonic mucosa. Cancer Lett 163(1):17–23, 2001.

49. Tu SP, Cui JT, Liston P, et al: Gene therapy for colon cancer by adeno-associated viral vector-mediated transfer of survivin Cys84Ala mutant. Gastroenterology 128(2):361–375, 2005.

50. Boman BM, Walters R, Fields JZ, et al: Colonic crypt changes during adenoma development in familial adenomatous polyposis: immunohistochemical evidence for expansion of the crypt base cell population. Am J Pathol 165(5):1489–1498, 2004.

51. Zhang T, Otevrel T, Gao Z, et al: Evidence that APC regulates survivin expression: a possible mechanism contributing to the stem cell origin of colon cancer. Cancer Res 61(24): 8664–8667, 2001.

52. Saleh HA, Jackson H, Banerjee M: Immunohistochemical expression of bcl-2 and p53 oncoproteins: correlation with Ki67 proliferation index and prognostic histopathologic parameters in colorectal neoplasia. Appl Immunohistochem Mol Morphol 8(3):175–182, 2000.

53. Ayhan A, Yasui W, Yokozaki H, et al: Loss of heterozygosity at the bcl-2 gene locus and expression of bcl-2 in human gastric and colorectal carcinomas. Jpn J Cancer Res 85(6):584–591, 1994.

54. Cheng L, Lai MD: Aberrant crypt foci as microscopic precursors of colorectal cancer. World J Gastroenterol 9(12): 2642–2649, 2003.

55. Lala PK, Chakraborty C: Role of nitric oxide in carcinogenesis and tumour progression. Lancet Oncol 2(3):149–156, 2001.

56. Dobrovolskaia MA, Kozlov SV: Inflammation and cancer: when NF-kappaB amalgamates the perilous partnership. Curr Cancer Drug Targets 5(5):325–344, 2005.

57. Itzkowitz SH, Yio X: Inflammation and cancer IV. Colorectal cancer in inflammatory bowel disease: the role of inflammation. Am J Physiol Gastrointest Liver Physiol 287(1):G7–G17, 2004.

58. van der Woude CJ, Kleibeuker JH, Jansen PL, Moshage H: Chronic inflammation, apoptosis and (pre-)malignant lesions in the gastro-intestinal tract. Apoptosis 9(2):123–130, 2004.

59. Crowley-Weber CL, Payne CM, Gleason-Guzman M, et al: Development and molecular characterization of HCT-116 cell lines resistant to the tumor promoter and multiple stress-inducer, deoxycholate. Carcinogenesis 23(12):2063–2080, 2002.

60. Colnot S, Niwa-Kawakita M, Hamard G, et al: Colorectal cancers in a new mouse model of familial adenomatous polyposis: influence of genetic and environmental modifiers. Lab Invest 84(12):1619–1630, 2004.

61. Greco C, Alvino S, Buglioni S, et al: Activation of c-MYC and c-MYB proto-oncogenes is associated with decreased apoptosis in tumor colon progression. Anticancer Res 21(5):3185–3192, 2001.

62. Smith DR, Myint T, Goh HS: Over-expression of the c-myc proto-oncogene in colorectal carcinoma. Br J Cancer 68(2): 407–413, 1993.

63. Finley GG, Schulz NT, Hill SA, et al: Expression of the myc gene family in different stages of human colorectal cancer. Oncogene 4(8):963–971, 1989.

64. Wong NA, Malcomson RD, Jodrell DI, et al: ERbeta isoform expression in colorectal carcinoma: an in vivo and in vitro study of clinicopathological and molecular correlates. J Pathol 207(1):53–60, 2005.

65. Martineti V, Picariello L, Tognarini I, et al: ERbeta is a potent inhibitor of cell proliferation in the HCT8 human colon cancer cell line through regulation of cell cycle components. Endocr Relat Cancer 12(2):455–469, 2005.

66. Maekawa M, Sugano K, Ushiama M, et al: Heterogeneity of DNA methylation status analyzed by bisulfite-PCR-SSCP and correlation with clinico-pathological characteristics in colorectal cancer. Clin Chem Lab Med 39(2):121–128, 2001.

67. McGivern A, Wynter CV, Whitehall VL, et al: Promoter hypermethylation frequency and BRAF mutations distinguish hereditary non-polyposis colon cancer from sporadic MSI-H colon cancer. Fam Cancer 3(2):101–107, 2004.

68. Wynter CV, Walsh MD, Higuchi T, et al: Methylation patterns define two types of hyperplastic polyp associated with colorectal cancer. Gut 53(4):573–580, 2004.

69. Chien CC, Chen SH, Liu CC, et al: Correlation of K-ras codon 12 mutations in human feces and ages of patients with colorectal cancer (CRC). Transl Res 149(2):96–102, 2007.

70. Takayama T, Miyanishi K, Hayashi T, et al: Aberrant crypt foci: detection, gene abnormalities, and clinical usefulness. Clin Gastroenterol Hepatol 3(7 Suppl 1):S42–S45, 2005.

71. Minamoto T: Detection and characterization of oncogene mutations in preneoplastic and early neoplastic lesions. Methods Mol Biol 291:263–278, 2005.

72. Okulczyk B, Kovalchuk O, Piotrowski Z, et al: Clinical usefulness of K-RAS mutation detection in colorectal cancer and in surgical margins of the colon. Rocz Akad Med Bialymst 49(Suppl 1):52–54, 2004.

73. Zhang J, Anastasiadis PZ, Liu Y, et al: Protein kinase C (PKC) betaII induces cell invasion through a Ras/Mek-, PKC iota/Rac 1-dependent signaling pathway. J Biol Chem 279(21): 22118–22123, 2004.

74. Yuan P, Sun MH, Zhang JS, et al: APC and K-ras gene mutation in aberrant crypt foci of human colon. World J Gastroenterol 7(3):352–356, 2001.

75. Dorer R, Odze RD: AMACR immunostaining is useful in detecting dysplastic epithelium in Barrett's esophagus, ulcerative colitis, and Crohn's disease. Am J Surg Pathol 30(7): 871–877, 2006.

76. Traka M, Gasper AV, Smith JA, et al: Transcriptome analysis of human colon Caco-2 cells exposed to sulforaphane. J Nutr 135(8):1865–1872, 2005.

77. Jiang Z, Fanger GR, Banner BF, et al: A dietary enzyme: alpha-methylacyl-CoA racemase/P504S is overexpressed in colon carcinoma. Cancer Detect Prev 27(6):422–426, 2003.

78. Zhou M, Chinnaiyan AM, Kleer CG, et al: Alpha-Methylacyl-CoA racemase: a novel tumor marker over-expressed in several human cancers and their precursor lesions. Am J Surg Pathol 26(7):926–931, 2002.

79. Kakar S, Aksoy S, Burgart LJ, Smyrk TC: Mucinous carcinoma of the colon: correlation of loss of mismatch repair enzymes with clinicopathologic features and survival. Mod Pathol 17(6):696–700, 2004.

80. Plevova P, Krepelova A, Papezova M, et al: Immunohistochemical detection of the hMLH1 and hMSH2 proteins in hereditary non-polyposis colon cancer and sporadic colon cancer. Neoplasma 51(4):275–284, 2004.

81. Muller A, Fishel R: Mismatch repair and the hereditary non-polyposis colorectal cancer syndrome (HNPCC). Cancer Invest 20(1):102–109, 2002.

82. Jiricny J: Mismatch repair and cancer. Cancer Surv 28:47–68, 1996.

83. Suzuki H, Gabrielson E, Chen W, et al: A genomic screen for genes upregulated by demethylation and histone deacetylase inhibition in human colorectal cancer. Nat Genet 31(2): 141–149, 2002.

84. Tang M, Torres-Lanzas J, Lopez-Rios F, et al: Wnt signaling promoter hypermethylation distinguishes lung primary adenocarcinomas from colorectal metastasis to the lung. Int J Cancer 119(11):2603–2606, 2006.

85. Aguilera O, Fraga MF, Ballestar E, et al: Epigenetic inactivation of the Wnt antagonist DICKKOPF-1 (DKK-1) gene in human colorectal cancer. Oncogene 25(29):4116–4121, 2006.

86. Gotley DC, Reeder JA, Fawcett J, et al: The deleted in colon cancer (DCC) gene is consistently expressed in colorectal cancers and metastases. Oncogene 13(4):787–795, 1996.

87. Mikami T, Mitomi H, Hara A, et al: Decreased expression of CD44, alpha-catenin, and deleted colon carcinoma and altered expression of beta-catenin in ulcerative colitis-associated dysplasia and carcinoma, as compared with sporadic colon neoplasms. Cancer 89(4):733–740, 2000.

88. Hedrick L, Cho KR, Fearon ER, et al: The DCC gene product in cellular differentiation and colorectal tumorigenesis. Genes Dev 8(10):1174–1183, 1994.

89. Stewenius Y, Gorunova L, Jonson T, et al: Structural and numerical chromosome changes in colon cancer develop through telomere-mediated anaphase bridges, not through mitotic multipolarity. Proc Natl Acad Sci U S A 102(15): 5541–5546, 2005.

90. Ikeguchi M, Makino M, Kaibara N: Telomerase activity and p53 gene mutation in familial polyposis coli. Anticancer Res 20(5C):3833–3837, 2000.

91. Krajewska WM, Stawinska M, Brys M, et al: Genotyping of p53 codon 175 in colorectal cancer. Med Sci Monit 9(5): BR188–BR191, 2003.

92. Iacopetta B, Russo A, Bazan V, et al: Functional categories of TP53 mutation in colorectal cancer: results of an International Collaborative Study. Ann Oncol 17(5):842–847, 2006.
93. Chang SC, Lin JK, Yang SH, et al: Relationship between genetic alterations and prognosis in sporadic colorectal cancer. Int J Cancer 118(7):1721–1727, 2006.
94. Soussi T: The p53 tumor suppressor gene: from molecular biology to clinical investigation. Ann N Y Acad Sci 910: 121–137; discussion 37–39, 2000.
95. Yamashita N, Minamoto T, Ochiai A, et al: Frequent and characteristic K-ras activation and absence of p53 protein accumulation in aberrant crypt foci of the colon. Gastroenterology 108(2):434–440, 1995.
96. Tendler Y, Reshef R, Cohen I, et al: Histochemical studies of progressive p53 mutations during colonic carcinogenesis in Sprague-Dawley rats induced by N-methyl-N-nitro-nitrosoguanidine or azoxymethane. Pathobiology 62(5–6):232–237, 1994.
97. Griffiths GJ, Koh MY, Brunton VG, et al: Expression of kinase-defective mutants of c-Src in human metastatic colon cancer cells decreases Bcl-xL and increases oxaliplatin- and Fas-induced apoptosis. J Biol Chem 279(44):46113–46121, 2004.
98. Windham TC, Parikh NU, Siwak DR, et al: Src activation regulates anoikis in human colon tumor cell lines. Oncogene 21(51):7797–7807, 2002.
99. Buban T, Schmidt M, Broll R, et al: Detection of mutations in the cDNA of the proliferation marker Ki-67 protein in four tumor cell lines. Cancer Genet Cytogenet 149(1):81–84, 2004.
100. Petrowsky H, Sturm I, Graubitz O, et al: Relevance of Ki-67 antigen expression and K-ras mutation in colorectal liver metastases. Eur J Surg Oncol 27(1):80–87, 2001.
101. Chung DC, Rustgi AK: The hereditary nonpolyposis colorectal cancer syndrome: genetics and clinical implications. Ann Intern Med 138(7):560–570, 2003.
102. Heinen CD, Schmutte C, Fishel R: DNA repair and tumorigenesis: lessons from hereditary cancer syndromes. Cancer Biol Ther 1(5):477–485, 2002.
103. Lynch HT, Smyrk T, Lynch JF: Overview of natural history, pathology, molecular genetics and management of HNPCC (Lynch syndrome). Int J Cancer 69(1):38–43, 1996.
104. Yamamoto H, Sawai H, Weber TK, et al: Somatic frameshift mutations in DNA mismatch repair and proapoptosis genes in hereditary nonpolyposis colorectal cancer. Cancer Res 58(5): 997–1003, 1998.
105. Plaschke J, Kruppa C, Tischler R, et al: Sequence analysis of the mismatch repair gene hMSH6 in the germline of patients with familial and sporadic colorectal cancer. Int J Cancer 85(5):606–613, 2000.
106. Plaschke J, Kruger S, Pistorius S, et al: Involvement of hMSH6 in the development of hereditary and sporadic colorectal cancer revealed by immunostaining is based on germline mutations, but rarely on somatic inactivation. Int J Cancer 97(5):643–648, 2002.
107. Maeda K, Nishiguchi Y, Onoda N, et al: Expression of the mismatch repair gene hMSH2 in sporadic colorectal cancer. Int J Oncol 13(6):1147–1151, 1992.
108. Liu T, Yan H, Kuismanen S, et al: The role of hPMS1 and hPMS2 in predisposing to colorectal cancer. Cancer Res 61(21):7798–7802, 2001.
109. Hendriks YM, Jagmohan-Changur S, van der Klift HM, et al: Heterozygous mutations in PMS2 cause hereditary nonpolyposis colorectal carcinoma (Lynch syndrome). Gastroenterology 130(2):312–322, 2006.
110. Esteller M, Toyota M, Sanchez-Cespedes M, et al: Inactivation of the DNA repair gene O6-methylguanine-DNA methyltransferase by promoter hypermethylation is associated with G to A mutations in K-ras in colorectal tumorigenesis. Cancer Res 60(9):2368–2371, 2000.
111. Esteller M, Risques RA, Toyota M, et al: Promoter hypermethylation of the DNA repair gene O(6)-methylguanine-DNA methyltransferase is associated with the presence of G:C to A: T transition mutations in p53 in human colorectal tumorigenesis. Cancer Res 61(12):4689–4692, 2001.
112. Shen L, Kondo Y, Rosner GL, et al: MGMT promoter methylation and field defect in sporadic colorectal cancer. J Natl Cancer Inst 97(18):1330–1338, 2005.
113. Cho KR, Vogelstein B: Genetic alterations in the adenoma—carcinoma sequence. Cancer 70(6 Suppl):1727–1731, 1992.
114. Nakamura Y, Nishisho I, Kinzler KW, et al: Mutations of the adenomatous polyposis coli gene in familial polyposis coli patients and sporadic colorectal tumors. Princess Takamatsu Symp 22:285–292, 1991.
115. Ahlquist DA: Molecular stool screening for colorectal cancer. Using DNA markers may be beneficial, but large scale evaluation is needed. Br Med J 321(7256):254–255, 2000.
116. Ahlquist DA, Harrington JJ, Burgart LJ, Roche PC: Morphometric analysis of the "mucocellular layer" overlying colorectal cancer and normal mucosa: relevance to exfoliation and stool screening. Hum Pathol 31(1):51–57, 2000.
117. Loktionov A, O'Neill IK, Silvester KR, et al: Quantitation of DNA from exfoliated colonocytes isolated from human stool surface as a novel noninvasive screening test for colorectal cancer. Clin Cancer Res 4(2):337–342, 1998.
118. Boland CR, Sato J, Saito K, et al: Genetic instability and chromosomal aberrations in colorectal cancer: a review of the current models. Cancer Detect Prev 22(5):377–382, 1998.
119. Rengucci C, Maiolo P, Saragoni L, et al: Multiple detection of genetic alterations in tumors and stool. Clin Cancer Res 7(3):590–593, 2001.
120. Tagore KS, Lawson MJ, Yucaitis JA, et al: Sensitivity and specificity of a stool DNA multitarget assay panel for the detection of advanced colorectal neoplasia. Clin Colorectal Cancer 3(1):47–53, 2003.
121. Calistri D, Rengucci C, Bocchini R, et al: Fecal multiple molecular tests to detect colorectal cancer in stool. Clin Gastroenterol Hepatol 1(5):377–383, 2003.
122. Syngal S, Stoffel E, Chung D, et al: Detection of stool DNA mutations before and after treatment of colorectal neoplasia. Cancer 106(2):277–283, 2006.
123. Traverso G, Diehl F, Hurst R, et al: Multicolor in vitro translation. Nat Biotechnol 21(9):1093–1097, 2003.

10

Radiologic Techniques: Virtual Colonoscopy

Karen M. Horton

KEY POINTS

- Virtual colonoscopy is an innovative application for computed tomography (CT) in which CT data and specialized three-dimensional (3D) software can be used to identify colon polyps.
- CT colonography requires complete colonic cleansing as well as stool-tagging agents in an attempt to "mark" any residual stool or fluid.
- To identify polyps in the colon with virtual colonoscopy, the colon must be adequately distended with either room air or carbon dioxide.
- The patient is imaged in the prone and supine positions, using low-dose radiation techniques.
- Interpretation strategies vary and include 3D review, 2D review, computer-aided diagnosis, and colon unraveling views.
- Virtual colonoscopy has limited sensitivity and specificity for lesions less than 5 mm, and polyps of this size are always benign. Therefore, radiologists report only polyps 6 mm or larger.
- The American Cancer Society has included virtual colonoscopy as an acceptable colon screening examination, to be carried out every 5 years. Insurance companies are now reviewing their policies and are likely to cover virtual colonoscopy for screening.

Introduction

Virtual colonoscopy (VC) is an innovative application for computed tomography (CT) in which CT data can be used to identify colon polyps. The technology has made significant advancements in recent years, but its exact role in colon cancer screening has not yet been determined. However, given encouraging results of recent screening trials and the inclusion of virtual colonoscopy in the American Cancer Society screening guidelines, virtual colonoscopy is likely to soon be a viable screening alternative to conventional colonoscopy.

Principles and Supporting Literature

Virtual colonoscopy is a method by which colon polyps can be detected using multidetector computed tomography (MDCT) scanners combined with specialized three-dimensional (3D) software. It requires bowel cleansing, colon insufflation, and careful review of the data. The method was first described in 1995, but although the concept was valid, early results were limited because of slow scanner speed, relatively thick collimation (3- to 5-mm slices), and lack of reliable high-speed 3D software.[1] Over the years, these limitations are no longer an obstacle. New MDCT scanners allow submillimeter slices, extremely fast scanning speeds, and now fast real-time software designed specifically for this application.

Most of the early published data from the 1990s and early 2000s involved only high-risk patients and patients with polyposis syndromes, but these studies did show encouraging results. However, virtual colonoscopy did not get widespread attention until the publication of the first large screening trial by Perry Pickhardt[2] in 2003. In this trial, 1233 asymptomatic adults underwent virtual colonoscopy and conventional colonoscopy in the same day. Virtual colonoscopy demonstrated a patient sensitivity of 94% and a specificity of 96%,[2] as seen in Table 10-1. In addition, the sensitivity of detecting polyps larger than 1 cm was 94% for the virtual colonoscopy and only 88% for the optical colonoscopy.[2] Although this difference was not statistically significant, this manuscript attracted a lot of attention from both the medical community and the lay community. This was the first large screening study to demonstrate high sensitivity and specificity for clinically significant polyps.

Table 10-1. Performance Characteristics of Virtual Colonoscopy and Optical Colonoscopy for the Detection of Adenomas*

Variable	Size Category No./Total No. (% [95% CI])				
	≥6 mm	≥7 mm	≥8 mm	≥9 mm	≥10 mm
Analysis According to Patient					
Virtual colonoscopy					
Sensitivity	149/168 (88.7 [82.9–93.1])	100/110 (90.9 [83.9–95.6])	77/82 (93.9 [86.3–98.0])	53/57 (93.0 [83.0–98.1])	45/48 (93.8 [82.8–98.7])
Specificity	848/1065 (79.6 [77.0–82.0])	981/1123 (87.4 [85.3–89.2])	1061/1151 (92.2 [90.5–93.7])	1116/1176 (94.9 [93.5–96.1])	1138/1185 (96.0 [94.8–97.1])
Accuracy	997/1233 (80.9 [78.6–83.0])	1081/1233 (87.7 [85.7–89.5])	1138/1233 (92.3 [90.7–93.7])	1169/1233 (94.8 [93.4–96.0])	1183/1233 (95.9 [94.7–97.0])
Test-positive rate†	366/1233 (29.7 [27.1–32.3])	242/1233 (19.6 [17.4–22.0])	167/1233 (13.5 [11.7–15.6])	113/1233 (9.2 [7.6–10.9])	92/1233 (7.5 [6.1–9.1])
Sensitivity of optical colonoscopy	155/168 (92.3 [87.1–95.8])	100/110 (90.9 [83.9–95.6])	75/82 (91.5 [83.2–96.5])	51/57 (89.5 [78.5–96.0])	42/48 (87.5 [74.8–95.3])
Analysis According to Polyp					
Sensitivity of virtual colonoscopy	180/210 (85.7 [80.2–90.1])	119/133 (89.5 [83.0–94.1])	88/95 (92.6 [85.4–97.0])	56/61 (91.8 [81.2–97.3])	47/51 (92.2 [81.1–97.8])
Sensitivity of optical colonoscopy	189/210 (90.0 [85.1–93.7])	120/133 (90.2 [83.9–94.7])	85/95 (89.5 [81.5–94.8])	55/61 (90.2 [79.8–96.3])	45/51 (88.2 [76.1–95.6])

*The data for optical colonoscopy are for the initial optical colonoscopy performed before the results on virtual colonoscopy were revealed. CI denotes confidence interval.
†Data are for the virtual colonoscopic studies that were deemed to be positive in each size category.
From Pickhardt PJ, Choi JR, Hwang I, et al: Computed tomographic virtual colonoscopy to screen for colorectal neoplasia in asymptomatic adults. N Eng J Med 349:2191–2200, 2003.

Two smaller studies of screening virtual colonoscopy were published in 2004 with less impressive results. The first was published by Cotton and colleagues,[3] and the second was published by Rockey and colleagues.[4] Both studies showed a significantly lower sensitivity and specificity for polyps, even in the centimeter range. These two studies had some limitations, especially involving training of the participating radiologists.[3,4] The Pickhardt study, however, showed that at least in that trial it was possible to get high sensitivity and specificity for colon polyps with high-quality data and experienced radiologists.[2] To confirm his results, the ACRIN National CT Colonography Trial was established. The trial enrolled over 2600 patients and was a multi-institutional trial involving 15 centers. Patients in this trial also underwent virtual colonoscopy and conventional colonoscopy on the same day. The results of this trial were published in September 2008.[5] In this study of asymptomatic adults, the CT colonography identified 90% of subjects with adenomas or cancers 10 mm or more in diameter.

Technique

Bowel Cleansing

As with other colon cancer screening examinations such as the barium enema and conventional colonoscopy, CT colonography requires complete colonic cleansing. The colon must be free of stool so that polyps and masses can be visualized with confidence. A variety of bowel preparations are available on the market, including magnesium citrate, and polyethylene glycol. Sodium phosphate has been recently discontinued due to an FDA warning of potential phosphate-induced nephropathy, even in healthy patients. When taken as directed, any of these agents can be used for CT colonography, and often the selection of the particular bowel preparation is based on the preference of the radiologist or referring physician. We prefer polyethylene glycol.

The bowel preparation begins the day before the examinations and consists of several steps. In addition to a clear liquid diet the day before the CT, the patient drinks 4 liters of polyethylene glycol mixture as directed. Two bisacodyl tablets are also given to the patient to clear some of the residual fluid remaining in the colon. In most patients, this preparation is adequate.

Stool Tagging

In addition to the bowel-cleansing agents, it is necessary to include stool-tagging agents in an attempt to "mark" any residual stool or fluid. Solid stool tagging is accomplished when the patient drinks a small quantity of barium during the bowel cleansing. This dilute barium mixes with residual solid stool, allowing quick identification on the CT (Fig. 10-1). A small quantity of iodinated oral contrast is also given to the patient just before bedtime (i.e., the night before the CT scan). This mixes with residual fluid increasing its density. Therefore, residual fluid also appears white (Fig. 10-2).

Both solid and liquid stool tagging are essential for high-quality CT colonography exams. It improves both the sensitivity and specificity of lesions by allowing the radiologist to easily distinguish small polyps from adherent stool and to identify polyps that may be submerged in fluid.

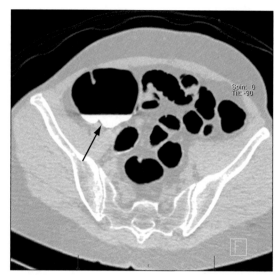

Figure 10-2. Axial image from virtual colonoscopy demonstrates high-density tagged fluid (*arrow*) in the cecum. Without liquid stool tagging, residual fluid may hide polyps.

Colonic Insufflation

To identify polyps in the colon, the colon must be adequately distended with air (Fig. 10-3). If the colon is collapsed, polyps and masses may be overlooked. Colonic insufflation can be

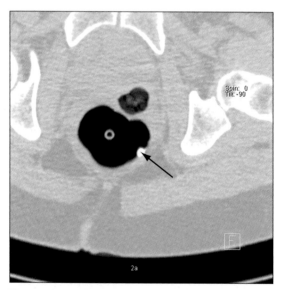

Figure 10-1. Axial image from virtual colonoscopy demonstrates focal adherent stool (*arrow*) in the rectum. The stool appears white as a result of the stool-tagging agent. This allows easy differentiation between adherent stool and polyps.

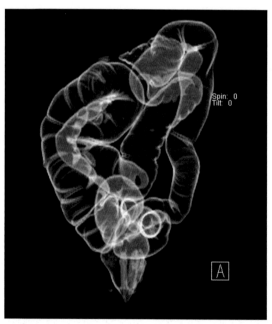

Figure 10-3. Rendered image of the colon from virtual colonoscopy shows a well-distended colon. The colon must be completely distended to enable detection of polyps.

Table 10-2. Clinical Adequacy of Distention for Individual Colon Segments According to Insufflation Method

Segment	Manual (n = 94) No. of Adequate (%)	Automated (n = 47) No. of Adequate (%)	P
Rectum	88 (94)	45 (96)	0.72
Sigmoid	48 (51)	28 (60)	0.37
Descending	85 (90)	45 (96)	0.34
Transverse	89 (95)	43 (91)	0.48
Ascending	92 (98)	45 (96)	0.60
Cecum	91 (97)	45 (96)	1.00

From Burling D, Taylor SA, Halligan S, et al: Automated insufflation of carbon dioxide for MDCT colonography: distension and patient experience compared with manual insufflation. AJR Am J Roentgenol 186:96–103, 2006.

accomplished with either room air or carbon dioxide. If room air is used, a small tube is inserted into the rectum and the colon is distended by manually pumping in room air, similar to the procedure used during a barium enema. However, many investigators and radiologists prefer to use an electronic insufflator pump and carbon dioxide. Carbon dioxide is absorbed by the body and exhaled by the patient. Therefore within minutes after the study the patient feels fine. The pump also maintains a steady colonic pressure during the study, automatically adding more gas when needed (Tables 10-2 and 10-3).

There is controversy in the literature as to the usefulness of administering glucagon before the CT colonography exam, we have found it to be helpful.[6,7] Glucagon relaxes the colon, thereby potentially allowing greater distention and reducing spasm and patient discomfort. However, it is expensive and has some risks. Therefore, we do not routinely use glucagon.

CT Scanning Parameters and Radiation Risk

After the colon is sufficiently distended with air, the patient is placed in the supine position and a scout topogram is performed. This allows the technologist to ensure adequate colon distention and to set the field of view. The patent is scanned twice, once supine and once prone. Both acquisitions are necessary to achieve high sensitivity. Also, certain parts of the colon are better distended in either position. For example, the transverse colon is typically better distended in the supine position, whereas the rectum is better distended in the prone position (Fig. 10-4). If necessary, a third acquisition, such as a decubitus, can be obtained in certain cases to make sure all segments are well distended.

Current MDCT scanners allow submillimeter collimation and thin slices, thus creating high-

Table 10-3. Effect of Increasing Total Volume of Carbon Dioxide Administered on Distention Score According to Patient Position

Position and Segment	Odds Ratio* (95% CI)	P†
Supine		
Rectum	0.69 (0.40–1.18)	.17
Sigmoid	0.65 (0.36–1.14)	.13
Descending	0.78 (0.44–1.34)	.37
Transverse	0.61 (0.27–1.34)	.22
Ascending	0.78 (0.45–1.75)	.55
Cecum	0.72 (0.36–1.46)	.37
Prone		
Rectum	0.56 (0.27–1.15)	.11
Sigmoid	0.47 (0.27–0.92)	.03
Descending	0.46 (0.21–0.98)	.04
Transverse	0.66 (0.37–1.17)	.16
Ascending	0.78 (0.22–2.70)	.52
Cecum	0.51 (0.28–0.92)	.03
Supine and prone combined		
Rectum	0.64 (0.41–1.02)	.06
Sigmoid	0.57 (0.34–0.94)	.03
Descending	0.66 (0.36–1.23)	.19
Transverse	0.64 (0.34–1.22)	.18
Ascending	0.78 (0.22–2.70)	.70
Cecum	0.59 (0.36–0.95)	.03

CI, confidence interval.
*Odds ratio is odds of being in next highest distention category for a 1-L increase in carbon dioxide volume.
†Values in boldface are statistically significant.
From Burling D, Taylor SA, Halligan S, et al: Automated insufflation of carbon dioxide for MDCT colonography: distension and patient experience compared with manual insufflation. AJR Am J Roentgenol 186:96–103, 2006.

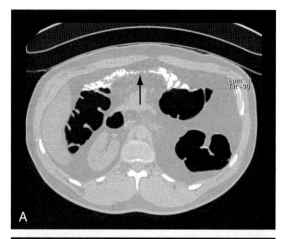

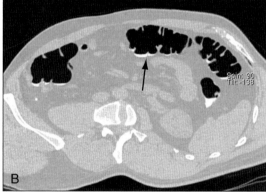

Figure 10-4. A, Axial image from virtual colonoscopy demonstrates collapse of the transverse colon (*arrow*) in the prone position. **B,** Axial image demonstrates better distention of the transverse colon (*arrow*) in the supine position.

resolution datasets, which maintain this high resolution in any imaging plan. MDCT offers several advantages over single-slice CT, including thinner collimation, shorter scan times, and higher resolution. For example, today's CT scanners can scan the entire abdomen and pelvis in less than 10 seconds.

Because there is a natural high contrast between the soft tissue density polyp and the air-filled colon, it is possible to decrease the radiation dose when performing CT colonography. For example, during a regular diagnostic CT of the abdomen and pelvis, we typically use 120 kV(p) and 200 mAs. However, for CT colonography, we use 120 kV(p) and decrease the effective mAs to 50, greatly reducing the radiation dose while maintaining diagnostic accuracy.

The overall radiation dose is comparable to the dose required to perform a barium enema. Reducing the mAs while maintaining sensitivity and specificity for polyp detection is well supported in the literature.[8]

Interpretation Strategies

After the CT data have been obtained, it is transferred to a 3D workstation with specially designed virtual colonoscopy software. Although software packages vary by vendor, they all offer the ability to review the data in both a 2D multiplanar format and a 3D endoluminal fly-through format, either separately or simultaneously. There are basically two approaches: the primary 2D read and the primary 3D read.

Radiologists utilizing the primary 2D read typically review the case primarily by scrolling through the axial, coronal, and/or sagittal images to identify and characterize polyps and masses. When a polyp is located, it is confirmed in the other planes and in the other dataset (Fig. 10-5). With this strategy, the endoluminal fly-through views are used only as needed for problem solving.

Radiologists performing a primary 3D review begin by flying through the colon using the endoluminal software, which simulates conventional colonoscopy (Fig. 10-6). The reviewer must fly forward and back in both the prone and supine dataset to ensure visualization of the entire colonic surface. Once a potential polyp is identified, it is confirmed in the axial, coronal, and/or sagittal views. Flat polyps can be especially challenging on both 2D and 3D (Fig. 10-7). Either approach is acceptable and the choice is really a matter of reviewer preference. With training and experience, most readers can become proficient in either method.

Initially, interpretation times were very long (45 to 60 minutes). However, improvements in software and the improved spatial resolution obtainable with MDCT have allowed a considerable reduction in interpretation times. Experienced readers can usually review a case in less than 15 minutes.

Reporting

In 2005, a group of radiologists highly experienced in virtual colonoscopy reviewed all the

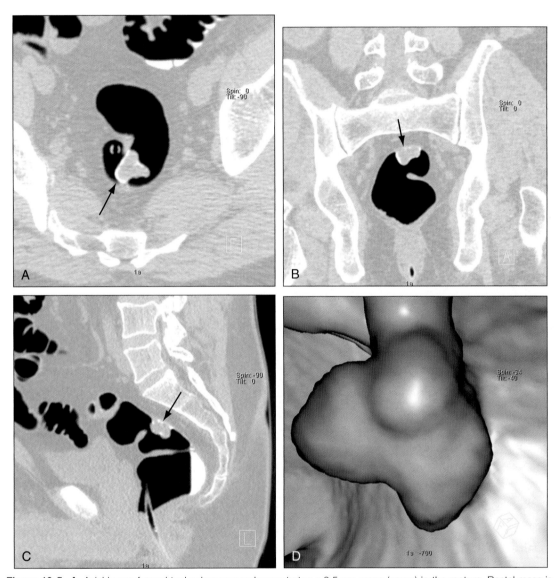

Figure 10-5. A, Axial image from virtual colonoscopy demonstrates a 2.5-cm mass (*arrow*) in the rectum. Rectal mass is also seen on coronal image (**B,** *arrow*), sagittal image (**C,** *arrow*), and endoluminal view (**D**).

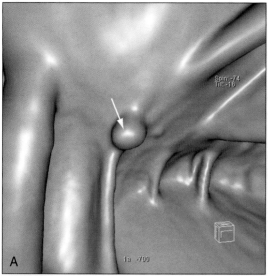

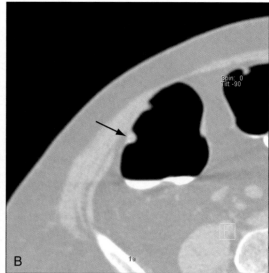

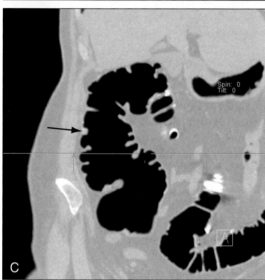

Figure 10-6. A, Endoluminal view from virtual colonoscopy shows an 8-mm polyp (*arrow*) in the ascending colon. Axial image (**B**) and coronal image (**C**) confirm the presence of a polyp (*arrows*) in the ascending colon.

relevant literature on colon polyps and colon cancer as well as the results of virtual colonoscopy trials. Their recommendations, published in *Radiology*,[9] are summarized in Boxes 10-1 and 10-2; the group recommended that radiologists not report lesions less than 5 mm. This is based on the fact that (1) virtual colonoscopy screening studies show limited sensitivity and specificity for detecting and characterizing these small lesions, (2) most polyps less than 5 mm are hyperplastic, (3) adenomatous polyps less than 5 mm are benign, and (4) only a small percentage of adenomatous polyps less than 5 mm grow and those that do can be safely

detected on the next screening exam.[9] Given these recommendations, radiologists are now reporting only polyps 6 mm or larger.

When a lesion 6 to 9 mm is detected on virtual colonoscopy, most radiologists recommend conventional colonoscopy for biopsy/ removal. However, there is growing evidence that it may be safe to monitor these lesions, since only 30% of polyps in this size range are adenomatous, and even these are almost invariably benign.[9]

Patients with lesions no more than 1 cm are always referred for conventional colonoscopy, because of the significant chance that there

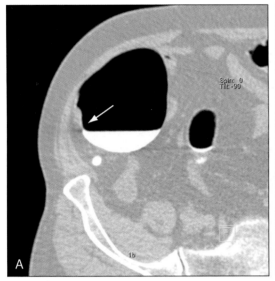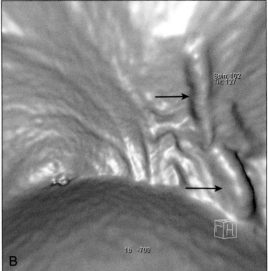

Figure 10-7. A, Axial image from virtual colonoscopy shows a subtle flat lesion (*arrow*) in the cecum. **B,** Endoluminal view confirms the presence of the flat cecal lesion (*arrows*).

Box 10-1. Suggested Feature Descriptors for Polyps and Masses

Lesion Size (mm)—For lesions 6 mm or larger, the single largest dimension of the polyp head (excluding stalk if present) on either multiplanar reconstruction (MPR) or 3D views. The type of view employed for measurement should be stated.

Morphology
- Sessile—broad-based lesion whose width is greater than its vertical height
- Pedunculated—polyp with separate stalk
- Flat—polyp with vertical height less than 3 mm above surrounding normal colonic mucosa

Location
- Refer to named standardized colonic segmental divisions: rectum, sigmoid colon, descending colon, transverse colon, ascending colon, and cecum.

Attenuation
- Soft tissue attenuation
- Fat

From Zalis ME, Barish MA, Choi JR, et al: CT colonography reporting and data system: a consensus proposal. Radiology 236:3–9, 2005.

Box 10-2. Suggested Categorization System for CT Colonography Findings and Follow-up Recommendations

C0. Inadequate Study/Awaiting Prior Comparisons
- Inadequate prep: cannot exclude lesions ≥10 mm owing to presence of fluid feces
- Inadequate insufflations: one or more colonic segments collapsed on both views
- Awaiting prior colon studies for comparison

C1. Normal Colon or Benign Lesion: Continue Routine Screening*
- No visible abnormalities of the colon
- No polyp ≥6 mm
- Lipoma or inverted diverticulum
- Nonneoplastic findings, e.g., colonic diverticula

C2. Intermediate Polyp or Indeterminate Finding: Surveillance or Colonoscopy Recommended[†]
- Intermediate polyp 6–9 mm, <3 in number
- Indeterminate findings, cannot exclude polyp ≥6 mm in technically adequate exam

C3. Polyp, Possibly Advanced Adenoma: Follow-up Colonoscopy Recommended
- Polyp ≥10 mm
- ≥3 polyps, each 6–9 mm

C4. Colonic Mass, Likely Malignant: Surgical Consultation Recommended[‡]
- Lesion compromises bowel lumen, demonstrates extracolonic invasion

*Every 5–10 years.
[†]Evidence suggests surveillance can be delayed at least 3 years, subject to individual patient circumstance.
[‡]Communicate to referring physician as per accepted guidelines for communication, such as ACR Practice Guideline for Communication: Diagnostic Radiology. Subject to local practice, endoscopic biopsy may be indicated.
From Zalis ME, Barish MA, Choi JR, et al: CT colonography reporting and data system: a consensus proposal. Radiology 236:3–9, 2005.

---

is high-grade dysplasia or carcinoma. It would be ideal if patients with significant findings on virtual colonoscopy could be referred for same-day conventional colonoscopy to avoid having to undergo an additional colon preparation. This, of course, would require timely interpretation of the study by the radiologists as well as cooperation between radiologists and gastroenterologists.

In addition to reporting the colonic findings, it is essential that the entire examination be reviewed and all extracolonic findings reported. In a study of extracolonic findings published by Hellstrom and colleagues[10] in the *American Journal of Roentgenology* in 2004, the review of extracolonic structures in patients undergoing virtual colonoscopy contributed to the detection of major, previously unknown disorders in 13% of patients.

Current Controversies

There has been some recent discussion in the literature with regard to who should be interpreting the colonoscopy exams. It is clear that abdominal and CT radiologists have developed the technique over the last 10 years and have the most experience. However, now that the virtual colonoscopy is well established and given the promising results in large screening trials as well as the potential for coverage by insurance companies, gastroenterologists are taking interest. The American Gastroenterological Association is now preparing training courses for gastroenterologists.

Obviously, gastroenterologists are well experienced in conventional colonoscopy and therefore may think that it would be reasonable for them to be able to interpret a virtual colonoscopy exam rather than radiologists. However, the CT virtual colonoscopy exam is basically a high-resolution CT scan of the abdomen and pelvis in which special software is used for reviewing the colon. The interpreting physician—whether a radiologist or gastroenterologist—needs to understand CT physics, radiation safety, and CT anatomy and pathology. The literature is clear that in 10% to 13% of patients undergoing virtual colonoscopy, significant findings will be present on the CT, outside of the colon. These extracolonic findings need to be reported in addition to the colon findings. Therefore, it makes sense for the reviewing physician to be able to review and interpret the entire study.

In my opinion, the radiologist should be the reviewing physician. However, to develop a successful program, radiologists and gastroenterologists need to work together to provide a comprehensive colon cancer screening program that includes both conventional and virtual colonoscopy.

Reimbursement Issues

In 2008 some carriers started to pay for symptomatic patients in whom conventional colonoscopy has not been successful or for patients for whom conventional colonoscopy may not be safe (e.g., those with coagulopathy, on anticoagulation, with drug allergies, or patients who cannot be safely sedated). For virtual colonoscopy to become a viable colon cancer screening option, it needs to be covered by insurance companies. In May 2009, CMS/Medicare issued a decision stating that the evidence is not sufficient to conclude that screening CT colonography would be beneficial for the Medicare population at this time. They encourage more research specifically addressing the Medicare population. Therefore, Medicare will not reimburse for screening CT colonography. However, other private insurance companies are stating to pay for CT colonography for screening.

Future Directions

Investigators are now evaluating image stool subtraction software, which combines thresholding, expansion, and convolution in an attempt to study the feasibility of performing virtual colonoscopy without the need for colonic cleansing. In a recent pilot study by Johnson and colleagues[11] using phantoms and patients, investigators concluded that laxative-free colon examination using barium for stool labeling could be performed with high accuracy with or without stool subtraction. However, further study is needed. When virtual colonoscopy is perfected, it will have a major advantage over conventional colonoscopy and will remove a major barrier to colon cancer screening.

A new method of reviewing the CT colonoscopy data called *virtual dissection* is being studied, but has not been validated.[12] In this method, the 3D model of the colon is unrolled and opened so it resembles a gross pathologic specimen. This technique has the potential to reduce interpretation times by allowing more rapid review of the 3D specimen and eliminating the need to fly forward and backward. However, this technique can distort colon lesions and normal pathology and therefore has not yet been accepted as a validated interpretation method.

Computer-aided diagnosis algorithms can be applied to virtual colonoscopy datasets and are now available from most vendors as a secondary reading tool.[13] It is designed as a second look to be reviewed after the radiologist has completed his/her review. The sensitivity and specificity of computer-aided diagnosis programs vary from vendor to vendor. As these programs are improved, they will likely be accepted as a "second read" and will be used in a similar fashion to the programs used in mammography.

Conclusions

Virtual colonoscopy has made significant improvements over the past 10 years. It is slowly being accepted as a potential colon cancer screening tool. Reimbursement issues are now being revised by major carriers. It is clear that radiologists and gastroenterologists will need to work together in order to determine which patients will benefit most from virtual colonoscopy as opposed to conventional colonoscopy.

References

1. Rex DK, Vining D, Kopecky KK: An initial experience with screening for colon polyps using spiral CT with and without CT colography (virtual colonoscopy). Gastrointest Endosc 50: 309–313, 1999.
2. Pickhardt PJ, Choi JR, Hwang I, et al: Computed tomographic virtual colonoscopy to screen for colorectal neoplasia in asymptomatic adults. N Engl J Med 349:2191–2200, 2003.
3. Cotton PB, Durkalski VL, Pineau BC, et al: Computed tomographic colonography (virtual colonoscopy): a multicenter comparison with standard colonoscopy for detection of colorectal neoplasia. JAMA 291:1713–1719, 2004.
4. Rockey DC, Koch J, Yee J, et al: Prospective comparison of air-contrast barium enema and colonoscopy in patients with fecal occult blood: a pilot study. Gastrointest Endosc 60:953–958, 2004.
5. Johnson CD, Chen MH, Toledano AY, et al: Accuracy of CT colonography for detection of large adenomas and cancers. N Engl J Med 359:1207–1217, 2008.
6. Yee J, Hung RK, Akerkar GA, Wall SD: The usefulness of glucagon hydrochloride for colonic distention in CT colonography. AJR Am J Roentgenol 173:169–172, 1999.
7. Morrin MM, Farrell RJ, Keogan MT, et al: CT colonography: colonic distention improved by dual positioning but not intravenous glucagon. Eur Radiol 12:525–530, 2002.
8. Hara AK, Johnson CD, Reed JE, et al: Reducing data size and radiation dose for CT colonography. AJR Am J Roentgenol 168:1181–1184, 1997.
9. Zalis ME, Barish MA, Choi JR, et al: CT colonography reporting and data system: a consensus proposal. Radiology 236:3–9, 2005.
10. Hellstrom M, Svensson MH, Lasson A: Extracolonic and incidental findings on CT colonography (virtual colonoscopy). AJR Am J Roentgenol 182:631–638, 2004.
11. Johnson KT, Carston MJ, Wentz RJ, et al: Development of a cathartic-free colorectal cancer screening test using virtual colonoscopy: a feasibility study. AJR Am J Roentgenol 188: W29–W36, 2007.
12. Silva AC, Wellnitz CV, Hara AK: Three-dimensional virtual dissection at CT colonography: unraveling the colon to search for lesions. Radiographics 26:1669–1686, 2006.
13. Taylor SA, Halligan S, Burling D, et al: Computer-assisted reader software versus expert reviewers for polyp detection on CT colonography. AJR Am J Roentgenol 186:696–702, 2006.

Preoperative Evaluation

11

Jerry Stonemetz, Nicole A. Phillips, and Susan L. Gearhart

KEY POINTS

- Several models for comprehensive preoperative assessment exist to assist the multidisciplinary team in the perioperative management of patients.
- Preoperative risk assessment and testing can be streamlined to ensure that the multidisciplinary team is providing efficient and safe care of their patients.
- Guidelines exist to assist the multidisciplinary team in the prevention of common postoperative complications, including venous thromboembolic events and surgical site infections.
- Several methods of pain control exist and should be utilized to provide optimal postoperative pain management.

Preoperative Preparation

The preoperative period is a critical time for the collection and collation of pertinent patient information that is relevant and necessary for any patient scheduled for surgery. Much of this information is important for the appropriate planning of resources and disposition of patients. For example, if patient comorbidity requires postoperative intensive care unit (ICU) monitoring, this information is useful because it is acquired proactively without waiting for the day of surgery for determination. Comprehensive collection of preoperative laboratory studies, tests, and consultant notes are critical for smooth workflow on the day of surgery, thus greatly reducing delays, cancellations, and frustration for all, including patients. The following four major types of preoperative models are in use today. (A more complete description of these models can be found in *Preoperative Systems* by Young and Gibby.[1])

1. *Surgeon's office evaluation and triage.* Typically, the surgeon's office has the sole responsibility for ordering specific preoperative tests, lab studies, and/or coordinating consultant evaluations. Not uncommonly, the surgeon may carry out "shot-gun" testing of patients to preclude surgical delays due to missing lab studies or tests—a common source of unnecessary lab testing.[2] In addition, even when the surgeon hand-carries information to the operating room, delays are common because this information is not available for review by anesthesia staff before the day of surgery. Faxing this information into the operating room or similar chart area is fraught with missing documentation and is a common source of frustration.

2. *Preoperative phone triage.* In this setting, hospital nurses most commonly telephone patients directly to capture health history. Under ideal situations, these nurses have had special training and work with the anesthesia team to identify high-risk or special-needs patients who can be allocated into alternative care plans or coordinated care that is more effectively accomplished before the day of surgery. Problems with this approach are dependency on patient information and the high costs associated with staffing nurses for this role. Surgical planning is typically independent and is managed predominantly through the operating room scheduling system that governs equipment and personnel.

3. *Nurse-managed preoperative clinics.* In a specific clinic typically within the hospital environment, patients may be required to visit to provide histories and some components of the physical exam. Frequently, lab tests and other tests are performed at these clinics and have been shown to reduce unnecessary

testing[3] and improve patient satisfaction.[4] Again, the high costs of staffing and managing preclude thorough dissemination of these clinics. Though more comprehensive than the telephone triage system, these clinics may be inconvenient for patients who do not need or want another visit to the hospital.

4. *Computerized physician-run clinics.* In a small minority of clinics, patients are required to complete a full history and questionnaire online, which feeds a specific rules-based engine that helps guide the triage process and may guide preoperative testing and consultations. An example of this type of clinic is the Cleveland Clinic, which has created a preoperative clinic manned by physicians and physician extenders. Each patient must complete a thorough questionnaire online, and if the patient is unable to interact with the system, the surgeon's office is responsible for guiding the patient through the process. This type of clinic appears to be a distinct possibility in the future because it helps to define preoperative testing based on evidence-based guidelines, thus reducing unnecessary testing and more effectively triaging patients to appropriate caregivers.

Effective preoperative preparation essentially helps to establish appropriate risk stratification of patients. Waiting until the day of surgery to define surgical risk stratification is too late. Creating specific care plans requires careful assignment to appropriate risk stratagems; presently even most pay-for-performance measures are pushing all providers to identify at-risk patients. It is impossible to adequately allocate patients into appropriate risk classification without an assessment of patient comorbidities as well as recognized surgical risk categories. The American Society of Anesthesia (ASA) has established a risk stratification system based on medical conditions that have intermediate benefit in proactively identifying a patient's surgical risk. Referred to as the ASA classification system, patients are classified from ASA I to ASA VI (Table 11-1). Unfortunately, this classification is very subjective and has not been shown to be extremely effective in assigning risk.[5] An alternative risk model was proposed by Pasternak[6] and defines five categories of risk based on predicted blood loss. Neither of these two categories has ever been demonstrated to correlate

Table 11-1. American Society of Anesthesia Classification System

ASA	Definition
I	Primarily healthy patients with no existing comorbid conditions; typically taking no medications and very active physically.
II	Patients with well-controlled medical problems. This may include patients on no medications but who are obese or smoke cigarettes. No acute exacerbations of their medical conditions prior to surgery.
III	Patients with established medical conditions that are not well controlled. May also include patients with multiple medical conditions such as patients with a previous myocardial infarction, diabetes, obesity, and renal insufficiency.
IV	Patients with extensive medical problems who have a definitive possibility of not surviving this operation or hospitalization.
V	Patients who are moribund and for whom heroic surgery may be the only option.
VI	Brain-dead organ harvest patients. No chance of survival.

with outcomes, but for purposes of risk stratification, some methodology is required. Most colorectal surgery should qualify as being associated with intermediate risk; however, certain patients may in fact have high surgical risk, particularly those with major vascular involvement. Patients' medical comorbidities are not as simply defined. The presence of major cardiac, pulmonary, renal, or other organ dysfunction has serious implications regarding the postoperative outcomes of patients. The next section identifies and discusses specific concerns regarding particular systems:

One of the authors (JS) has created a preoperative roadmap that has been deployed at the Johns Hopkins Medical Institutions and that provides some guidance for surgeons regarding how to order preoperative testing as well as how to determine which patients should be seen in a preoperative evaluation clinic (PEC). This roadmap contains sections that define generic testing guidelines (Box 11-1). Additional recommendations based on types of comorbidities are provided in Table 11-2. This roadmap also has recommendations regarding which medications to hold versus medications to instruct patients to take on the morning of surgery (Table 11-3). More and more often, we are advocating that

Box 11-1. Recommended Testing for All Patients Scheduled for Low- or Intermediate-Risk Surgery

Do

- Hb/HCT (hemoglobin/hematocrit) on any menstruating female. For minor procedures on healthy patients, Hb may be checked on the morning of surgery.
- Urine pregnancy test on any menstruating female on the morning of surgery.
- Electrocardiogram on any patient older than 50, unless a previous normal tracing is provided within 1 year. For a patient with a cardiac history or whose previous tracing is remarkable for abnormal findings, then a comparison tracing is required within 1 month of surgery.

Do Not

- No chest x-ray unless a history of pulmonary dysfunction with no previous chest x-ray for 1 year.
- No PT/PTT (prothrombin time/partial thromboplastin time) except in patient with a history of bleeding or easy bruising. If ordering these tests, order only PT, not PTT (reserved for patients on heparin).

patients take their morning medications before surgery, specifically medications such as cardiac medication, statins, and proton pump inhibitors. Other medications such as oral hypoglycemic agents are currently being recommended to be held on the morning of surgery. In fact, one of the new Surgical Care Improvement Project (SCIP) measures targets the administration of beta blockers within 24 hours of surgery to patients currently taking these medications.[7]

Specific Medical Considerations

Cardiac Risk

The risks of intra- or postoperative cardiac morbidity are associated with the type of surgery being conducted. According to guidelines established by the American Heart Association (AHA), abdominal surgeries are classified as intermediate-risk procedures.[8] Of more importance than the type of surgery being considered, however, is the individual's complex medical history, physical capacity, and the circumstances under which the surgery is to be performed. Patients with major cardiovascular risk include those with current or recent ischemic heart disease, significant arrhythmias, or severe vascular disease. In some cases, these factors may prove too significant to pursue a surgical course, and alternative treatment methods should be considered. Patients with an intermediate level of cardiovascular risk can be classified as such through examination of their medical history. Indications of past ischemic heart disease, heart failure, diabetes mellitus, renal insufficiency, or cerebrovascular disease place patients in this

Table 11-2. Medical Conditions with Specific Testing Recommendations

Condition	Testing Recommendation
Diabetes	Fasting basic metabolic profile (BMP); electrocardiogram (ECG) for all patients older than 20 years
Hypertension or cardiac disease	BMP; ECG; consider echocardiography (ECHO), stress test, and/or cardiac evaluation if symptoms significant
Chronic obstructive pulmonary disease	Pulmonary function tests (PFTs) if symptoms are significant
Anemia and/or bleeding history	Heme 8; Consider prothrombin time (PT). Auto-donors need to have hemoglobin/hematocrit (Hb/HCT) after donation (morning of surgery should be adequate)
Liver dysfunction or malnutrition	Comprehensive metabolic profile (CMP), Heme 8, PT
High-risk surgical procedures (major blood loss expected)	Heme 8; CMP, PT; consider ECHO, stress test, and/or cardiac evaluation if medical condition warrants
Poor exercise tolerance	Heme 8; CMP; ECG; primary medical doctor evaluation; consider ECHO, stress test, and/or cardiac evaluation
Morbid obesity	BMP; CMP; ECG; consider ECHO (must rule out pulmonary hypertension), stress test, and/or cardiac evaluation
End-stage renal disease (dialysis patient)	Postdialysis lab tests to include Heme 8 and BMP at a minimum; sodium/potassium (Na/K) on morning of surgery
Pacemaker	*Must be interrogated within 6 months, and have report on chart.* Pacer-dependent patients and those with implantable cardioverter defibrillator (ICD) devices must be interrogated within 3 months. ICD patients need device turned off morning of surgery

Table 11-3. Medications to Hold on Day of Surgery

Class	Medication	Recommendation
Oral hypoglycemic agents	Metformin (Glucophage), pioglitazone (Actos), glyburide, tolazamide (Tolinase), rosiglitazone (Avandia), glimepiride (Amaryl), all others	Hold at least 8 hours before surgery. Recommend holding morning dose on day of surgery
Diuretics	Furosemide (Lasix), hydrochlorothiazide (HCTZ)	Hold on morning of surgery, *unless* prescribed for congestive heart failure (CHF) (CHF patients should take their morning dose of diuretics)
ACE inhibitors/ARBs	Lisinopril, amlodipine/benezepril (Lotrel) captopril, hydrochlorothiazide/benazepril, (Lotensin), fosinopril (Monopril), lisinopril/hydrochlorothiazide (Prinzide), candesartan cilexetil (Atacand), olmesartan medoxomil (Benicar), valsartan (Diovan), irbesartan/hydrochlorothiazide (Avalide)	Hold on morning of surgery, *unless* prescribed for CHF (CHF patients should take their morning dose of medications)
Insulin	NPH, Regular	Hold insulin on morning of surgery. Bring insulin with patient to hospital
Alternative therapies	Herbal supplements	Stop at least 24 hours before surgery

ACE, angiotensin-converting enzyme; ARBs, angiotensin receptor blockers.

intermediate-risk category. Among such patients, beta blockage is recommended for those with ischemic heart disease or for those who present with more than one cardiovascular risk factor.[8,9] Additional cardiac testing may be of benefit in assessing current status and further delineating interventional procedures.[10]

Cardiac testing and cardiologic consultation may also prove necessary for patients presenting without a history of disease but whose physical examination indicates the possibility of undetermined disease or other risk factors. Several of these factors can be assessed directly; advanced age, low functional capacity, and obesity all accompany a low-risk stratification for the patient, which is independent of possible comorbidities.[8] If other previously undiagnosed conditions are discovered on examination, a higher level of risk classification may be assigned. According to AHA guidelines, other factors that should be taken into account include abnormal electrocardiogram (ECG), rhythm other than sinus, history of stroke, and uncontrolled systemic hypertension. Such factors have been classified as minor risk indicators.[8]

Special consideration needs to be given to patients who present for surgery with a history of cardiac stents. It has been clearly demonstrated that these stents are associated with an increased risk of re-thrombosis resulting in myocardial infarction and a high mortality rate.[11]

Current AHA guidelines stipulate that patients with bare metal stents have elective surgery delayed for at least 6 months and for 1 year for those with drug-eluting stents.[8] In addition, these patients need to remain on antiplatelet therapy (81 mg aspirin at a minimum) for the remainder of their lives. This poses a dilemma in that we have typically required aspirin to be stopped at least 1 week before surgery. There have been many case reports of intraoperative and immediate postoperative myocardial infarction in these patients. Consequently, there are strong recommendations that antiplatelet therapy be continued until the day of surgery. If there are concerns about surgical morbidity as a result, a conversation should occur among the surgeon, the patient's cardiologist, and, ideally, the anesthesiologist regarding the appropriate care of these patients. Compromises such as holding aspirin and/or clopidogrel may be reasonable. Primarily, we recommend that clopidogrel be held at least 5 days, possibly 7, since the presence of this drug in the system cannot be reversed. Conversely, we recommend that 81 mg aspirin be continued up to the day of surgery. Exceptions can be made, and stopping 81 mg aspirin even 5 days preoperatively is likely to result in a return of about 50% of platelet function, which should help to control surgical oozing and still provide some antiplatelet benefit. It is probably *more* important that antiplatelet therapy be resumed as soon after surgery as possible—certainly within 24 hours and ideally within 12 hours. This should allow for adequate hemostasis and provide protection from stent thrombosis in addition to potential deep venous thrombosis/pulmonary embolism (DVT/PE).

Pulmonary Risk

It is equally important to consider pulmonary risk factors, since the dangers presented by pulmonary complications have a significant impact on the efficacy of surgical intervention and postoperative recovery.[12] In a recent review of the literature on preoperative risk factors for noncardiothoracic surgery, Smetana and associates[12] presented a comprehensive analysis of pulmonary risk stratification. Of particular interest is their determination that advanced age is a noteworthy predictor of pulmonary risk, independent of the comorbid conditions with which it may be associated. Furthermore, other significant indicators of increased risk for postoperative complications included chronic lung disease, functional dependence, and congestive heart failure. The authors determined that the ASA classification system can also serve as an accurate predictor of pulmonary complications; higher ASA class levels correspond to increased risks of perioperative pulmonary morbidities. It is surprising that obesity was not found to be a factor in the development of significant pulmonary complications, although it is associated with diminished lung volume capacity.[12]

Venous Thrombotic Events

Affecting nearly 25% of all hospitalized patients, DVT hinders the recovery of many surgical patients.[13] PE is considered one of the major causes of preventable deaths in hospitalized patients; as such, care should be taken to assess the patient's risk status with regard to DVT and PE in all potential surgical cases. Furthermore, up to 30% of patients suffering from a venous thrombotic event (VTE) develop post-thrombotic swelling and recurrent DVT.[14] Many clinical risk factors are associated with VTEs, as listed in Box 11-2. Cancer patients face increased risks of VTE. Anaya and Nathens[13] found that among patients facing major oncologic surgery, the risk of DVT is

---

Box 11-2. Common Risk Factors for Venous Thrombotic Events (VTEs)

Surgery
Trauma
Immobility
Malignancy
Previous VTE
Advanced age
Pregnancy and postpartum
Estrogen-containing contraceptives or hormone
    replacement therapy
Selective estrogen receptor modulators
Inflammatory bowel disease
Nephrotic syndrome
Myeloproliferative disease
Paroxysmal nocturnal hemoglobinuria
Obesity
Smoking
Central venous catheterization
Inherited or acquired hypercoagulability
Acute medical illness
Respiratory failure
Heart failure

---

double that of other surgical patients. According to the same study, the risk of fatal PE is approximately three times greater among this patient population than among their cancer-free peers.[14] More specifically, adenocarcinoma of the colon has been perceived in several recent studies to be associated with even higher VTE risk than that of other malignancy types.[15] Furthermore, cancer therapies themselves (hormonal, chemotherapy, and radiation therapy) serve as clinical risk factors for DVT. Because of the pelvic nature of the surgery and the positioning frequently required, the authors indicate a risk of DVT as high as 40% for patients undergoing colorectal cancer surgery.[16] Laparoscopic surgery—although thought to be associated with a higher risk of VTE because of the use of a pneumoperitoneum, which results in decreased venous return—has been shown to result in an equivalent or lower incidence of VTE than open surgery.[16–18] Despite these findings, guidelines for prevention of VTE are the same for laparoscopic or open surgery and are shown in Table 11-4. Adherence to these guidelines has not been shown to have any adverse effects with regard to bleeding. However, specific recommendations regarding epidural catheters and VTE prophylaxis are listed in Table 11-2 as well. Furthermore, the ENOXACAN

Table 11-4. Guidelines for Prevention of Venothrombotic Events (VTEs) in Surgical Patients

Risk Category	Recommended Prophylaxis
Low risk Age <40 years, no risk factors, minor surgery	Aggressive and early mobilization
Moderate risk Presence of *one* of the following • Age 40–60 • Major surgery • Risk factors present	LDUH every 12 hr or LMWH or if bleeding risk GCS and IPC
High risk Age >60 years Age >40 + major surgery + risk factor	LDUH every 8 hr or LMWH or if bleeding risk GCS and IPC
Highest risk Age >40 years + major surgery and: 1. Previous VTE or cancer or hypercoagulable condition 2. Major trauma 3. Spinal cord injury 4. Hip/knee arthroplasty 5. Hip surgery	LMWH (spinal cord injury, trauma) LDUH every 8 hr + GCS/IPC or LMWH + GCS/IPC Consider extended prophylaxis for cancer or spinal cord injury

GCS, graduated compression stockings; IPC, intermittent pneumatic compression; LDUH, low-dose unfractionated heparin; LMWH: low-molecular-weight heparin.

II study demonstrated that extended prophylaxis after surgery for up to 4 weeks may also decrease the incidence of VTE, especially in patients with a known history of VTE.[19]

Bowel Preparation and Surgical Site Infection

Historically, it was thought that a strict bowel cleansing regimen associated with the use of oral antibiotics was necessary to prevent postoperative wound and anastomotic complications. Presently, studies have demonstrated that bowel preparation is not associated with a decreased risk for infectious complications.[20] In fact, performing a left-sided colonic anastomosis in an unprepped bowel is now acceptable. However, for aesthetic reasons, most surgeons request a mechanical bowel preparation for colonic surgery using either Golytely for patients with electrolyte concerns or Fleet Phospho-Soda preparation for those without concern. An additional day of clear liquids before bowel preparation helps with tolerance of the preparation. In addition, an oral antibiotic neomycin and erythromycin base may be given along with the mechanical bowel preparation. Although this practice has led to a decrease in surgical site infection, the oral antibiotic regimen is not well tolerated by patients. Currently, intravenous

antibiotic coverage with a dose of cefoxitin or ampicillin-sulbactam (or a quinolone or monobactam plus metronidazole for the penicillin-allergic patient) is preferentially given within 1 hour before skin incision.[20]

Elective colorectal surgery is considered to be a clean-contaminated procedure in which a hollow viscus has been opened under a controlled circumstance. When compared with a clean procedure, a clean-contaminated procedure is associated with twice the risk of surgical site infection. Other risk factors known to contribute to the development of postoperative surgical site infection include obesity, advanced age, malnutrition, diabetes mellitus, tobacco use, and anemia. In particular recently, perioperative hypothermia and poor glycemic control have been demonstrated to increase the risk of surgical site infection and worsen outcomes in patients with sepsis. In a large randomized trial of critically ill postoperative patients, tight blood glucose control to less than 110 mg/dL with the use of exogenous insulin was associated with a 40% decrease in mortality rate, fewer nosocomial infections, and less organ dysfunction.[21]

Postoperative Analgesia

Perioperative pain control is aimed at the regulation of the pain response initiated by nociceptors throughout the body, and appropriate pain management should be considered during the preoperative planning of surgery. In addition to being one of the National Patient Safety Goals of the Joint Commission,[22] good pain management provides for better surgical outcomes for patients. Nociceptors respond to direct stimuli as well as mediators released during surgical trauma, inflammation, and stress (Fig. 11-1). The mediators known to stimulate nociceptors and implicated in the development of chronic pain, phantom pain, and hypersensitization include prostaglandins, bradykinins, histamine, and serotonin. More important, pain and the subsequent neurogenic inflammation have the same effects as surgical stress. These effects include an increase in heart rate, high blood pressure, increased oxygen consumption, myocardial ischemia, lung injury, and the release of other pro-inflammatory mediators. Once the pain impulse to the brain is activated, descending pain fibers modulate the response. Certain neurotransmitters including opioids bind to receptors, which results in an inhibition of the perception of painful stimuli and the associated physiologic effects. Therefore, methods of postoperative pain management use opioid analgesia to directly inhibit the pain response and nonopioid analgesia to decrease mediator release from inflammation.

Because most opioid receptors are located within the central nervous system, opioids must be lipid soluble and must cross the blood-brain barrier to have an effect. The dose of opioid analgesia may be escalated to eliminate pain but at the risk of inducing respiratory depression. Presently, opioids are given intravenously or through a catheter placed in the epidural space. The intravenous opioid is given through a pump, which allows administration of a preset dose of medication at a present time interval and is given only when the patient presses the medication button (patient-controlled anesthesia, or PCA). The most common forms of opiates administered through a PCA include morphine, fentanyl, and hydormorphine. Fentanyl is favored over the other two because of its rapid onset and its association with less nausea and vomiting.

Another option for perioperative pain management is regional anesthesia. Epidural catheters, when placed preoperatively, can be used for postoperative pain management. In addition,

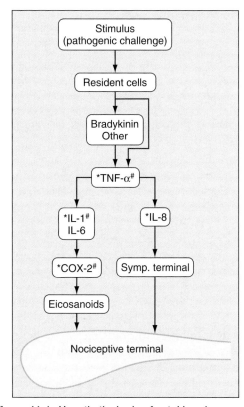

Figure 11-1. Hypothetical role of cytokines in sensitization of nociceptors during inflammation and the underlying putative peripheral mechanisms leading to hyperalgesia. Pathogenic stimuli activate resident cells and lead to release of inflammatory mediators (e.g., bradykinin). Pro-inflammatory cytokines are synthesized and released by macrophages and other immune or immune-related cells. Nociceptors are postulated to be sensitized by two pathways involving the cytokines: (1) Tumor necrosis factor α (TNF-α) induces synthesis and release of interleukin 1 (IL-1) and IL-6, which, in turn, induce the release of eicosanoids (prostaglandin E_2 and I_2 [PGE_2, PGI_2]) by activating cyclooxygenase-2 (COX-2). (2) TNF-α induces synthesis and release of IL-8. IL-8 activates sympathetic terminals that sensitize nociceptors via β_2-adrenergic receptors. Glucocorticoids inhibit the synthesis of the cytokines and the activation of COX-2 (indicated by *). Anti-inflammatory cytokines (e.g., IL-4 and IL-10) that are also synthesized and released by immune cells inhibit the synthesis and release of pro-inflammatory cytokines (indicated by #). This scheme is fully dependent on behavioral experiments and pharmacologic interventions. The different steps need to be verified experimentally using neurophysiologic experiments. Symp. terminal, sympathetic terminal. (From Jänig W: Autonomic nervous system and pain. In Basbaum AI, Kaneko A, Shepherd GM, et al [eds]: The Senses: A Comprehensive Reference, vol. 5, Chapter 17. San Diego: Academic Press, 2008, Figure 12; modified from Poole S, Cunna FQ, Ferreira SH: Hyperalgesia from subcutaneous cytokines. In Watkins LR, Maier SF [eds]: Cytokines and Pain. Basel: Birkhäuser Verlag, 1999, pp 59–87, Figure 8.)

the intraoperative use of this catheter may decrease the amount of anesthetic necessary to perform surgery and, as a result, reduce ileus and postoperative nausea and vomiting.[23] Postoperatively, the administration of analgesia through an epidural catheter is regulated by the patient; however, a continuous low dose is usually provided. Recently, several studies have evaluated the use of regional perfusion catheters placed directly into the wound at the time of surgery. These were found to be a useful adjunct to reducing postoperative pain.[24] When using local anethetics to provide analgesia, it is important to be aware of their adverse reactions, which include cardiac arrhythmias, hypertension, direct tissue toxicity, central nervous system toxicity, methemoglobinemia, and allergic reactions. Arrhythmia associated with the use of local anesthetic can rapidly degenerate into ventricular fibrillation, and care must be taken not to inject any local anesthetic intravascularly. Methemoglobinemia is usually associated with prilocaine, which is a topical anesthetic used in a eutectic mixture of local anesthetic (EMLA) cream or the throat spray benzocaine (Cetacaine). This condition is the result of the high affinity of oxygen for the hemoglobin molecule and results in lack of oxygen dissociation in the periphery with resulting cyanosis. Methylene blue reduces the ferric ion to the ferrous form, thereby allowing for oxygen to dissociate. This must be administered immediately in doses of 1 to 2 mg/kg.

Nonopioid analgesia can be separated into two categories: nonsteroidal anti-inflammatory drugs (NSAIDs) and acetaminophen. NSAIDs are useful for the treatment of mild to moderate pain. The most infamous of the NSAIDs are the cyclooxygenase 2 (COX-2) inhibitors. COX-2 is produced during inflammation and serves as the enzyme for production of prostaglandins that mediate pain and fever. Unlike COX-1, COX-2 has no gastrointestinal side effects. Unfortunately, COX-2 inhibitors have been associated with adverse cardiovascular events, including myocardial infarction and cerebrovascular accident,[25] and these inhibitors are no longer available for use. For perioperative pain, intravenous ketorolac is a nonselective COX inhibitor that can be given intravenously and is a useful adjunct to opioid analgesia. The adverse effects of ketorolac include nephrotoxicity and bleeding. In addition, acetaminophen has an excellent

safety profile and is often used for its antipyretic effects.

On discharge, oral analgesia is provided with either oxycodone or hydrocodone. These are usually used in conjunction with acetaminophen to reduce inflammation. Oxycodone and hydrocodone are effective in mild to moderate pain and can be dosed either every 4 hours or in a longer-acting form of oxycodone, every 12 hours.

Conclusion

The preoperative evaluation of the patient with primary colorectal cancer is essential in the surgical management of this disease. Information regarding the stage of the disease may assist the surgeon in determining the best course of therapy. Details of the patient's history and physical exam can be useful in preparing the patient for surgery in the hope of achieving the best outcome. Careful discussion of the expectation of the surgery and perioperative care are essential for preparing the patient for his cancer treatment.

References

1. Young D, Gibby G: Preoperative systems. In Stonemetz J, Ruskin K (eds): Anesthesia Informatics. New York: Springer, 2008, pp 167–189.
2. Smetana GW, Macpherson DS: The case against routine preoperative laboratory testing. Med Clin North Am 87:7–40, 2003.
3. Tsen LC, Segal S, Pothier M, et al: The effect of alterations in a preoperative assessment clinic on reducing the number and improving the yield of cardiology consultations. Anesth Analg 95(6):1563–1568, 2002.
4. Hepner DL, Bader AM, Hurwitz S, et al:. Patient satisfaction with preoperative assessment in a preoperative assessment testing clinic. Anesth Analg 98:1099–1105, 2004.
5. Macario A, Vitez TS, Dunn B, et al: Hospital costs and severity of illness in three types of elective surgery. Anesthesiology 86:92–100, 1997.
6. Pasternak LR: Preoperative assessment: guidelines and challenges. Acta Anaesthesiol Scand Suppl 111:318–320, 1997.
7. Quality Net web site,. http://www.qualitynet.org/dcs/Content Server?cid=1147977084781&pagename=Medqic%2FMeasure %2FMeasureTemplate&c=Measure. Accessed November 20, 2008.
8. Fleisher LA, Beckman JA, Brown KA, et al: ACC/AHA 2007 Guidelines on Perioperative Cardiovascular Evaluation and Care for Noncardiac Surgery: a report of the American College of Cardiology/American Heart Association Task Force on Practice Guidelines (Writing Committee to Revise the 2002 Guidelines on Perioperative Cardiovascular Evaluation for Noncardiac Surgery). J Am Coll Cardiol 50:159–241, 2007.
9. Maddox T: Preoperative cardiovascular evaluation for noncardiac surgery. Mt Sinai J Med 72(3):185–192, 2005.
10. Schouten O, Bax J, Poldermans D: Assessment of cardiac risk before noncardiac general surgery. Heart 92:1866–1872, 2006.
11. Nuttall GA, Brown MJ, Stombaugh JW, et al: Time and cardiac risk of surgery after bare-metal stent percutaneous coronary intervention. Anesthesiology 109(4):588–595, 2008.
12. Smetana G, Lawrence V, Cornell J: Preoperative pulmonary risk stratification for noncardiothoracic surgery: systemic review for the American College of Physicians. Ann Intern Med 144(8): 581–595, 2006.

13. Anaya D, Nathens A: Thrombosis and coagulation: deep vein thrombosis and pulmonary embolism prophylaxis. Surg Clin North Am 85(6):1163–1177, ix–x, 2005.

14. Cinello M, Nucifora G, Bertolissi M, et al: American College of Cardiology/American Heart Association perioperative assessment guidelines for noncardiac surgery reduces cardiologic resource utilization preserving a favourable clinical outcome. J Cardiovasc Med (Hagerstown) 8(11):882–888, 2007.

15. Borly L, Willie-Jorgensen P, Rasmussen MS: Systemic review of thromboprophylaxis in colorectal surgery—an update. Colorectal Dis 7(2):122–127, 2005.

16. Catheline JM, Turner R, Gaillard JL, et al: Thromboembolism in laparoscopic surgery: risk factors and prevention measures. Surg Laparosc Endosc Percutan Tech 9(2):135–139, 1999.

17. Lindberg F, Bergqvist D, Rasmussen I: Incidence of thromboembolic complications after laparoscopic cholecystectomy: review of the literature. Surg Laparosc Endosc Percutan Tech 7(4): 324–331, 1997.

18. White RH, Zhou H, Romano PS: Incidence of symptomatic venous thromboembolism after different elective or urgent surgical procedures. Thromb Haemost 90(3):446–455, 2003.

19. Bergqvist D, Agnelli G, Cohen AT, et al: Duration of prophylaxis against venous thromboembolism with enoxaparin after surgery for cancer. N Engl J Med 346(13):975–980, 2002.

20. Lewis RT: Oral vs. systemic antibiotic prophylaxis in elective colon surgery: a randomized study and meta-analysis send a message from the 1990's. Can J Surg 45:173–180, 2002.

21. van den Berghe G, Wouters P, Weekers F, et al: Intensive insulin therapy in the critically ill patients. N Engl J Med 345: 1359–1367, 2001.

22. The Joint Commission. 2008 National Patient Safety Goals (NPSGs). http://www.jointcommission.org/PatientSafety/NationalPatientSafetyGoals. Accessed December 4, 2008.

23. Holte K, Kehlet H: Effect of postoperative epidural analgesia on surgical outcome. Minerva Anesthesiol 68(4):157–161, 2002.

24. Schurr MJ, Gordon DB, Pellino TA, Scanlon TA: Continuous local anesthetic infusion for pain management after outpatient inguinal herniorrhaphy. Surgery 136(4):761–769, 2004.

25. Drazen JM: Cox-2 inhibitors—a lesson in unexpected problems. N Engl J Med 352(11):1092–1102, 2005.

12 Limited Resection: Indications, Techniques, and Outcomes of Transanal Excision and Transanal Endoscopic Microsurgery

Elizabeth C. Wick

KEY POINTS

- Local excision is applicable in a select subset with early rectal cancer.
- Meticulous preoperative staging, including endorectal ultrasound and magnetic resonance imaging (MRI), is important for patient selection.
- Unexpected findings on the final pathology report such as higher T level or lymph node involvement may warrant immediate radical resection in medically fit patients.
- Close follow-up after local excision is important. Local recurrences usually occur within 2 years.
- Salvage surgery after local or distant recurrence is frequently challenging and associated with poor prognosis.

Introduction

Total mesorectal excision is the standard operation for rectal cancer. In this procedure referred to as *radical resection* in this chapter, the rectum is excised together with the mesorectum, which contains lymphatic tissue draining the rectum.[1] More proximal rectal tumors (upper and mid rectum) can be removed by an anterior resection of the rectum with sphincter preservation. However, very distal rectal tumors may require an abdominal perineal resection with permanent colostomy to achieve a wide excision of the tumor. Patients who undergo radical resection of stage I rectal cancers can expect excellent long-term results (4.5% 5-year local recurrence rate and 90% 5-year disease-free survival rate).[2] However, anterior and abdominal perineal resections of the rectum constitute major abdominal surgery and thus carry risk of postoperative mor-

bidity and mortality including anastomotic leak, which could require re-operation; injury to pelvic nerves leading to sexual and/or urinary dysfunction; and the chance of suboptimal long-term bowel function (clustering of bowel movements and incomplete evacuation). Local excision of the tumor is an attractive alternative to radical resection for early rectal cancer because (1) it is a more straightforward surgical procedure, (2) it preserves bowel function, and (3) it carries less risk of perioperative morbidity. Nevertheless, the role of local excision in the treatment of rectal cancer continues to be debated. During the past 10 years, a series of retrospective studies has reported higher than expected rates of pelvic recurrences after local excision of rectal tumors.[2-5] There is concern about the adequacy of the local excision as a cancer operation because the procedure addresses only the primary tumor and does not assess for lymphatic spread by removing the regional lymph nodes. In addition, because of the nature of the procedure, locally excised rectal tumors frequently have closer margins and are more prone to spillage of tumor cells into the surgical field. Thus, at this time, local excision is best suited for selected early rectal cancer (T1N0)—tumors associated with a low risk of lymphatic spread.

Local excision is sometimes used to treat patients with more advanced tumors (T2 and T3), but these patients generally have medical comorbidities that make radical excision risky, or they adamantly desire sphincter preservation for very low rectal cancers. Neoadjuvant and adjuvant chemotherapy and radiation therapy treatments continue to improve, and this has prompted interest in using local excision combined with concurrent neoadjuvant chemoradiation to treat certain T2 rectal cancer. At this time, local excision of T2 tumors should be considered only in the setting of a clinical trial.

Long-term Outcomes After Local Excision

The procedure of local excision gained momentum after Morson and colleagues[6] (1977) reported that radical resection and local excision have similar oncologic results. During the past decade a number of centers have retrospectively reviewed their results with local excision for rectal cancer and discovered higher than anticipated rates of local recurrence and lower than anticipated rates of long-term survival (Table 12-1). Although the studies have been limited by the sample size and heterogeneity of the study population, by variable preoperative staging strategies, and by disparate surgical technique, the results have curbed some of the enthusiasm for local excision. To date, there has been no prospective comparison of local excision and radical resection for early rectal cancer. However, in the retrospective studies comparing local excision with radical resection, local excision of T1 and T2 rectal cancer is found to be associated with higher rates of pelvic recurrences, At this time, however, it is not clear whether this ultimately influences 5-year survival rates. Based on retrospective studies with variable follow-up of T1 and T2 cancers, local recurrence rates range from 7% to 18% and from 13% to 37%. In T1 and T2 cancers, disease-free survival rates range from 77% to 93% and from 63% to 87%, respectively.

Analysis of the available studies demonstrates that local excision incurs a higher risk of pelvic recurrence, and the trend is toward decreased 5-year disease-free survival after local excision. Nevertheless, the difference between local excision and radical resection with respect to disease-free survival is less clear-cut.

Patient Selection

Local excision is appropriate treatment for tumors limited to the rectal wall without evidence of lymph node metastasis. Curative local excision hinges on patient selection. Tumors that have microscopically spread to the perirectal fat or lymphatics are inadequately treated by local excision alone. At present, the most accurate way to predict tumor spread to the lymphatic tissue is depth of invasion of the primary tumor. Unfortunately, this information is available only after excision. The goals of preoperative staging in patients under consideration for local excision are (1) to identify early rectal cancers that are limited to the bowel with no lymphatic involvement and (2) to determine technical feasibility of the procedure.

First, digital examination is used to determine the mobility of the tumor, the distance from the anal verge, and the strength of the internal and external anal sphincter. An immobile, fixed tumor predicts invasion through the bowel wall. After digital examination, the proctoscope is inserted to document the tumor size

Table 12-1. Outcomes After Local Excision of T1 and T2 Rectal Cancer

Study (Year)	Number of Patients	5-Year Local Recurrence (%)	5-Year Disease-free Survival (%)
T1 Rectal Cancer			
Chakravarti et al (1999)[20]	44	11	80
Steele et al (1999)[5]	59	7	87
Garcia-Aguilar (2000)[3]	55	18	77
Paty et al (2002)[4]	45	14	92
You et al (2007)[21]	601	12.5	77.4
T2 Rectal Cancer			
Garcia-Aguilar (2000)[3]	27	37	55
Paty et al (2002)[4]	51	28	87
You et al (2007)[21]	164	22.1	67.6

Box 12-1. Criteria for Local Excision

Physical Examination

Tumor < 4 cm in diameter

Tumor < 40% bowel circumference

Tumor within 10 cm of dentate line (<5 cm for transanal excision and 5–10 cm for TEM)

Tumor freely mobile on digital rectal exam

Imaging (EUS/MRI)

Tumor limited to submucosa (T1)

No lymph node involvement

EUS, endoscopic ultrasonography; MRI, magnetic resonance imaging; TEM, transanal endoscopic microsurgery.
From Greenberg J, Bleday R: Local excision of rectal cancer. Clin Colon Rect Surg 16(1):40–46, 2005.

and distance from the dentate line. This determines whether local excision is technically feasible. Tumors best suited for local excision are smaller than 4 cm in diameter and involve less than 40% of the rectal wall. Distance from the anal verge is important for determining whether transanal techniques are adequate for resection or whether transanal endoscopic microsurgery (TEM) excision should be considered. Proximal tumors can be challenging to excise through the transanal approach. Frequently, radical resection can be accomplished with sphincter preservation in these proximal cancers, and thus the benefits of local excision may not outweigh the increased risk of local recurrence after local excision. General criteria for local excision are listed in Box 12-1.

Radiology studies complement physical examination in the preoperative planning evaluation of low tumors. Computed tomography (CT) scan and conventional magnetic resonance imaging (MRI) can identify metastatic disease and tumor infiltration into the perirectal fat but do not have fine resolution to discern the depth of tumor invasion into the bowel wall or involvement of mesenteric lymph nodes and are not part of the *local staging* of rectal cancer. Endorectal ultrasound (ERUS) and MRI with an endorectal coil provide detailed images of the rectal wall and perirectal fat and can reliably predict the T and N stage of the tumor. A meta-analysis of ERUS and MRI reported that ERUS accurately predicted T and N stage in 90% and 67% of cases, respectively, whereas MRI was correct in 82% and 66% of cases.[7] The accuracy of ERUS in particular is operator dependent. Despite clinical and radiologic staging to the contrary, up to 14% of T1 and 23% of T2 tumors have occult lymph node metastasis found at the time of radical resection.[8] We can expect that, as radiologic staging techniques are refined, more occult lymphatic metastases will be discovered preoperatively. In the interim, a system of substratification of T1 lesions based on certain pathologic features noted on biopsy slides has been devised to identify T1 tumors with a high risk of lymphatic involvement. Lymphatic or vascular invasion, high-grade histology, and poor cellular differentiation on the biopsy specimen portend a more aggressive tumor and a greater probability of lymph node metastases. Thus, tumors with these findings are generally better suited for radical resection. Furthermore, for sessile tumors, the Kikuchi classification stratifies T1 rectal cancers based on the depth of submucosal invasion: sm1, sm2, sm3 (Fig. 12-1). Each level correlates with increased frequency of lymph node involvement (sm1: 1%–3%; sm2: 8%; sm3: 23%).[9] Given the high likelihood of lymph node involvement, sm3 lesions should generally be treated with radical resection. sm1 lesions are well suited to local excision, but sm2 lesions with ominous characteristics such as poor differentiation or lymphatic invasion may be better served with radical resection.

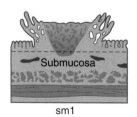
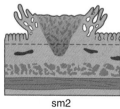
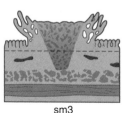

sm1　　　　sm2　　　　sm3

Figure 12-1. Depth of submucosal invasion in malignant polyps. (From Nivatvongs S: Surgical management of malignant colorectal polyps. Surg Clin North Am 82:1052–1055, 2000, Fig. 2.)

Operative Techniques

Transanal Excision

Currently, transanal excision is the most common technique to locally excise rectal cancers. Older techniques included transcoccygeal and transphincteric resections, but they have fallen out of favor because of associated morbidity (postoperative fistulas and fecal incontinence, respectively). Transanal excision is undertaken with the intent of excising the tumor with (1) a 1- to 2-cm margin circumferentially and (2) a full-thickness rectal wall (perirectal fat should be visible after the specimen is excised) (Fig. 12-2). The patient receives a mechanical bowel preparation before the procedure, and, depending on the location of the tumor, the patient can be placed either in lithotomy (posterior tumors) or prone (anterior or posterior tumors) position. An anal retractor is used to dilate the anus to facilitate access to the lesion; exposure can be enhanced with a ring and hook retractor (Lone Star Retractor, Lone Star Medical Products, Stafford, Texas).

The intended 1-cm resection margin is marked with cautery before beginning the excision. Stay sutures are placed on the four quadrants of what will be the residual defect to help with closing the defect. When the tumor is removed, it should be pinned and oriented for the pathologist. Usually, the defect should be closed transversely to prevent obstructing or narrowing the rectal lumen with the closure. Postoperative complications are infrequent after transanal excision; the most common complication is urinary tract infection. Rarely, rectovaginal fistula (after the resection of an anterior tumor), rectal stricture, local sepsis, and fecal incontinence can occur.

Transanal Endoscopic Microsurgery

Originally developed for the management of benign rectal tumors, transanal endoscopic microsurgery (TEM) is increasingly being used in the management of early rectal cancers. It has expanded the number of tumors eligible for local excision, since TEM improves visibility and allows transanal access to tumors up to 20 cm from the anal verge. Buess and colleagues[10] introduced TEM in 1983 with a specially designed rectoscope manufactured by Wolff (Knittlingen, Germany). Currently, an operating rectoscope (12 or 20 cm long and 4 cm in diameter) is used with a high-quality binocular magnifying system (×6) faceplate (Fig. 12-3). The system allows for up to 10 mm Hg rectal distention. Instruments are introduced via gas-

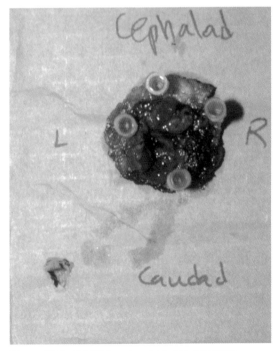

Figure 12-2. Full-thickness rectal tumor specimen oriented for the pathologist.

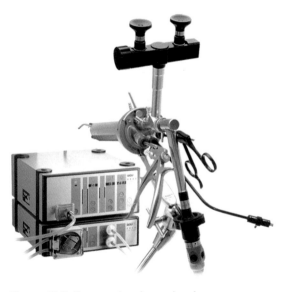

Figure 12-3. Transanal endoscopic microsurgery proctoscope and operating instruments. (Courtesy of Richard Wolf Medical Instruments.)

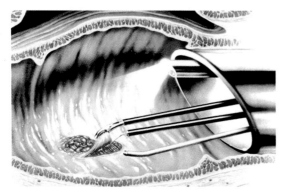

Figure 12-4. Transanal endoscopic microsurgery resection of rectal tumor. Specially designed long graspers and cautery are used to remove tumors. (Courtesy of Richard Wolf Medical Instruments.)

tight operating ports on the faceplate. The resection is done with grasping instruments and cautery (Fig. 12-4). The defect is then closed with a running suture using a specially designed needle driver and metallic clip "anchor" in place of a knot to secure the ends of the suture. Assembly and use of the TEM equipment are complex, and additional training is necessary before starting the procedure. Experience with TEM and rectal cancer is limited. To date, there has been only one randomized, controlled trial comparing TEM with anterior resection for early rectal cancer. Although the study showed no difference in local recurrence or long-term survival between the two treatments, it was limited by small sample size, relatively short follow-up period, and lack of details about the tumors studied.[11]

Radical Resection Immediately After Local Excision

As previously mentioned, it is not infrequent for early rectal cancers to be understaged preoperatively. A T1N0 tumor by ultrasound and MRI may be a T2 or T3 or N1 tumor when the final pathology is evaluated after local excision. In addition, a positive margin on a local excision specimen is strongly associated with rapid recurrence and should be addressed immediately.[4] Radical "re-resection" should be considered in medically fit patients if any of the latter circumstances arise. If done within 30 days after local excision, radical re-resection results are similar to initial radical resection results compared stage by stage.[12]

Follow-up and Salvage Therapy After Local Excision

Most patients (81% in one series) with recurrent rectal cancer are asymptomatic.[13] Thus, close follow-up is important after local excision and should include both physical examination with digital rectal examination and visualization of the scar using a proctoscope. Local recurrence may be extraluminal, probably as a result of tumor cells seeding the perirectal fat at the time of initial resection. ERUS can detect up to one third of patients with local recurrences that were missed by physical examination and proctoscopy.[12] ERUS, MRI, and positron emission tomography (PET) scan should complement the physical and endoscopic examinations as concerning features arise on the physical examination. The appropriate frequency of postoperative imaging has not been established. The follow-up schedule should be more aggressive (every 4 months for 3 years, then every 6 months for 2 years, then yearly) for local excision patients than for radical excision patients.[14]

Pelvic recurrences after local excision of rectal tumors are challenging to identify, and despite close follow-up, there can be significant tumor progression before an abnormality is detected. Many patients with locally recurrent rectal cancer are not candidates for surgical treatment, and patients who are able to be treated surgically with complete excision frequently require extended operations with en bloc resection of adjacent organs. A series from the University of Minnesota reported that only 79% of patients with recurrent disease were able to undergo resection, and only 59% were disease-free at 39 months.[15]

It important to remember when analyzing the results of salvage surgery that early rectal cancers treated with radical resection are associated with up to a 90% chance of 5-year disease-free survival.

Local Excision Followed by Adjuvant Chemoradiation

There has been considerable interest in using adjuvant chemoradiation treatment (the sandwich approach) to improve the disease-free survival and decrease the local recurrence rate after local excision, particularly in patients who have a high-risk pathology, are medically unfit for salvage surgery, or refuse radical resection. In theory, adjuvant therapy addresses some of the drawbacks of local excision: close resection margins and concern for either seeding of tumor cells. Initially, this strategy was described in small retrospective series, and it was difficult to identify a clear benefit from adjuvant therapy. The Cancer and Leukemia Group B (CALGB) organized a multi-institutional prospective study of local excision alone for T1 tumors and local excision followed by adjuvant chemotherapy and radiation for T2 tumors. The results were recently published, and at a median follow-up of 7 years, the local recurrence rate in the T1 group was 7% and in the T2 group 14%—similar to results observed in the earlier single-institution studies but not as good as the outcomes noted after radical resection of early rectal cancers.[16]

Neoadjuvant Chemoradiation Followed by Local Excision

Neoadjuvant therapy decreases pelvic recurrence after radical resection of more advanced rectal cancers (stages II and III). Furthermore, several retrospective series of neoadjuvant therapy followed by local excision for T2 and T3 tumors have observed lower rates of local recurrence than usually seen after local excision alone, but conclusions from these studies are limited by the short patient follow-up.[17,18] This led to increased interest in the use of neoadjuvant chemoradiation to decrease the rate of pelvic recurrences after local excision of early rectal cancers. Currently, the American College of Surgeons Oncology Group (ACOSOG) is completing a phase II study of T2N0 rectal cancer (staged by ERUS or MRI with endorectal coil) to determine whether the neoadjuvant chemoradiation (i.e., oxaliplatin and capecitabine plus radiation for 5 weeks) followed by local excision will be equivalent to the results of radical resection of similar tumors followed in the National Cancer Database.[19] The results of this study may establish a subset of more advanced tumors that can be successfully treated with neoadjuvant therapy followed by local excision with results comparable to radical resection.

Conclusion

Radical surgery affords the best oncologic operation and long-term outcome for early rectal cancer, but the push for sphincter preservation in rectal surgery has led to a renewed interest in local excision for rectal cancer. Local excision has less perioperative morbidity and better long-term bowel function compared with radical excision, but it is associated with a higher risk of local recurrence. Local excision in medically fit patients is appropriate for T1 rectal cancer without aggressive features such as lymphovascular invasion or poor cellular differentiation. At this time, local excision of T2, particularly in combination with neoadjuvant or adjuvant chemoradiation therapy, should be considered only in the setting of a clinical trial. Newer modalities of preoperative imaging and improved neoadjuvant and adjuvant therapies are hoped to expand the indications for local excision for early rectal cancers.

References

1. Heald RJ, Moran BJ, Ryall RD, et al: Rectal cancer: the Basingstoke experience of total mesorectal excision, 1978–1997. Arch Surg 133(8):894–899, 1998.
2. Mellgren A, Sirivongs P, Rothenberger DA, et al: Is local excision adequate therapy for early rectal cancer? Dis Colon Rectum 43(8):1064–1071; discussion 1071–1074, 2000.
3. Garcia-Aguilar J, Mellgren A, Sirivongs P, et al: Local excision of rectal cancer without adjuvant therapy: a word of caution. Ann Surg 231(3):345–351, 2000.
4. Paty PB, Nash GM, Baron P, et al: Long-term results of local excision for rectal cancer. Ann Surg 236(4):522–529; discussion 529–530, 2002.
5. Steele GD Jr, Herndon JE, Bleday R, et al: Sphincter-sparing treatment for distal rectal adenocarcinoma. Ann Surg Oncol 6(5):433–441, 1999.
6. Morson BC, Bussey HJ, Samoorian S: Policy of local excision for early cancer of the colorectum. Gut 18(12):1045–1050, 1977.
7. Kwok H, Bissett IP, Hill GL: Preoperative staging of rectal cancer. Int J Colorectal Dis 15(1):9–20, 2000.
8. Nascimbeni R, Burgart LJ, Nivatvongs S, Larson DR: Risk of lymph node metastasis in T1 carcinoma of the colon and rectum. Dis Colon Rectum 45(2):200–206, 2002.
9. Kikuchi R, Takano M, Takagi K, et al: Management of early invasive colorectal cancer. Risk of recurrence and clinical guidelines. Dis Colon Rectum 38(12):1286–1295, 1995.
10. Saclarides TJ, Smith L, Ko ST, et al: Transanal endoscopic microscopy. Dis Colon Rectum 35(12):1183–1191.
11. Winde G, Nottberg H, Keller R, et al: Surgical cure for early rectal carcinomas (T1). Transanal endoscopic microsurgery vs. anterior resection. Dis Colon Rectum 39(9):969–976, 1996.
12. Hahnloser D, Wolff BG, Larson DW, et al: Immediate radical resection after local excision of rectal cancer: an oncologic compromise? Dis Colon Rectum 48(3):429–437, 2005.
13. de Anda EH, Lee SH, Finne CO, et al: Endorectal ultrasound in the follow-up of rectal cancer patients treated by local excision or radical surgery. Dis Colon Rectum 47(6):818–824, 2004.
14. Garcia-Aguilar J, Cromwell JW, Marra C, et al: Treatment of locally recurrent rectal cancer. Dis Colon Rectum 44(12):1743–1748, 2001.
15. Friel CM, Cromwell JW, Marra C, et al: Salvage radical surgery after failed local excision for early rectal cancer. Dis Colon Rectum 45(7):875–879, 2002.
16. Greenberg JA, Shibata D, Herndon JE Jr, et al: Local excision of distal rectal cancer: an update of cancer and leukemia

group B 8984. Dis Colon Rectum 51(8):1185–1191; discussion 1191–1194, 2008. Epub 2008 June 7.

17. Kim CJ, Yeatman TJ, Coppola D, et al: Local excision of T2 and T3 rectal cancers after downstaging chemoradiation. Ann Surg 234(3):352–358; discussion 358–359, 2001.

18. Schell SR, Zlotecki RA, Mendenhall WM, et al: Transanal excision of locally advanced rectal cancers downstaged using neoadjuvant chemoradiotherapy. J Am Coll Surg 194(5):584–590; discussion 590–591, 2002.

19. American College of Surgeons Oncology Group (ACOSOG). www.acosog.org/studies/index.jsp. Accessed February 13, 2009.

20. Chakravarti A, Compton CC, Shellito PC, et al: Long-term follow-up of patients with rectal cancer managed by local excision with and without adjuvant irradiation. Ann Surg 230(1):49–54, 1999.

21. You YN, Baxter NN, Stewart A, Nelson H: Is the increasing rate of local excision for stage I rectal cancer in the United States justified: a nationwide cohort study from the National Cancer Database. Ann Surg 245(5):726–733, 2007.

13 Endoscopic Techniques in Colorectal Neoplasia

Eun Ji Shin and Samuel A. Giday

KEY POINTS

- Endoscopic techniques that are discussed include endoscopic resection and colonic stenting.
- Endoscopic resections are primarily used in the management of premalignant lesions such as polyps and noninvasive carcinomas (carcinoma in situ and intramucosal carcinomas). Endomucosal resections can be performed in highly selected invasive cancers that have penetrated through the submucosa and are thought to have minimal to no risk of lymph node metastases.
- Endoscopic techniques discussed in this chapter include polypectomy, endoscopic mucosal resection, and endoscopic submucosal dissection.
- Colorectal self-expandable metal stents are an option to allow emergent decompression in patients who present with obstruction. Colonic stents can serve as a bridge intervention to elective surgery by allowing a bowel preparation and then elective resection of the tumor with anastomosis as a single-step procedure.
- Colonic stents also can be used as an effective palliative intervention in patients with end-stage disease and impending obstruction.

Introduction

Treatment modalities for colorectal malignancy used to be the exclusive domain of surgery. However, with the recent development and advancement in the field of therapeutic endoscopy, gastroenterologists have played an increasingly larger role in the treatment of colorectal neoplasia. This chapter focuses on two endoscopic modalities—endoscopic resection and colonic stenting—which are aimed at the opposite spectrum of the colorectal malignancy management. Endoscopic resection is intended as a treatment modality for the premalignant precursors (polyps) and early superficial stages of colorectal neoplasia, whereas the colonic stent is focused on the management of devastating sequelae of the later stages of colorectal cancer, that is, colonic obstruction.

Endoscopic Resection

Endoscopic resection is gaining increasing acceptance as a viable management option for early gastrointestinal malignancy. For the purpose of this chapter, early gastrointestinal malignancy refers to lesions confined within the submucosal layer with no or low risk of lymph node metastasis, such that the endoscopic resection is potentially curative, obviating the need for more invasive surgical therapy.[1]

Superficial lesions have been classified into three main types by the Japanese Gastric Cancer Association: type I polypoid, type II nonpolypoid and nonexcavated, and type III nonpolypoid with an ulcer. Type I lesions are further subclassified into type Ip (pedunculated) and type Is (sessile) lesions. Type II lesions are further subclassified into type IIa (slightly elevated), type IIb (completely flat), and type IIc (slightly depressed) lesions.[1] In general, type IIc lesions tend to be more invasive at smaller tumor size when compared with type IIa lesions. Furthermore, the larger diameter of type II lesions is associated with deeper depth of invasion.

Submucosal lesions in the colon are divided into sm1, sm2, and sm3 lesions, based on depth of invasion. Submucosal lesions in the upper third sector (sm1) are further subdivided into a, b, and c, based on the horizontal spread of the lesion. In the colon, the risk of lymph node metastasis is directly correlated with the depth of invasion and has not been shown to occur before the penetration of the submucosal layer.[1] The cut-off commonly used for safe endoscopic resection of early colonic neoplasia is depth of invasion into the submucosal layer of less than 500 μm.[2]

Indications

The currently accepted indications for endoscopic resection in early colorectal cancers include: (1) well- or moderately differentiated adenocarcinoma; (2) cancer confined to the mucosa layer or intramucosal cancer type IIa less than 20 mm; (3) cancer confined to the mucosa layer or intramucosal cancer type IIb or IIc less than 10 mm; (4) cancer superficially invading the submucosal layer (sm1a and b, less than 500 μm from the muscularis mucosa layer); and (5) laterally spreading tumor.[3]

Techniques

Many techniques are currently used for endoscopic resection of early colorectal neoplasia. To simplify the discussion, the techniques are divided into three broad classifications: polypectomy, endoscopic mucosal resection, and endoscopic submucosal dissection.

Polypectomy

The most fundamental technique in endoscopic resection is simple polypectomy, also known as the "just-cut" method with a standard polypectomy snare. This technique is most useful for lesions with a small stalk, in which the polypectomy snare is advanced through the working channel of the endoscope and enclosed around the stalk.[4] Then, either as cold guillotine or with electrocautery, the lesion is transected off the stalk.

A modification of the just-cut method is the "lift-and-cut" method. The variations of this technique all require a double-channel endoscope. In the first variation, the first snare is used to "grasp and lift" the lesion, while the second snare is passed down to the base to resect the lesion. In the second variation, the grasping-and-lifting function is performed by a grasping forceps rather than an endoscopic snare. This technique is useful for slightly elevated lesions.

Although the technique of polypectomy is adequate for most polypoid lesions, there are obvious limitations in the endoscopic resection of flat and sessile lesions. In response, techniques of endoscopic mucosal resection (EMR) and endoscopic submucosal dissection (ESD) were developed extensively in Japan. Often, EMR is used for lesions less than 2 cm or is used in piecemeal fashion for larger lesions, whereas ESD is amenable to lesions of variable sizes.

Endoscopic Mucosal Resection

The techniques of EMR can be further divided into those that require suction and those that do not. Two subtypes of EMR techniques do not require suction. The first is the inject-and-cut method, which is akin to a saline-assisted polypectomy (Fig. 13-1). Submucosal injection is performed with creation of a submucosal cushion under the lesion, and a standard endoscopic polypectomy snare is used to cut the lesion. The second variation is the inject lift-and-cut method, which is a combination of the submucosal injection with the lift-and-cut technique of polypectomy. Submucosal injection is performed by creating a cushion, and then a grasping forceps or a snare is used to grasp and lift the lesion, where a second snare is passed through the second working channel of the double-channel endoscope to resect the lesion.

Two subtypes of EMR techniques require endoscopic suction to be applied for resection. However, both methods, which were adopted from the upper gastrointestinal tract, require judicious use of the suction because the wall of the colon is significantly thinner than the wall of the stomach. EMR-cap involves fixing a transparent cap at the end of the endoscope.[5] A specially designed snare is positioned on the inner lip of the cap, while the endoscope is away from the lesion. The cap with the preloaded snare is then positioned over the lesion, and suction is applied to bring the lesion into the cap. The snare is enclosed around the lesion within the cap, and electrocautery is applied to cut the lesion. In EMR ligation, a standard variceal band ligation device is used with a submucosal injection.[6,7] The band ligation device is positioned above the lesion and

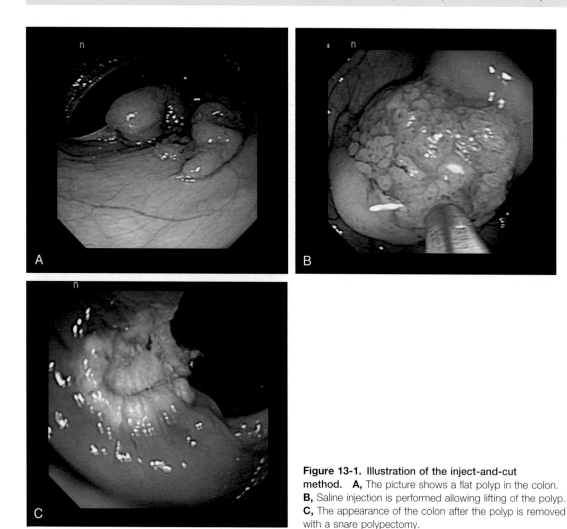

Figure 13-1. Illustration of the inject-and-cut method. A, The picture shows a flat polyp in the colon. **B,** Saline injection is performed allowing lifting of the polyp. **C,** The appearance of the colon after the polyp is removed with a snare polypectomy.

the submucosal cushion; after suction is applied bringing the lesion into the cap, the band is deployed around the lesion as in the standard variceal banding technique. Then, a specially designed hexagonal electrocautery snare is advanced through the banding cap device to cut the lesion either just above or below (Fig. 13-2).

Endoscopic Submucosal Dissection

Although EMR techniques are simple for smaller lesions, the ability of EMR to resect en bloc large, flat lesions is limited by size, especially if one of the cap-suction–based EMR techniques is used. ESD involves marking the margins of the lesion with electrocautery and generous sub-

mucosal injections. A circumferential submucosal incision is made with specialized endoscopic electrocautery knives, and dissection of the lesion from the underlying layers is performed to complete the resection. Various electrocautery knives have been developed for ESD, including needle knife, insulated-tip diathermic knife, flex knife, hook knife, triangle-tipped knife, and splash needle, each of which has specific advantages and limitations. ESD is a highly specialized technique that is not yet widely available outside of Japan and other Asian countries, but it is increasingly gaining momentum. ESD is generally more time-consuming and labor-intensive compared with other methods of endoscopic resections, but it is more reliable in allowing complete en bloc resection of lesions with a lower likelihood of local recurrence. ESD

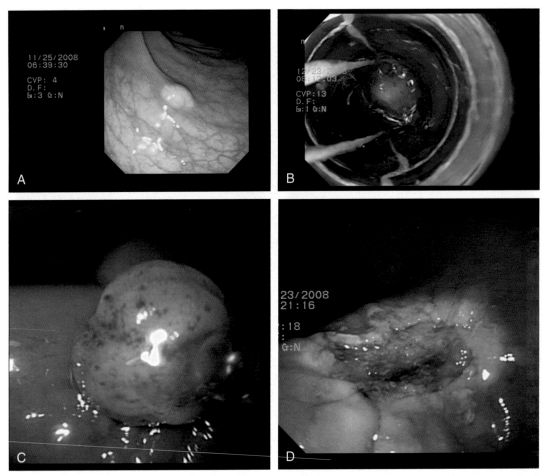

Figure 13-2. Illustration of the endoscopic mucosal resection (EMR) ligation or the inject, band, and cut method. **A,** A 1-cm carcinoid tumor injected with saline with excellent lifting. **B,** Banding of target area is performed using the Duette multibanding system. **C,** The elevated target area after banding. **D,** The post-endoscopic mucosal resection (EMR) site within the colon.

is also associated with a potential for higher risk of complications, including perforation. Review of the literature indicates a perforation rate of around 4% to 10% for ESD and 0.3% to 0.5% for EMR.[8,9]

Submucosal Injection. In endoscopic resection—regardless of the technique—it is critical to maintain an adequate submucosal cushion during the procedure to decrease complication rate. Furthermore, mucosal resection of the lesion should not be attempted if the lesion does not "lift" during the submucosal injection, since this is a good predictor of deeper invasion of the tumor into the submucosal layer. Various solutions that have been studied for submucosal injection during EMR and ESD include normal saline, hypertonic sodium chloride solution, hyaluronic acid, hydroxypropyl methylcellulose, glycerol, dextrose, albumin, fibrinogen, and autologous blood.[10]

The ideal agent should be inexpensive, readily available, nontoxic, and easy to inject, while creating a longlasting cushion.

Outcomes

Kudo[11] reported his experience with 674 cases of early colorectal cancer, of which endoscopic resections were performed in 633 cases.[11] Ten patients underwent surgical resection following endoscopic resection because of deep submucosal invasion. None of the patients who successfully underwent complete endoscopic resection developed local recurrence or distant metastasis during the follow-up period.[1,11]

Tanaka and colleagues[12] reported their experience in 81 patients with large laterally spreading tumors (mean diameter of 31 mm) who underwent endoscopic resection, half of whom underwent en bloc resections. Submucosal invasions (less than 400 μm) were detected in seven patients, three of whom went to surgery. Locally recurrent disease occurred in 6 of the 78 endoscopic resection follow-up group, and all were successfully treated with repeat endoscopic resection. None of the 78 endoscopic resection patients developed lymph node or distant metastatic disease after a mean follow-up of 5 years.[1,12]

Colorectal Self-Expandable Metal Stents

Despite increased awareness of the benefits of routine colorectal cancer screening, up to one third of patients with colorectal cancer present with acute obstruction.[13–15] Of those who present with acute obstruction, up to one third will be unresectable owing to local tumor infiltration, metastatic disease, or severe medical comorbidities.[14,16,17]

Acute colonic obstruction is considered a surgical emergency, since persistent obstruction may lead to colonic ischemia, sepsis, and perforation. Traditionally, the management involved a three-stage process: (1) emergent surgical decompression of the acute colonic obstruction with decompressing colostomy, (2) primary resection of the tumor, and (3) reestablishing bowel continuity with colostomy take-down.[18] The current surgical standard of care for acute malignant obstruction of the distal colon involves Hartmann's procedure,[15,19] in which a colostomy is formed for decompression with the resection of the primary tumor. The diversion colostomy is crucial because of the concern for the disintegration of the surgical anastomosis by the fecal stream from an unprepped colon.[20] Thus, the patient must wait at least 8 weeks after the initial surgery before the colostomy can be safely reversed. However, many have to wait much longer to ensure integrity of the colonic mucosa and the surgical anastomosis, since most of these patients also require adjuvant chemotherapy. Furthermore, 25% to 50% of the patients are not even able to undergo the second surgery for the colostomy take-down procedure on the basis

of medical comorbidities and remain with a permanent colostomy.[15,21] Other surgical options include radical resection with an ileo-rectal anastomosis and intraoperative colonic lavage.[20]

Regardless of which surgical technique is adopted, emergency surgical decompression of acute malignant colonic obstruction is associated with a mortality rate of 15% to 20% and a morbidity rate of 39% to 50%.[14,22–25] In contrast, if elective surgery is performed, the mortality rates can decrease to 0.9% to 6.0%.[22] Furthermore, emergent surgery is more likely to result in a temporary or permanent colostomy, given that the poorly prepped, dilated colon makes primary anastomosis imprudent.[14] In fact, rates of primary anastomosis were almost twice as high for patients who underwent elective surgery after colonic stenting decompression compared with patients who underwent emergency surgery.[26]

Given the high mortality and morbidity rates associated with emergent surgical decompression of the colon, the technique of colonic stenting as a bridge intervention to elective surgery and as a palliative intervention was introduced. As a natural extension of the techniques of stenting of esophageal, gastric outlet, and biliary obstruction, endoscopic stenting for malignant colonic obstruction was first reported in 1992 by Spinelli and colleagues.[27] Since that time, the use of endoscopically placed colorectal self-expandable metal stents has been gaining widespread acceptance as a viable and effective management option for malignant colonic obstruction.

Several studies have compared the outcomes of patients with acute malignant colonic obstruction who underwent a colorectal self-expandable metal stent decompression followed by elective colonic resection and those who underwent an emergency surgical decompression and resection. A meta-analysis of 10 studies compared colonic stents with emergent surgery for malignant large bowel obstruction.[28] The meta-analysis included 451 patients, of whom 244 (54.1%) had undergone a colonic stent placement attempt. Colonic stent placement was successful in 226 patients (92.6%) with individual reported success rates ranging from 88% to 100%. There were 25 deaths in the surgical group (12.1%), compared with 14 deaths in the stent group (5.7%). In patients with primary colorectal cancer, patients in the stent group had significantly lower rates of mortality (odds ratio [OR] 0.40; $P = .02$) and medical complications (OR 0.17; $P < .001$). The average length of hospital stay was almost 7 days less in the stent group (-6.59 days; $P < .001$), and significantly fewer patients in the stent group required an intensive care unit (ICU) stay after the decompression intervention (OR 0.07; $P < .001$). The rate of long-term need for stoma was also significantly lower in the stent group (OR 0.04; $P < .001$).

Indications

Endoscopically placed colorectal self-expandable metal stents (SEMS) for acute malignant colonic obstruction are indicated in patients with resectable disease who need a temporary decompression as a bridge to definitive curative resection and in patients with unresectable disease who need long-term palliative intervention.[29] SEMS decompression transforms an emergent colonic surgery to an elective surgery with the ability to adequately prep the bowel and to better assess the disease status before proceeding with curative intent. Thus, for patients who undergo colorectal stent placement as a bridge to surgical therapy, the endoscopic decompression may allow for a one-stage colonic resection operation with a primary anastomosis.[29] Furthermore, although colonic segmental resection for malignancy following decompression was traditionally reserved for the open laparotomy approach, several studies have shown that successful laparoscopic resections can be performed after adequate decompression with SEMS in this population.[30–33]

Techniques

Stents are usually placed by a gastroenterologist under endoscopic and/or fluoroscopic guidance.[20] Endoscopically guided placement of SEMS with or without fluoroscopy has several advantages over fluoroscopic guidance alone: the ability to access the entire colon, the ability to visually inspect the malignant obstruction, the ability to obtain tissue samples, and the improved mechanics of being able to pass some colorectal SEMS directly through the biopsy channel of the endoscope[20] (Fig. 13-3).

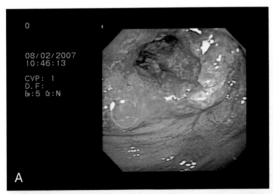
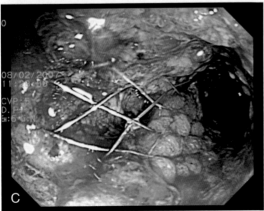
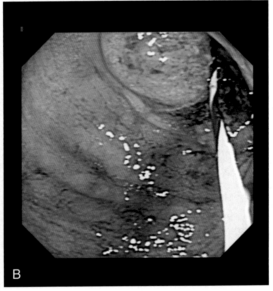

Figure 13-3. Steps involved in the insertion of a self-expandable metal stent (SEMS). A, A near-obstructing colon cancer. **B,** Placement of a guidewire beyond the obstructive lesion. **C,** The endoscopic view after deployment of SEMS.

Currently, four self-expandable colorectal stents have been approved by the U. S. Food and Drug Administration (FDA) for malignant colonic obstruction[20] (Table 13-1). Two of the currently approved colorectal SEMS have a smaller diameter (10 F) predeployment, which allows the system to be deployed through the working channel of a therapeutic endoscope (a working channel less than 3.8 mm in diameter is required to allow passage of the Enteral Wallstent or the Wallflex stent).[20] A theoretical advantage of non–through-the-scope (TTS) stents is the lack of foreshortening of the stent during and after deployment.[31]

Preprocedural Preparation and Positioning

Colonic perforation is considered to be a contraindication to colonic SEMS placement. Thus, a plain radiograph is obtained to exclude the presence of a perforation. Often, a retrograde contrast study (water-soluble or barium enema) is obtained to better delineate the anatomy and the character of the malignant stricture (length, location, and degree of obstruction). It is also important to determine whether there are any additional sites of obstruction, since relieving only one site of obstruction will not be of clinical benefit to the patient.[31]

Once a perforation has been ruled out, the patient may require bowel preparation for the procedure. If a patient has a complete obstruction, often the bowel distal to the lesion is free of stool and a bowel preparation is usually not necessary. In patients with partial distal colon obstruction, one or two enemas are usually sufficient. In patients with partial proximal colon obstruction, a gentle oral bowel preparation can be attempted.[31] For patients with complete obstruction and significantly dilated colon, prophylactic antibiotics should be given because air insufflation during the colonoscopy may induce microperforation and bacteremia.[31,34]

The patient should be placed in the traditional left lateral decubitus position. Conscious sedation is often adequate for most patients with colonic lesions, and no sedation may be needed for distal lesions.

The next section describes in detail the techniques of insertion of SEMS. Currently, two of the commercially available colonic stents are deployed through the scope (TTS), whereas the diameters of the deployment systems of the remaining stents are too large to allow passage through the working channel of the therapeutic endoscope. Furthermore, there are endoscopic, fluoroscopic, and endoscopic/fluoroscopic guided methods of colonic SEMS deployment. We describe here the deployment techniques of both the TTS and non-TTS colonic SEMS.

Table 13-1. US FDA-approved Colorectal SEMS

	Enteral Wallstent	Enteral Wallflex Colonic Stent	Precision Colonic Ultraflex Stent	Colonic Z Stent
Company	Boston Scientific	Boston Scientific	Boston Scientific	Wilson-Cook
Material	Elgiloy (monofilament wire, braided in a tubular mesh)	Nitinol wire	Nitinol wire, diamond configuration	Stainless-steel wire
Diameter before deployment	10F	10F	16F	30F
Diameter after deployment	20 or 22 mm	25 mm	30 mm flared proximal end; 25 mm body	30 mm ends; 25 mm body
Length	60 or 90 mm	60, 90, or 120 mm	57, 87, or 117 mm	40, 60, 80, 100, or 120 mm
Features	No flared ends TTS	Flared ends TTS	Flared proximal end Non-TTS Deployment from distal end	Flared ends Non-TTS Deployment from proximal end

FDA, Food and Drug Administration; SEMS, self-expandable metal stent; TTS, through the scope.
Modified from Baron TH: Acute colonic obstruction. Gastrointest Endosc Clin N Am 17:323–339, vi, 2007.

Non–Through-the-Scope Colonic Stent Deployment Technique

In distal left-sided obstruction, a non–fluoroscopic-guided placement is feasible with a non-TTS stent. The endoscope is advanced to the site of the obstruction. The endoscope needs to be advanced beyond the lesion; thus, the lesion must be within the reach of a 10-mm endoscope. If the lumen is not initially large enough to allow passage of the endoscope, a gentle dilation with a balloon or laser therapy to recanalize the lumen can be performed.[27,31] However, great care must be used with recanalization of the lumen, since balloon dilatation and laser therapy of the stricture before stent placement have been associated with an increased risk of perforation and bleeding. When the endoscope is beyond the malignant stricture, a stiff 0.035-inch guidewire is advanced as high as possible beyond the lesion. The endoscope is then carefully withdrawn while the position and length of the stricture are evaluated. The stent is advanced over the guidewire beyond the lesion, and the endoscope is reinserted to confirm the placement of the stent endoscopically.[31]

If the endoscope is unable to pass safely beyond the malignant obstruction, a biliary catheter preloaded with a hydrophilic guidewire is used to navigate the stricture. The biliary catheter is positioned at the point of luminal narrowing, and the guidewire is advanced carefully beyond the stricture under endoscopic and fluoroscopic guidance. Once the guidewire has safely passed beyond the stricture, as confirmed by the presence of the guidewire in a dilated air-filled proximal bowel on fluoroscopic images, the biliary catheter is advanced over the guidewire beyond the lesion. The biliary hydrophilic guidewire is removed, and water-soluble contrast is injected to better delineate the lesion and to confirm correct position of the catheter. Then, a stiff 0.035-inch guidewire is reintroduced and the catheter is removed. Next, the endoscope is carefully withdrawn while leaving the guidewire in place. The stent is advanced over the guidewire beyond the lesion and deployed under fluoroscopic guidance. One can also reinsert the endoscope next to the stent to endoscopically visualize the stent placement in addition to the fluoroscopic imaging.[31]

It is crucial to check a postdeployment fluoroscopic image to confirm that the stent is adequately expanded, as evidenced by a waist within the body of the stent with the ends flared open. If the deployed stent does not exhibit a waist within the stent, there should be a suspicion that the stent may not have been long enough to adequately bridge the entire lesion. After injection of contrast through the stent to assess patency, an overlapping second (or rarely, a third) stent may need to be placed to fully bridge the obstructive lesion. It is advised that the stent chosen should be 4 to 6 cm longer than the stricture to ensure optimal placement, with the center of the stent across the stricture and open ends on both the proximal and distal margins of the lesion.

Through-the-Scope Colonic Stent Deployment Technique

Using the same technique to recanalize the lumen as previously described,[27,31] the endoscope is advanced beyond the lesion at least 20 cm, and a stiff 0.035-inch guidewire is placed through the working channel of the endoscope. Next, the TTS stent is passed over the guidewire through the therapeutic endoscope channel beyond the point of obstruction. Then, the endoscope is removed just below the distal margin of the obstruction while leaving the stent and guidewire in place, and the stent is deployed under endoscopic guidance without the need for fluoroscopic guidance[31] (see Fig. 13-3).

If the endoscope is unable to traverse the lesion, the technique to introduce the guidewire and biliary catheter beyond the mass, as previously described, is used. Once the stiff 0.035-inch guidewire is advanced and the biliary catheter is removed, the TTS SEMS is advanced over the guidewire through the working channel of the therapeutic endoscope and advanced beyond the lesion. When proper positioning is confirmed, the stent is deployed under both endoscopic and fluoroscopic guidance. The post-stent placement images are also required after deployment as with the non-TTS SEMS.

Complications

Given the dearth of data from a randomized controlled trial examining the efficacy and safety of colorectal SEMS, a pooled analysis was per-

> **Box 13-1.** Complications of Colonic SEMS Placement
>
> | Early Complications (<30 days) | Late Complications (>30 days) |
> | --- | --- |
> | Perforation | Re-obstruction |
> | Bleeding (self-limited) | Stent migration |
> | Stent migration | Tenesmus |
> | Re-obstruction | |
> | Pain | |
> | Tenesmus | |

SEMS, self-expandable metal stent.

formed by Sebastian and associates[35] in 2004. Potential complications after colorectal SEMS placement include perforation, bleeding, stent migration, re-obstruction, and pain (Box 13-1). Perforation occurred in 3.8% of patients, and pre-stent placement balloon dilatation of the malignant obstruction site was associated with a higher risk of perforation.[29,35] In a systematic review of 29 studies (with 598 total patients), the non-balloon dilation group had a perforation rate of 2%, whereas the balloon dilation group had a rate of 10% ($P < .05$).[36,37] Guidewire manipulation could also contribute to the risk of perforation.

Bleeding can be seen in 0% to 5% of patients. Fortunately, bleeding is usually minor, and most patients do not require additional treatment.[36,38]

Stent migration occurred in 11.8% of patients with most occurring within the first week of placement.[29,35] Migration may be due to the small diameter of the stent, angulation of the colon, inadequate length of the stent to bridge the stricture, and postoperative chemoradiation therapy with subsequent tumor debulking.[36] Stents placed as a long-term palliative intervention migrated more frequently than those placed as a bridge to curative surgical resection (116/791 versus 16/407; $P = .010$).[35] Stent migration may manifest with signs of re-obstruction or symptoms of tenesmus.[36] If the stent migrates distally, removal can be relatively simple, although special care must be taken with any free edges to decrease the risk of perforation.

Re-obstruction occurred in about 10% of patients at a median time of 24 weeks, most frequently in the patients undergoing colonic stenting as a palliative intervention.[29,36,37] Tumor overgrowth was the most common cause, followed by stent migration, tumor ingrowth, and

fecal impaction of the stent.[36] Tumor overgrowth can be treated endoscopically with additional stenting to overlap the margins of the previous stent. Tumor ingrowth can be treated locally with laser therapy or with repeat stenting within the previously placed stent.[28] Because of the concern for fecal impaction of the stent, patients are advised to maintain a low-residue diet and to take stool softeners or laxatives if necessary.

Pain, both abdominal and rectal, is not uncommon, but usually resolves without specific intervention.[36] Tenesmus can occur with stents placed very low in the rectum, and special care should be made to avoid placing the stent within 2 cm from the squamocolumnar junction.

A topic of concern is the theoretical risk of tumor dissemination due to the expansile force of the SEMS in patients with localized disease who undergo colonic stenting as a bridge to curative resection. A study by Saida and colleagues[39] demonstrated no significant difference in long-term survival between patients who underwent preoperative colonic stenting and those who underwent surgical decompression for malignant obstruction at 3 years (48% versus 50%) and at 5 years (40% versus 44%).[28] Furthermore, a meta-analysis also showed no significant difference in long-term survival rates between patients with colonic stent and those with surgical decompression.[28]

Cost-Effectiveness

Osman and colleagues[40] found that the cost for a patient who underwent colonic stenting (£1445 [$2110]) was less than half that for a patient who underwent surgical decompression (£3205 [$4681]) for palliation. For those undergoing curative resection, there was a 12% reduction in overall cost in the group who received a colonic stent before proceeding with single-stage surgical resection (£5035 [$7353]) compared with the traditional two-stage surgical procedure (£5720 [$8354]). A 19.7% decrease in the overall cost of treatment was seen in the stent group compared with the traditional surgical group in a study by Binkert and colleagues.[41] The lower cost seen in both studies was attributed to the shorter length of stay, shorter duration of ICU stay, fewer surgical procedures, and reduced operating room time.[35,37] A decision analysis comparing two competing strategies (emergent colonic stent followed by elective resection with primary anastomosis versus emergent surgical resection followed by diversion [Hartmann's procedure] or primary anastomosis) in a patient presenting with acute malignant colonic obstruction was performed. It revealed that the strategy with colonic stent placement resulted in 23% fewer operative procedures, 83% reduction in stoma requirement, 50% decrease in procedure-related mortality, and lower mean cost per patient.[15,42]

References

1. Larghi A, Waxman I: Endoscopic mucosal resection: treatment of neoplasia. Gastrointest Endosc Clin N Am 15:431–454, viii, 2005.
2. Rembacken BJ, Gotoda T, Fujii T, Axon AT: Endoscopic mucosal resection. Endoscopy 33:709–718, 2001.
3. Gotoda T: Endoscopic resection for premalignant and malignant lesions of the gastrointestinal tract from the esophagus to the colon. Gastrointest Endosc Clin N Am 18:435–450, viii, 2008.
4. Williams C, Muto T, Rutter KRP: Removal of polyps with fiberoptic colonoscope: a new approach to colonic polypectomy. Br Med J 1:451–452, 1973.
5. Inoue H, Endo M, Takeshita K, et al: A new simplified technique of endoscopic esophageal mucosal resection using a cap-fitted panendoscope (EMRC). Surg Endosc 6:264–265, 1992.
6. Masuda K, Fukjisaki J, Suzuki H, et al: Endoscopic mucosal resection using a ligating device (EMRL). Endoscopia Digestiva 5:58–62, 1993.
7. Suzuki Y, Ishida M, Kanke K, et al: Endoscopic mucosal resection for gastric adenoma and carcinoma using a ligating device for variceal ligation [abstract]. Gastrointest Endosc 43:305, 1996.
8. Tanaka S, Oka S, Chayama K: Colorectal endoscopic submucosal dissection: present status and future perspective, including its differentiation from endoscopic mucosal resection. J Gastroenterol 43:641–651, 2008.
9. Tanaka S, Oka S, Kaneko I, et al: Endoscopic submucosal dissection for colorectal neoplasia: possibility of standardization. Gastrointest Endosc 66:100–107, 2007.
10. Kantsevoy SV, Adler DG, Conway JD, et al: Endoscopic mucosal resection and endoscopic submucosal dissection. Gastrointest Endosc 68:11–18, 2008.
11. Kudo S: Endoscopic mucosal resection of flat and depressed types of early colorectal cancer. Endoscopy 25:455–461, 1993.
12. Tanaka S, Haruma K, Oka S, et al: Clinicopathologic features and endoscopic treatment of superficially spreading colorectal neoplasms larger than 20 mm. Gastrointest Endosc 54:62–66, 2001.
13. Deans GT, Krukowski ZH, Irwin ST: Malignant obstruction of the left colon. Br J Surg 81:1270–1276.
14. Aitken DG, Horgan AF: Endoluminal insertion of colonic stents. Surg Oncol 16:59–63, 2007.
15. Farrell JJ: Preoperative colonic stenting: how, when and why? Curr Opin Gastroenterol 23:544–549, 2007.
16. Repici A, Reggio D, De Angelis C, et al: Covered metal stents for management of inoperable malignant colorectal strictures. Gastrointest Endosc 52:735–740, 2000.
17. Griffith RS: Preoperative evaluation. Medical obstacles to surgery. Cancer 70:1333–1341, 1992.
18. Adler DG, Baron TH: Endoscopic palliation of colorectal cancer. Hematol Oncol Clin North Am 16:1015–1029, 2002.
19. Koruth NM, Hunter DC, Krukowski ZH, Matheson NA: Immediate resection in emergency large bowel surgery: a 7 year audit. Br J Surg 72:703–707, 1985.
20. Baron TH: Acute colonic obstruction. Gastrointest Endosc Clin N Am 17:323–339, vi, 2007.
21. Riedl S, Wiebelt H, Bergmann U, Hermanek P Jr: [Postoperative complications and fatalities in surgical therapy of colon carcinoma. Results of the German multicenter study by the Colorectal Carcinoma Study Group]. Chirurg 66:597–606, 1995.
22. Seitz U, Seewald S, Bohnacker S, Soehendra N: Advances in interventional gastrointestinal endoscopy in colon and rectum. Int J Colorectal Dis 18:12–18, 2003.
23. Buechter KJ, Boustany C, Caillouette R, Cohn I Jr: Surgical management of the acutely obstructed colon. A review of 127 cases. Am J Surg 156:163–168, 1988.
24. Mulcahy HE, Skelly MM, Husain A, O'Donoghue DP: Long-term outcome following curative surgery for malignant large bowel obstruction. Br J Surg 83:46–50, 1996.
25. Tekkis PP, Poloniecki JD, Thompson MR, Stamatakis JD: Operative mortality in colorectal cancer: prospective national study. Br Med J 327:1196–1201, 2003.
26. Watt AM, Faragher IG, Griffin TT, et al: Self-expanding metallic stents for relieving malignant colorectal obstruction: a systematic review. Ann Surg 246:24–30, 2007.
27. Spinelli P, Dal Fante M, Mancini A: Self-expanding mesh stent for endoscopic palliation of rectal obstructing tumors: a preliminary report. Surg Endosc 6:72–74, 1992.
28. Tilney HS, Lovegrove RE, Purkayastha S, et al: Comparison of colonic stenting and open surgery for malignant large bowel obstruction. Surg Endosc 21:225–233, 2007.
29. Simmons DT, Baron TH: Endoluminal palliation. Gastrointest Endosc Clin N Am 15:467–484, viii, 2005.
30. Balague C, Targarona EM, Sainz S, et al: Minimally invasive treatment for obstructive tumors of the left colon: endoluminal self-expanding metal stent and laparoscopic colectomy. Preliminary results. Dig Surg 21:282–286, 2004.
31. Baron TH: Colonic stenting: technique, technology, and outcomes for malignant and benign disease. Gastrointest Endosc Clin N Am 15:757–771, 2005.
32. Law WL, Choi HK, Lee YM, Chu KW: Laparoscopic colectomy for obstructing sigmoid cancer with prior insertion of an expandable metallic stent. Surg Laparosc Endosc Percutan Tech 14: 29–32, 2004.
33. Morino M, Bertello A, Garbarini A, et al: Malignant colonic obstruction managed by endoscopic stent decompression followed by laparoscopic resections. Surg Endosc 16:1483–1487, 2002.
34. Baron TH, Dean PA, Yates MR III, et al: Expandable metal stents for the treatment of colonic obstruction: techniques and outcomes. Gastrointest Endosc 47:277–286, 1998.
35. Sebastian S, Johnston S, Geoghegan T, et al: Pooled analysis of the efficacy and safety of self-expanding metal stenting in malignant colorectal obstruction. Am J Gastroenterol 99:2051–2057, 2004.
36. Dharmadhikari R, Nice C: Complications of colonic stenting: a pictorial review. Abdom Imaging 33:278–284, 2008.
37. Khot UP, Lang AW, Murali K, Parker MC: Systematic review of the efficacy and safety of colorectal stents. Br J Surg 89: 1096–1102, 2002.
38. Suzuki N, Saunders BP, Thomas-Gibson S, et al: Colorectal stenting for malignant and benign disease: outcomes in colonic stenting. Dis Colon Rectum 47:1201–1207, 2004.
39. Saida Y, Sumiyama Y, Nagao J, Uramatsu M: Long-term prognosis of preoperative "bridge to surgery" expandable metallic stent insertion for obstructive colorectal cancer: comparison with emergency operation. Dis Colon Rectum 46:S44–S49, 2003.
40. Osman HS, Rashid N, Sathananthan N, Parker MC: The cost effectiveness of self-expanding metal stents in the management of malignant left-sided large bowel obstruction. Colorectal Dis 2:233–237, 2000.
41. Binkert CA, Ledermann H, Jost R, et al: Acute colonic obstruction: clinical aspects and cost-effectiveness of preoperative and palliative treatment with self-expanding metallic stents—a preliminary report. Radiology 206:199–204, 1998.
42. Targownik LE, Spiegel BM, Sack J, et al: Colonic stent vs. emergency surgery for management of acute left-sided malignant colonic obstruction: a decision analysis. Gastrointest Endosc 60:865–874, 2004.

14 Open Surgical Techniques in Colorectal Cancer

Vanita Ahuja

KEY POINTS

- Variations in surgical techniques exist in the treatment of colorectal cancer. Following the National Cancer Institute (NCI) guidelines helps minimize inconsistencies in staging and enhances surgical quality control.
- Operative planning for resection should include radical en bloc removal of the blood supply and draining lymphatics at the level of feeding arterial vessel.
- NCI recommends that at least 12 lymph nodes be evaluated to determine prognosis and further treatment.
- In rectal cancer surgery, all effort should be made to obtain a negative circumferential margin of at least 2 mm. In most cases, a distal margin of 2 cm removes all microscopic disease.
- The recurrence rate can be lowered if total mesorectal excision, with a negative circumferential and distal margin, is part of the rectal cancer surgery.

Introduction

Surgery remains the primary modality of treatment for malignancies of the lower gastrointestinal tract. Based on experience, an estimated 90% to 92% of patients with colon cancer and 84% of patients with rectal cancer are treated surgically. The chance of cure with surgery as the sole treatment modality decreases with increasing tumor depth penetration and lymph node involvement.[1] Variations in surgical techniques exist in the treatment of colorectal cancer and can be best evaluated by studying rates of local recurrence and survival. The wide range in recurrence rate (4%–55%) is evidence that the type of surgical technique significantly affects cancer outcome, especially for rectal cancer. Based on the latter findings, the National Cancer Institute ([NCI] Bethesda, Maryland) systematically reviewed the literature and drafted guidelines to reduce surgical variation and to help standardize

documentation. These guidelines helped minimize inconsistencies in staging patients with colorectal cancer and enhanced surgical quality control in 2001. Along with the surgical principles governing them, these guidelines are incorporated into the remainder of this chapter.

Surgical Oncologic Principles: Historical Perspective

In the 1960s, the idea that modifying surgical techniques to consider oncologic principles can have a positive influence on survival in colorectal cancer began to formulate. Turnball and associates,[2] in a much-criticized study in 1967 at the Cleveland Clinic Hospital, retrospectively compared the outcomes of patients who had resections for malignancy using the no-touch isolation technique with the outcomes of patients who underwent more traditional resections. The no-touch isolation technique involves the ligation of the draining vessels at their origin early in the dissection, then the proximal and distal bowel to the lesion is ligated, and finally the tumor is mobilized. This procedure isolates the tumor, which prevents intraluminal and hematogenous spillage that would otherwise occur during manipulation of the tumor. The study concluded that patients with no-touch oncologic resection had a better 5-year survival rate.

In 1998, Wiggers and associates[3] compared the no-touch technique with the conventional technique in a randomized prospective trial. The trial found no significant difference in 5-year survival rates between the no-touch group and the conventional group, but there was a trend toward better cancer-related survival in the former group. The trials emphasized the fact that operative techniques and following oncologic principles are essential; however, the no-touch technique is no longer followed. Since then, evidence increasingly suggests that the quality of the oncologic outcome is directly proportional to the surgical team's adherence to NCI oncologic guidelines. Most of the evidence comes from rectal cancer, but the correlation holds for colon cancer. The German Study Group Colo-Rectal Carcinoma trial showed that the surgeon is a critical variable in determining locoregional recurrence rate and morbidity.[4]

The oncologic principles involving resection include:

■ High ligation of all draining mesenteric vessels
■ Minimal trauma during mobilization
■ Adequate margins
■ Clearance of tumors from invading organs
■ Complete intraoperative exploration

Oncologic Principles for Bowel Resection and Margins

Operative planning for resection for colonic malignancy ideally should include radical en bloc removal of the blood supply and the draining of lymphatics at the level of the origin of the primary feeding arterial vessel. The vascular supply to the colon is demonstrated in Figure 14-1. The ultimate length of the resected bowel segment is dictated by the lymphovascular resection. Enker and associates[5] recommend that resection of the distal and proximal margin should be at least 5 cm from the tumor, since the local recurrence rate is 6.9% for margins greater than 5 cm and 20% for those less than 5 cm in Dukes stage B. The bowel margins should be wide enough to limit intraluminal and pericolic recurrence. Generally accepted surgical principles recommend resection margin distance of 5 to 10 cm.

Guidelines in the United States recommend ligation of the primary feeding artery at the level of its origin. Although the level of ligation of the primary feeding artery is still under debate, high ligation is favored based on results of studies that show improvement of 5-year survival rates with high versus low ligation. The following studies showed favorable 5-year survival rates with high ligation—all found in the article by Hida and colleagues[6]: Rosi and colleagues showed 77% versus 63% with low ligation, Bacon and colleagues found 73.6% versus 63.2%, and Slanetz and Grimson found 74.5% versus 65.8%. It is recommended that when the primary tumor is equidistant from two feeding vessels, both vessels should be excised at their origin.[6]

The drainage of the lymphatic system mirrors that of the vascular system. In colon carcinoma, there are two possible directions for lymphatic drainage: central along the mesenteric vessels

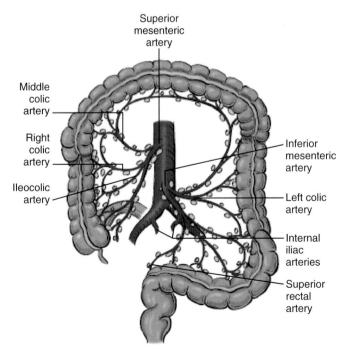

Figure 14-1. Lymph node and blood supply of colon and rectum. (From Greene FL, Page DL: AJCC Cancer Staging Manual, 6th ed. Philadelphia: Lippincott Williams & Wilkins, 2002, p 123.)

and para-intestinal. Divide the major draining mesenteric vessel(s) at the point of origin with the accompanying lymphatic network to prevent regional lymphatic recurrence. For right colon resections, the length of ileum resected does not appear to affect local recurrence. Therefore, the shortest length of ileum should be resected to prevent malabsorption syndromes while ensuring adequate blood supply to the anastomosis.

Staging the Extent of Cancer Resection

The extent of tumor not resected intraoperatively strongly influences prognosis and therapy. The absence or presence of residual tumor after surgical treatment is described by the letter R. Accepted guidelines from the American Joint Committee on Cancer (AJCC) Prognostic Factors Consensus Conference were recommended to describe the extent of resection. Resections should be categorized as follows:

R0—All gross disease resected by en bloc resection with margins histologically free of disease

R1—All gross disease resected by en bloc resection with margins histologically positive for disease

R2—Residual gross disease remains unresected

The radial margins should be tumor-free and histologically free of disease for the resection to be considered curative. Patients who do not have histologic assessment of radial tumor margin or who had an R1 or R2 resection are considered to have an incomplete resection for cure. Incomplete resection R1 and R2 does not change the TNM stage, but it does affect curability. This is well seen in rectal cancer when the local recurrence rate after resection of a rectal cancer was approaching 80% in those with margins positive for disease and less than 10% in those with margins negative for disease.

Lymphadenectomy

Lymph node resection carries prognostic and therapeutic implications. The lymph node resection should be radical and removed en bloc. The lymph node dissection should be carried to the level of the origin of the primary feeding vessel. Colon cancer staging requires adequate analysis of lymph nodes to determine prognosis and

further treatment. The 1990 Working Party report of the World Congress of Gastroenterology recommends that at least 12 lymph nodes must be evaluated. This recommendation was reiterated by an NCI sponsor panel of experts.[7]

A systemic review of evidence for the association between lymph node evaluation and surgical outcome in patients with colon cancer showed that the number of lymph nodes evaluated after surgical resection was positively associated with survival of patients with stage II and stage III colon cancer.[8] Because of the high risk for recurrence of colon cancer, adjuvant chemotherapy is recommended for patients with lymph node metastases (stage III).

However, a population-based study by Baxter and associates[9] found that only 37% of patients with colon cancer receive adequate lymph node evaluation during colon cancer staging. The two potentially modifiable influences are the completeness of lymph node evaluation by the examining pathologist and the adequacy of the surgical resection. The number of lymph nodes recovered has been identified as a potentially important measure of the quality of cancer care by many organizations. The proficiency of the surgeon and total hospital case volume are positively associated with the number of lymph nodes recovered. Patients in lower-volume hospitals were more likely to have fewer than seven lymph nodes detected. The experience of the pathologist and the technique of pathologic evaluation have also been shown to be important in lymph node recovery after adjusting for surgeon and tumor-related factors.

Guidelines in the United States recommend that nodes at the origin of the primary feeding artery (apical node) should be tagged for pathologic evaluation because the apical nodes have prognostic significance in addition to the number of nodes positive for disease in the specimens. The apical lymph node is defined as the "most proximal lymph node within 1 cm of vessel ligation at apex of vascular pedicle."[6,7,10] Multivariate analysis has shown that involvement of the apical lymph node is significantly associated with adverse outcome. The general recommendation for surgical resection of the colon is to ligate the primary feeding arterial vessel at the level of its origin and resect at least 5 cm of bowel on both sides. This technique should produce better patient prognosis and more accurate staging. A smaller extent of resection decreases the number of recovered nodes and increases the risk of under-staging.[11,12]

The concept of sentinel lymph node examination has been studied for colon cancer, but there is no uniformity in the definition of cellular burden, nor is there common agreement on how to clinically define relevant metastatic disease. Some studies have shown that the detection of immunohistochemistry (IHC) cytokeratin-positive cells in stage II (N0) colon cancer indicates a worse prognosis, whereas other studies have failed to show a survival difference. Until the use of sentinel lymph nodes and the detection of cancer cells by immunohistochemistry have been standardized and proved more effective than nodal dissection, the procedures recommended herein should be used.[13,14]

Colon

Surgical Preparation

Intraoperative identification of the tumor may be difficult in patients who have small or flat tumors or who are undergoing resection after a polypectomy. This is especially true with laparoscopic procedures, in which the bowel often cannot be palpated. Preoperative localization with marking during endoscopy can assist in intraoperative identification of the tumor. If the lesion is in the cecum, the ileocecal valve and the appendiceal orifice should be viewed endoscopically; then the localization of the tumor is simple. Distal lesion can be measured from the anus; however, estimates of the location of the tumor may be inaccurate.

In our practice, endoscopic tattooing, a process in which an agent is injected into the bowel wall submucosally at or near the site of the lesion, has been used to facilitate intraoperative identification of the tumor site. The most common agent for achieving this goal is India ink, which generally yields excellent results. As an alternative, many institutions use a commercially available sterile suspension of carbon particles, which is also very safe and effective. Intraoperative endoscopy is another option for locating lesions and to confirm small tumors.

Be thorough during the endoscopy to locate all lesions. The rate of synchronous colon cancers ranges from 2% to 11%, and the incidence of synchronous adenomatous polyps may be greater than 30%. In this case, as much colon length as possible should be preserved without compromise to the cancer resection. An alternative is subtotal colectomy with an ileorectal or ileosigmoid anastomosis rather than a multiple anastomosis.[15]

Extent of Resection

Right Colon

Right colon cancers account for up to 15% of primary colorectal cancers. Patients with adenocarcinoma involving the cecum or ascending colon who do not have hereditary nonpolyposis colorectal cancer (HNPCC) or other synchronous lesions should be treated with a right hemicolectomy. The standard extent of resection for various colon cancers has been defined. The ileocolic, right colic, and right branch of the middle colic arteries and veins should be ligated near their origin to ensure an adequate lymphadenectomy. For tumors of the cecum and the ascending colon, a right hemicolectomy that includes the right branch of the middle colic artery at its origin should be performed. For tumors of the hepatic flexure, an extended right colectomy that includes the entire middle colic artery is indicated (Fig. 14-2).

Step 1: Incision. The patient is placed in a supine position, and the abdomen is prepped and draped after intubation. A midline incision centered on the umbilicus is made; another excellent option is a transverse incision just above the level of the umbilicus. Then a self-retaining Bookwalter retractor is placed and the abdomen is explored. First, the abdomen should be examined visually, and then the liver palpated for metastasis; the periaortic, celiac, and portal regions should be examined for adenopathy; and lastly the pelvis should be examined for any possible metastases in the rectal cul-de-sac and ovaries. The lesion of the right colon is inspected and palpated to determine whether it is resectable. The entire small and large intestines should be examined for any synchronous lesions.

Step 2: Mobilization of the Right Colon. Once the resectability is determined, the peritoneal, ileal, and lateral colonic attachments are incised. An incision is made in the peritoneal reflection attached to the lateral wall of the bowel, starting from the tip of the cecum upward to the region of the hepatic flexure. Sometimes the full thickness of the abdominal wall may require excision because of local spread

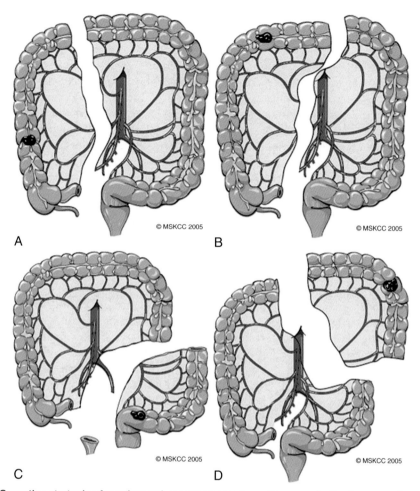

Figure 14-2. Operative strategies for colorectal cancer by location of tumor. **A,** Cecal or ascending colon cancer. **B,** Proximal transverse colon cancer. **C,** Sigmoid colon cancer. **D,** Splenic flexure colon cancer. (From Weiser MR, Posner MC, et al: Adenocarcinoma of the colon and rectum. In Yeo CJ [ed]: Shackelford's Surgery of the Alimentary Tract, 6th ed. Philadelphia: Elsevier, 2007, Fig 156–6.)

of tumor. The entire hepatic flexure is mobilized as part of right hemicolectomy. The hepatocolic ligament contains small blood vessels, which can be divided with electrocautery. After the lateral attachments are divided, the right colon is lifted medially, and the loose areolar tissue lying under is dissected off gently. The right ureter should be identified when elevating the right colon. Care is also taken to avoid injury to the third portion of the duodenum toward the top of ascending colon. The greater omentum is then dissected off the right transverse colon.

Step 3: Division of the Ileocolic Pedicle.
After mobilization of the colon is achieved, the next step is to incise the mesentery. A unique feature of the right colon mesentery is the presence of large avascular windows within the mesentery. There is an avascular mesentery between

the ileocolic artery and the right branch of the middle colic artery and between the ileocolic artery and the last ileal branch. The peritoneum over the avascular mesentery is skeletonized with a Bovie cautery, and then the ileocolic artery and vein are dissected to their origin at the base of the mesentery. Proximal and distal ties are placed on artery and vein and ligated twice. The avascular mesentery to the right branch of the middle colic artery is then incised by electrocautery. The right branch of the middle colic artery and vein is dissected, and then transected after proximal and distal ties are placed. The anatomy of the ileocolic artery is a constant structure, and in 90% of patients the right colic artery branches off from the ileocolic artery. Occasionally, the right colic artery is a separate branch off the superior mesenteric artery and is encountered when the mesentery is incised to the right branch of the middle colic artery.

Step 4: Margin Resection and Anastomosis.

The terminal ileum is prepared about 10 cm from the ileocecal valve, and an intestinal stapler is used to transect the ileum. The stapler is reloaded and used to transect the right transverse colon. Both the stapled edges are invaginated (serosa meets serosa) by oversewing with 3-0 silk interrupted Lembert sutures. Atraumatic clamps are then placed on the proximal ileum and transverse colon. A side-to-side anastomosis or end-to-side anastomosis may be performed, either hand-sewn or stapled. In our practice, a two-layered, hand-sewn anastomosis is preferred with an outer interrupted nonabsorbable serosal layer, and an inner layer of absorbable continuous Connell sutures being placed. The mesenteric defect is then closed traditionally with either running or interrupted sutures. The retroperitoneum is then inspected for any bleeding. Drains are not needed in this case. The bowel should be laid into the abdominal cavity, ensuring correct position, and the anastomosis can be covered with the omentum.

The fascia is then closed, followed by irrigation of the wound. The skin edges are approximated and stapled. The nasogastric tube is discontinued on extubation.

Step 5: Postoperative Care.

Postoperatively, the patient is maintained on intravenous fluids and is started on ice chips on postoperative day 1 and on a clear diet on postoperative day 2. The diet is advanced to regular diet on passing flatus. The patient is usually discharged 4 to 6 days after the operation if the bowel functions and pain control have been achieved.[16,17]

Transverse Colon

Transverse colon cancer is uncommon, accounting for approximately 8% of primary colorectal cancers. Lesions at the proximal and mid-transverse colon are best treated with an extended right hemicolectomy. This involves ligation of the ileocolic, right colic, and middle colic vessels. Generally, an anastomosis between the hepatic and splenic flexure is not done. The ascending and descending colons tend to migrate to their respective lateral gutters, causing tension at the anastomosis and limiting blood supply.

Left Colon

Tumors of the splenic flexure region and descending colon account for less than 5% of colorectal primaries. A left hemicolectomy is performed for a splenic flexure cancer. Cancers in the descending colon may be managed with a left hemicolectomy, which involves division of the left colic artery near its origin and preservation of the left branch of the middle colic artery. The anastomosis is made between the distal transverse colon to the sigmoid after a full splenic flexure mobilization. A left hemicolectomy may also be performed with ligation of the inferior mesenteric vessels, and an anastomosis is done between the transverse colon and the upper rectum.

Step 1: Patient Positioning.

The patient is placed in a supine position, and a nasogastric tube and Foley catheter are inserted after general anesthesia has been induced. If it is known preoperatively that formation of a colostomy is likely, then an appropriate location for the stoma should be selected by an endostoma nurse preoperatively. Prophylaxis against deep vein thrombosis is accomplished by pneumatic decompression devices and subcutaneous heparin.

Step 2: Incision and Exposure.

A midline incision extending cephalad to the xiphoid process for the splenic flexure lesion is made for exploration. Adhesions from previous abdominal surgery are carefully lysed. A thorough abdominal exploration is performed with careful inspection to the liver, omentum, and parietal peritoneal surfaces. The ovaries are inspected, and routine prophylactic oophorectomy is not recommended unless the patient is postmenopausal. The small bowel is examined and the colon inspected for the primary lesion and palpated for any synchronous lesions. Optimal exposure is obtained by retracting the small bowel cephalad and to the right in a moist towel, using a self-retaining retractor.

Step 3: Colon Mobilization.

The dissection is started with the sigmoid colon being retracted to the right and the peritoneal reflection along the white line of Toldt proximal to the splenic flexure and distal to the pelvic inlet. The ureter should be identified as it crosses the iliac artery, and the operator should be careful that the ureter is not drawn up with the mesentery and accidentally divided.

The self-retaining retractor is then repositioned, and the left costal margin is vigorously retracted to provide adequate exposure of the left upper quadrant. The splenic flexure is mobilized by gently retracting inferiorly and to the right while the gastrocolic omentum distal to the gastroepiploic arcade is divided. The splenocolic ligament is more vascular, and vessels running through it should be ligated and then divided. This should be done carefully, since forceful handling of the spleen can produce splenic capsule tear. If a splenic tear or injury occurs, splenic salvage should be carried out unless hemostasis cannot be established.

Step 4: Margins Resection and Anastomosis. The proximal and distal sites of colonic transection are identified and divided with a GIA (gastrointestinal anastomosis) stapling device. The left colon is now affixed by the mesocolon, and the peritoneum overlying the mesentery is scored to outline the path of transection. The left colic vessels should be doubly ligated with a high ligation to sample enough nodes adequately. The specimen is delivered once complete division of the vessels and mesentery are obtained. The specimen is opened off the field to identify the tumor and inspect the margins. The colonic re-anastomosis may be end-to-end, end-to-side, or side-to-side, depending on the caliber, blood supply, and mobility of the proximal and distal segments as well as on the surgeon's preference. Complete mobilization of the proximal segment is required to ensure that the two segments of bowel are approximated

without tension. The mesenteric defect is closed with interrupted 3-0 silk sutures. The fascia is then closed, and skin is closed either by staples or by subcutaneous sutures. The skin is left opened when there is gross contamination and closed via delayed primary closure.[18]

Sigmoid Colon

Sigmoid colon tumors, among the most common tumors, are treated by sigmoid colectomy. This involves division of the sigmoid and superior rectal vessels with anastomosis of the descending colon to the upper rectum. However, important structures such as the ureter, hypogastric nerve, and iliac vessels have to be identified during dissection of sigmoid tumors. Ureteral stent should be considered for surgeries involving large bulky tumor or in a previously radiated field. A review published by Bothwell and associates[19] showed that experienced surgeons performed prophylactic ureteral catheter placement in 16.4% of their sigmoid and rectosigmoid colectomies. The risk of ureteral injury (1.1%) as a direct result of catheter insertion is small, but not insignificant. Prophylactic ureteral catheters do not ensure the prevention of transmural ureteral injuries, but may assist in their immediate recognition.[19]

Step 1: Mobilization of Colon. The patient is placed in the supine position with arms abducted on arm boards and legs in a low lithotomy position (Fig. 14-3). After abdominal exploration, the small bowel is packed into the upper abdomen, and the patient is placed in a slight Trendelenburg position. The rectosigmoid

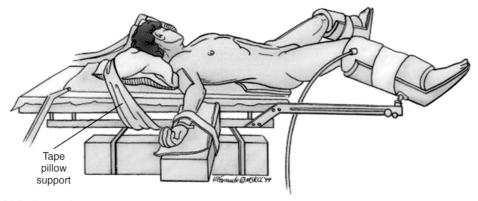

Figure 14-3. Appropriate patient position for sigmoid resection. (From Cohen AM: Operation for colorectal cancer: low anterior resection. In Yeo CJ [ed]: Shackelford's Surgery of the Alimentary Tract, 6th ed. Philadelphia: Elsevier, 2007, Fig 158-1.)

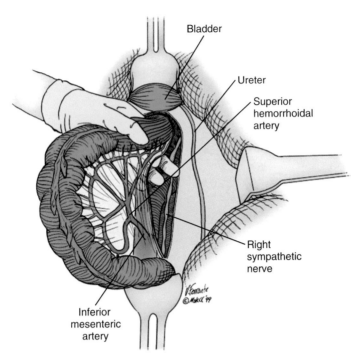

Bladder

Ureter

Superior
hemorrhoidal
artery

Right
sympathetic
nerve

Inferior
mesenteric
artery

**Figure 14-4. Mobilization of the
sigmoid colon from the right.** (From
Cohen AM: Operation for colorectal
cancer: low anterior resection. In Yeo CJ
[ed]: Shackelford's Surgery of the
Alimentary Tract, 6th ed. Philadelphia:
Elsevier, 2007, Fig 158-6.)

is retracted to the right, and the peritoneal attachments to the left of the sigmoid colon are incised along the avascular plane. The peritoneum is incised along the left side of the descending colon as far as the splenic flexure. Adhesions to the spleen are divided, and the splenic flexure is taken down. The colon mobilization extends proximally to the left transverse colon.

The splenic flexure may need to be fully mobilized for a tension-free anastomosis (Fig. 14-4). A mid-sigmoidal lesion can be removed, as described previously for left/descending colectomy, with a primary anastomosis between the proximal descending colon and the distal sigmoid colon. The lesion in the distal sigmoid requires additional distal dissection carried inferiorly into the anterior rectal recess. The left ureter and gonadal vessels are identified and preserved by using sharp and gentle blunt dissection to separate the retroperitoneal tissues from the sigmoid mesentery. The proximal colon margin is selected and divided with the GIA stapler. For resections involving the sigmoid colon and proximal rectum tumors, ligate the inferior mesenteric artery (for sigmoidal lesion) and superior hemorrhoidal artery (for proximal rectal lesion). The superior hemorrhoidal artery is identified by palpation within the mesentery, doubly clamped with Kelly clamps, and ligated (Fig. 14-5). The divided sigmoid is now used as a

handle to facilitate division of the relatively avascular mesorectum. Dissection is carried distally with care being taken to avoid entry into the presacral venous plexus. Once sufficient distal margin is obtained, the specimen is divided and removed from the field.

Step 2: Anastomosis. A low-colonic anastomosis may then be performed using a double-staple, end-to-end anastomosis technique to minimize fecal contamination. The size of the stapling device should be based on the caliber of the anal opening, which must accommodate the stapler itself (Fig. 14-6). A purse-string suture is placed in the cut edge of the distal descending with a 0-prolene suture. The anvil of the circular stapler is placed within the proximal bowel and secured in place. The assistant, seated between the patient's legs, introduces the circular stapler through the anus and pierces the top of the rectal pouch through the midportion of the staple line. The proximal bowel is then engaged to the circular stapler, and the stapler is closed and fired. The device is removed, and the proximal and distal donuts of tissue are checked to ensure that the anastomosis is completely circumferential.

Step 3: Anastomotic Leak. The anastomosis is checked for leaks by insufflating air into the

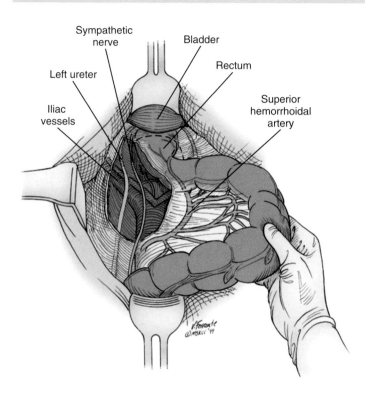

Sympathetic nerve

Bladder

Rectum

Left ureter

Iliac vessels

Superior hemorrhoidal artery

Figure 14-5. Mobilization of the sigmoid colon from the left. (From Cohen AM: Operation for colorectal cancer: low anterior resection. In Yeo CJ [ed]: Shackelford's Surgery of the Alimentary Tract, 6th ed. Philadelphia: Elsevier, 2007, Fig 158-5.)

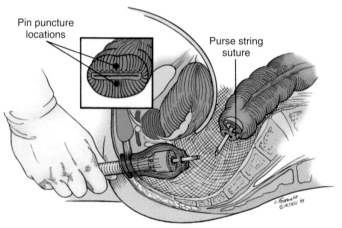

Pin puncture locations

Purse string suture

Figure 14-6. Double stapling technique. (From Cohen AM: Operation for colorectal cancer: low anterior resection. In Yeo CJ [ed]: Shackelford's Surgery of the Alimentary Tract, 6th ed. Philadelphia: Elsevier, 2007, Fig 158-15.)

rectum via a proctoscope while the anastomosis is submersed in saline and the proximal bowel is occluded. Any air bubbles that appear within the pool of irrigation indicate lack of anastomotic integrity, and the anastomosis should be investigated. The incidence of anastomotic complications increases the lower the anastomosis is in the rectum. Other factors that increase the incidence of leakage include previous radiation therapy, immunosuppression, and underlying vascular insufficiency or diabetes.

Many surgeons perform routine temporary fecal diversion for patients undergoing low anastomosis, especially for those subjected to preoperative irradiation or to those receiving steroid treatment. Loop ileostomy is the most commonly performed temporary diversion to diminish the morbidity resulting from leakage and to reduce the likelihood of an emergency operation. Our practice is to perform diversion for patients with a colorectal or coloanal anastomosis within 5 cm of the anus, especially if they have undergone preoperative radiation therapy or are immunosuppressed.

The alternative to a stapled anastomosis is a hand-sewn colorectal end-to-end anastomosis, which may be done in one or two layers with interrupted or continuous sutures. Hand-sewn anastomosis may be required in complete disruption of the stapled line. Hand-sewn colorectal anastomosis is typically performed from the abdominal field. It is often easiest to place all of the sutures first, then "parachute" the proximal bowel down to the rectal cuff as the sutures are tied. The knots are generally tied on the inside to produce mucosal inversion.[20]

Step 4: Postoperative Care. The nasogastric tube may be removed within 24 hours after the operation; however, it may need to be replaced in 10% of patients. Patients are usually started on ice chips after 24 hours and advanced to clear liquids in 48 hours. Advancement to a regular diet occurs when patients are doing well with clear liquids and are passing flatus.

Postoperative Complications

The return of bowel function may be delayed by intra-abdominal sepsis or mechanical obstruction. Postoperative mechanical obstruction initially should be managed conservatively with prolonged nasogastric intubation and intravenous fluids. If the obstruction does not resolve in 10 to 14 days, the patient may require operative re-exploration. Postoperative fever may increase the concern for anastomotic leak; however, other common sources should be ruled out. All colonic anastomoses carry a 3% to 5% rate of anastomotic leak. The anastomosis may be safely studied with Gastrografin contrast if the patient is stable. A small leak may be treated conservatively, but large disruptions need to be treated with operative intervention and a temporary colostomy.

Special Circumstances

Inadvertent perforation of the rectum during the operation should be documented. These patients are still considered to have a complete R0 resection. Inadvertent perforation is seen especially in resection of rectal carcinoma. The reported rate ranges from 7.7% to 25.6%. Retrospective data show negative implication for local recurrence and survival with statistically significant reduction in 5-year survival rates and an increase in local recurrence rates. Patients with rectal perforation may be candidates for adjuvant chemotherapy to reduce rates of local recurrence.

The ideal method to manage locally advanced, adherent colorectal tumors is en bloc resection. If a tumor is transected at the site of local adherence rather than en bloc, then resection is incomplete. Tumors are considered to be R0 when en bloc resection is achieved and when the margins are not found to be involved on histologic examination. Direct extension of the tumor to the ovary or a grossly abnormal ovary should follow with an en bloc or complete resection of the ovary. Data do not support prophylactic routine oophorectomy.

In patients presenting with perforation and peritonitis, surgical management includes removal of the diseased segment and irrigation of the peritoneal cavity. Options for subsequent management include creation of a mucous fistula/Hartmann pouch or primary anastomosis with proximal diversion via loop ileostomy. Perforated colon cancer is associated with a high rate of local recurrence and a low rate of overall survival.

Cancer remains the most common cause of large bowel obstruction. Obstructing right and transverse colon cancers are usually managed with a right hemicolectomy and primary anastomosis. Left-sided colon cancer can be managed with a one- or two-stage procedure. Colonic stenting has become an option for patients with malignant colonic obstruction. Stenting allows transient relief of obstruction and bowel preparation with or without evaluation of the proximal colon with colonoscopy before planned resection.

Rectum

There are many discrepancies in literature for defining the junction of the colon and rectum. These variations lead to inconsistencies when assigning colon or rectal protocols for patients.

The rectum is defined as the area 12 cm or less from the anal verge by rigid proctoscopy. This definition is based on research that demonstrates that lesions located more than 12 cm from the anal verge have a local recurrence rate more consistent with patterns of recurrence in the colon than the rectum. Pilipshen and associates[21] have shown that the local recurrence rate was 9.6% for lesions located more than 12 cm compared with 30.1% and 30.7% for mid-rectal and low-rectal cancers, respectively.

Chapter 14 Open Surgical Techniques in Colorectal Cancer | **155**

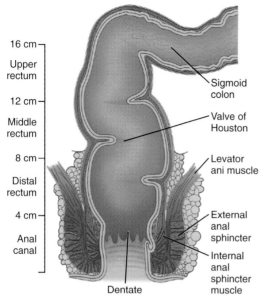

Figure 14-7. Anatomy of the rectum. (From Schaffzrin DM, Smith LE: Rectal cancer. In Cameron JL [ed]: Current Surgical Therapy. Philadelphia: Elsevier, 2004, Fig 3.)

Traditionally, the rectum has been defined intraoperatively as beginning at the end of taeniae coli or peritoneal reflection. This can be highly variable owing to differences in age, gender, and gynecologic and obstetric conditions. However, the anal verge is the preferred anal landmark, since the edge of the tumor and the verge can be visualized simultaneously during rigid proctoscopy (Fig. 14-7).

Therapy

Patients with early-stage, distal rectal cancers limited to the submucosa (T1N0M0) without high-risk features can be treated by local excision. Local excision techniques include transanal, trans-sphincteric, and transcoccygeal (Kraske resection). However, the trans-sphincteric and transcoccygeal resections have been abandoned because they are associated with high rates of complications, including fecal fistulas and incontinence. Local palliative procedures, including fulguration and radiation, are options for patients who are medically unfit or unwilling to undergo major surgery. High T1 rectal tumors and rectal tumors that have invaded the muscularis propria (T2N0M0) in medically fit patients are not amenable to a

transanal approach and are treated with radical rectal surgery. Patients with locally advanced disease (T3/T4 and/or N1) are generally treated preoperatively with chemoradiation followed by radical resection. In patients with resectable metastatic disease, a variety of factors including patient comorbidities, resectability of metastases, and the patient's symptoms must be considered in planning the timing of chemotherapy and surgery. In selected circumstances, surgical resection of the primary rectal lesion can be done for palliative purposes on patients with unresectable metastatic disease. Careful preoperative staging with the modalities, including surgical biopsy and endorectal ultrasound (ERUS), is important to appropriately stratify patients.

Radical Resection

Several important principles for all radical surgery for rectal cancers include total mesorectal excision (TME), circumferential and distal resection margins, and autonomic nerve preservation.

Circumferential and Distal Margins

Recently, the importance of the circumferential margin in rectal cancer surgery has been highlighted. The circumferential margin is assessed by serial slicing and evaluation of multiple coronal sections of the tumor and mesorectum. Circumferential margins less than 2 mm may be associated with higher local recurrence, distant metastases, and death; thus, all efforts should be made to obtain a negative circumferential margin of at least 2 mm, including en bloc resection of adjacent structures.[22]

Traditionally, distal margins of 2 to 5 cm were considered standard in surgery for rectal cancers. In most cases, a distal margin of 2 cm removes all microscopic disease. Recent studies have shown that distal margins less than 2 cm are not associated with higher local recurrence or reduced survival in patients with small cancers of the lower rectum without adverse histologic features or in those who received neoadjuvant chemoradiation therapy.[23] Distal spread more than 1 cm beyond the mucosal edge of the rectal cancer was seen in only 10% of patients and was associated with poor differentiation and node-positive lesions.

Total Mesorectal Excision

Total mesorectal excision (TME) is the excision of the tumor en bloc with its blood and lymphatic supply, that is, the mesorectum. TME was described in 1982 by Heald and colleagues[24] and is now considered the gold standard for surgical treatment of middle and lower third rectal cancers. TME has evolved from principles originated from observations of Moynihan[25] in 1908 regarding potential pathways for lymphatic spread and the hypothesis of Heald and colleagues[26] that the mesorectum represents embryologic advantages conferring protection against tumor dissemination until the terminal stages. TME reduces the rate of locoregional recurrence in rectal cancer. Heald and colleagues documented a 0% 2-year local recurrence rate, without the benefit of adjuvant radiation therapy, in their initial series of 100 cases and 8% at 10 years among patients who had curative resection.

TME facilitates obtaining a negative circumferential and distal margin and lowers the local recurrence rates, which approximate 6.5% from multiple published series (Table 14-1). This is in contrast to local recurrence rates of 14% to 40% in series published before the use of TME dissection. TME also allows preservation of the autonomic nerve function and reduces the likelihood of postoperative genitourinary dysfunction, such as impotence, retrograde ejaculation, and urinary incontinence. However, TME dissection may be associated with an increase in the rate of anastomotic leak.

TME dissection occurs in the areolar plane between the visceral fascia that envelops the rectum and mesorectum and the parietal fascia that envelops the pelvic wall structures (Figs. 14-8 and 14-9). TME dissection in conjunction with either a low anterior resection (LAR) or abdominoperineal resection (APR) requires en bloc removal of the entire mesorectum, including the mesorectal distal to the tumor, which contains the draining lymph nodes of the rectum as an intact unit.

Autonomic Nerve Preservation

The hypogastric nerve arises from the ventral nerve roots of T12 to L3 and supplies sympathetic nerve innervation. The hypogastric nerve may be associated with the visceral fascia of the mesorectum. Injury to the hypogastric plexus results in increased bladder tone, impaired ejaculation, and dyspareunia. The parasympathetic innervation (nervi erigentes) arises from the S2 to S4 ventral nerve roots and is found on the pelvic sidewall. Injury to these nerves can lead to erectile dysfunction, voiding issues, and impaired vaginal lubrication. During TME, sharp meticulous dissection facilitates identification and preservation of the autonomic nerves.

Table 14-1 Long-term Outcomes with TME from Selected Series

Study	No. of Patients	Follow-up	Study Design	Local Recurrence Rate (%)
Heald et al (1982)[24]	113	2 yr	Retrospective	0
McAnena et al (1990)[27]	57	4.8 yr	Retrospective	3.5
Macfarlane et al (1993)[28]	135	7.7 yr	Retrospective	5
Enker et al (1995)[29]	246	5 yr	Retrospective	7.3
Zaheer et al (1998)[30]	514	5 yr	Retrospective	5.7
Heald et al (1998)[31]	519	10 yr	Retrospective	8 at 10 yr
Havenga et al (1999)[32]	1411	5 yr	Retrospective	7.6
Bolognese (2000)[33]	71	73.5 mo	Retrospective	12.6
Martling et al (2000)[34]	381	24 mo	Prospective with historical controls	6
Bissett et al (2000)[35]	124	5 yr	Retrospective with controls	10
Kapiteijn et al (2001)[36]	1748	2 yr	Randomized control trial	8.2
				2.4 with preop XRT
Tocchi et al (2001)[37]	53	68.9 mo	Retrospective	9
Wibe et al (2002)[38]	686	14–60 mo	Retrospective	7

XRT, radiotherapy.
Adapted from Ridgway P, Darzi AW: The role of mesorectal excision in the management of rectal cancer. Cancer Control 10:205–211, 2003, Table 2.

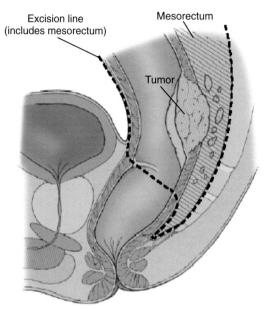

Figure 14-8. Total mesorectal excision. The dashed lines indicate the extent of mesorectal excision. (From Nelson H, Sargent DJ: Refining multimodal therapy for rectal cancer. N Engl J Med 345:690, 2001, Fig 1.)

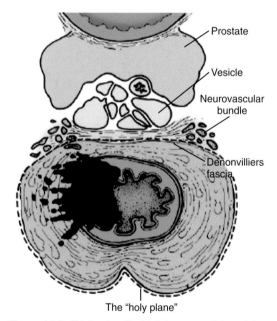

Figure 14-9. "Holy plane" of total mesorectal excision in relation to anterior anatomy in a male. (From Heald RJ, Moran BJ: Embryology and anatomy of the rectum. Sem Surg Oncol 15[2]:66–71, 1998. Copyright 1998. Reprinted with permission of John Wiley & Sons, Inc, Fig 6.)

Sphincter Salvage Procedures

In most patients, the decision to perform a sphincter-saving operation or an APR is already made. However, in distal rectal cancers, this determination may not be made until the rectum has been fully mobilized and the distal margin has been assessed.

All radical resections for rectal cancer use the same technique for mobilizing the rectum and achieving proximal, lateral, and radial margin clearance. Anterior resections are classified as high, low, or extended low, depending on the extent of rectal mobilization and resection and the level of the anastomosis. Sphincter preservation is usually possible in patients who have rectal cancers located more than 1 cm above the uppermost portion of the anorectal ring and who have acceptable preoperative anorectal function and reasonable pelvic anatomy. However, in patients with preexisting anorectal dysfunction, a colostomy may often provide better quality of life than persistent postoperative perineal morbidity. In general, sphincter-preserving operations are more likely to occur in a thin patient with a wide pelvis compared with an obese patient with a narrow pelvis.

The possibility of a permanent or temporary diverting stoma should be discussed at length with the patient. Patients should be seen by an enterostomal therapist for counseling and for marking the abdominal wall for either a colostomy or an ileostomy.

Patients should receive an intravenous antibiotic agent before induction of anesthesia. An epidural catheter is often placed for postoperative analgesia. A Foley catheter is placed in all patients. In selected patients with a large bulky rectal tumor or in re-operative procedures, ureteral stents may be placed to facilitate intraoperative identification of the ureters. The patient is placed in the modified lithotomy position with the legs in stirrups using Allen or Yellofin-style stirrups (Allen Medical Systems, Acton, MA) with the hips minimally flexed and abducted, knees flexed, and the feet flat in the stirrups. The surgeon should confirm that there is no pressure on the peroneal nerve or bony prominences. In addition, the buttocks should be positioned at the edge of the table on a roll that elevates them; this allows access to the anus. The positioning in stirrups is invaluable in allowing an assistant to be positioned in between the legs to help with retraction of the bladder and vagina. In addition, it allows access to the anus for placement of a circular stapler for sphincter restorative procedures. All patients should also have compression stockings with pneumatic compression devices with heparin, unless contraindicated.

Once the patient is under anesthesia, a digital rectal examination and rigid proctoscopy are performed to empty the rectum and reassess the rectal cancer. The involvement of the sphincter is assessed, and the distal edge of the tumor is noted. In addition, a rectal washout is performed using a large Foley catheter with a 30-mL balloon inflated and with normal saline mixed with diluted povidone-iodine solution.

A low midline incision is made avoiding any potential ostomy sites and extending inferiorly to the pubis. The operating surgeon should be positioned on the patient's left side. A self-retaining retractor, such as the Bookwalter, is placed, and an abdominal exploration is performed to evaluate for presence of metastatic disease. The small bowel is then packed away.

Step 1: Mobilization of the Colon. The sigmoid and left colon are mobilized by incising the white line of Toldt up to the splenic flexure while retracting the rectosigmoid to the right. The left ureter and gonadal vessels are identified using sharp and blunt dissection, and the sigmoid mesentery is separated from the retroperitoneum. The right ureter is usually easier to find in its typical location as it crosses the iliac artery. The mobilization of the splenic flexure is continued and extended proximally to the left transverse colon. This process may be facilitated by the surgeon moving in between the legs to increase the exposure of the splenic attachments, which should be taken with sharp meticulous dissection. Injury to the spleen can occur at this point from traction being applied to the omentum rather than to the spleen itself.

Step 2: Ligation of Inferior Mesenteric Artery. The surgeon now continues mobilization of the rectosigmoid anteriorly and to the left to identify the base of the inferior mesenteric artery (IMA) and vein. Once the IMA is identified, it is helpful to define an avascular plane on either side of the base of the artery (Fig. 14-10). Ligation of the IMA can then be performed after confirming that there is adequate collateral blood flow through the marginal artery of Drum-

mond. A high ligation of the IMA is performed approximately 1 cm from its origin from the aorta to preserve the para-aortic sympathetic plexus. The right and left ureters should have been identified before ligating the IMA. High ligation of the IMA is preferred, since it ensures adequate reach of the proximal colon without tension when the anastomosis is performed. When this is done, we usually divide the sigmoid–descending colon junction with a linear stapler. The mesentery to the sigmoid-descending colon is scored, and then the marginal arcades are clamped, divided, and ligated. If a pouch is planned, the surgeon must ensure that the proximal end of the colon reaches beyond the pubis symphysis without tension.

Step 3: TME with Autonomic Nerve Preservation. The TME dissection is continued by exposing the avascular plane posterior to the rectum and anterior to the sacral promontory (Fig. 14-11A). This is facilitated by retracting the rectosigmoid anteriorly and inferiorly. Sharp dissection under direct visualization should be performed to separate the shiny posterior surface of the mesorectum from the sacrum. The patient may also be placed in Trendelenburg position. The hypogastric nerves should be identified at the sacral promontory as they descend into the presacral space. These nerves must be preserved posteriorly and laterally to maintain postoperative genitourinary function. Both ureters should be identified and retracted laterally. The presacral fascia is incised down to the retrosacral or Waldeyer's fascia. Waldeyer's fascia is a thickened band attaching the rectum to the endopelvic fascia at the S4 level. Once the Waldeyer's fascia is incised, the dissection continues beyond the coccyx, and attention is paid to the anterior curve of the coccyx to prevent injury to the presacral veins. A lighted St. Mark's retractor facilitates this dissection.

The posterior dissection is done as far as possible, and then the lateral dissection is begun. The surgeon must identify the nervi erigentes on the lateral pelvic sidewalls or "stalks" and preserve them (Fig. 14-11B). The lateral dissection is again facilitated by having the assistant standing between the legs and using the St. Mark's retractor to retract the lateral side wall while the surgeon retracts the rectum and mesorectum medially. Adequate tension is essential during this lateral dissection to stay within the "holy

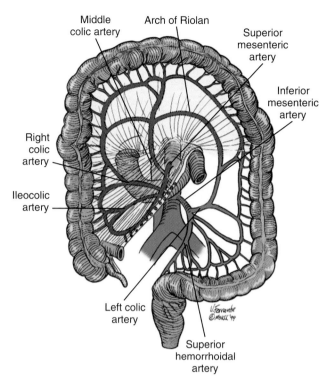

Middle colic artery

Arch of Riolan

Superior mesenteric artery

Inferior mesenteric artery

Right colic artery

Ileocolic artery

Left colic artery

Superior hemorrhoidal artery

Figure 14-10. Arterial supply to the rectum and colon. (From Cohen AM: Operation for colorectal cancer: low anterior resection. In Yeo CJ [ed]: Shackelford's Surgery of the Alimentary Tract, 6th ed. Philadelphia: Elsevier, 2007, Fig 158-4.)

plane" as defined by Heald (see Fig. 14-9). The middle rectal artery can generally be cauterized, although if it is present as a large vessel, it should be ligated during the lateral dissection. The integrity of the endopelvic fascia should be maintained at all times during the dissection. The lateral dissection ends at the levator muscles, which form the inferior boundary of the pelvic cavity.

The anterior dissection is now begun. This dissection is often the most difficult, since the planes of dissection are less discrete and the mesorectum is thin. Placing the patient in some reverse Trendelenburg position may facilitate this dissection. The dissection is continued by incising the cul-de-sac and incising Denonvilliers fascia. The dissection is performed in a plane parallel with Denonvilliers fascia between the rectum and the posterior wall of the seminal vesicles in men (Fig. 14-11C) or the vagina in women (Fig. 14-11D). The assistant can again use the lip of St. Marks retractor to elevate these structures anteriorly while the surgeon retracts posteriorly. Dissection is continued to the levator ani muscles, which then indicates that the entire mesorectum has been mobilized. The involvement of any of the structures in the

pelvis, such as bladder, ovary, prostate or sacrum, by contiguous involvement from the tumor requires en bloc removal of these organs. In patients with a narrow pelvis, the anterior dissection can be facilitated by having the assistant between the patient's legs apply cephalad pressure to the anus to elevate the levator ani and distal rectum towards the surgeon.

Step 4: Margin Assessment and Anastomosis. After the TME is complete, the point of transaction is chosen distal to the tumor. Recent studies have shown that a 2-cm margin is adequate for an oncologic resection. The level of transection can be confirmed by digital examination or rigid sigmoidoscopy. However, if an adequate distal margin cannot be attained, the surgeon needs to proceed with an APR. In addition to the distal margin, clearance of the circumferential margin is important, as previously discussed, and may require resection of en bloc structures. Once the point of transection is decided, electrocautery is used to dissect off the mesorectal fat until the rectum is cleared circumferentially. The bowel is clamped with a noncrushing clamp distal to the tumor to perform another rectal washout. A transverse

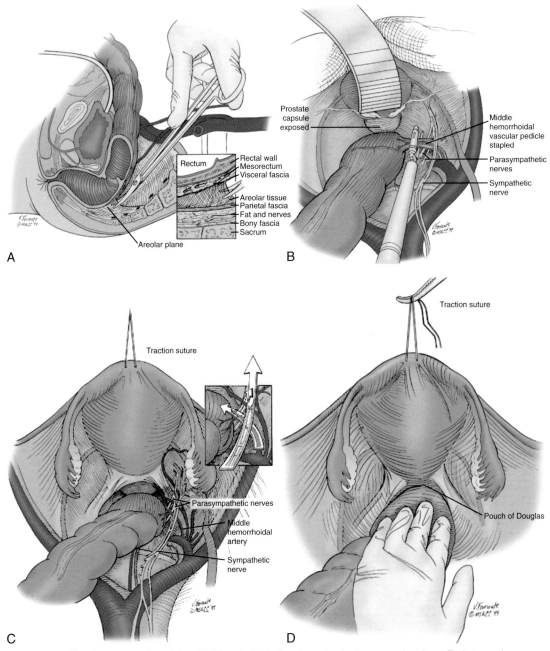

Figure 14-11. Total mesorectal excision (TME). **A,** Posterior dissection in the avascular plane. **B,** Autonomic nerves and the lateral vascular stalks. **C,** Anterior anatomy. **D,** Anterior dissection during TME in a female. (Adapted from Cohen AM: Operation for colorectal cancer: low anterior resection. In Zuidema GD [ed]: Shackelford's Surgery of the Alimentary Tract, 5th ed., 2002, Figs 18-8, 18-9, 18-10, and 18-12.)

anastomosis (TA) stapler is then placed distal to the clamp. The stapler is fired and the rectum divided sharply and handed off the field, leaving a closed rectal stump for anastomosis. The size of the transverse anastomosis stapler (30, 45, or 60 mm) depends on the depth and diameter of the pelvis.

The surgeon should inspect the distal and radial margins of the resected specimen to determine the integrity of the mesorectal dissection. The specimen should be oriented for the pathologist, and frozen sections of the margins can be performed if necessary. If the margins are inadequate, the surgical plan must be altered to improve clearance of the margin and reduce the risk of local recurrence.

After the specimen is removed, the pelvis should be irrigated with normal saline, and hemostasis should be ensured. Posterior bleeding may be seen secondary to injury to the sacral veins and is usually controlled by direct pressure.

Of the many choices of anastomosis, the end-to-end is the traditional choice. Most surgeons use the double-stapled end-to-end anastomosis, although a hand-sewn anastomosis can be performed (Fig. 14-12). The operating field is isolated with towels in preparation for manipulation of the proximal colon. The proximal end of the colon is prepared by clearing off the residual fat, and then the staple line is excised. Sizers are used to select a staple diameter. A purse-string suture of 2-0 or 3-0 polypropylene is placed using full-thickness bites at 2-mm intervals. The anvil of the appropriate-sized circular stapler is inserted, and the purse-string suture is tied around the shaft. The head of the circular stapler is inserted into the anus and advanced proxi-mally to the apex of the closed rectal stump. The trocar is introduced through or adjacent to the staple line. The anvil and stapler are joined. At this point, the colon is inspected to ensure that no adjacent tissue is entrapped and that the mesentery of the bowel is not twisted. The stapler is fired, opened slightly, and then removed. This is the second stapling line in the double-staple technique. The stapler is then inspected on a separate table to see that the tissue from the proximal and distal bowel is intact in two rings, that is, "the donuts."

The integrity of the anastomosis is confirmed by insufflating air into the rectum with a proctoscope while the anastomosis is submersed in saline to look for air leaks. The proximal bowel should be clamped during this test. In addition, the proctoscope allows direct visualization of the anastomosis to look for bleeding.

In patients with a low coloanal anastomosis and patients who have received neoadjuvant chemoradiation, we routinely perform a diverting loop ileostomy at a site marked preoperatively. The ileostomy can usually be reversed within 12 weeks of surgery. The ileostomy is created by making a 2-cm skin opening. The dissection is then carried down to the anterior rectus sheath. The fascial sheath is opened in a cruciate fashion with muscle-splitting and then opening the posterior peritoneum. The ileum is brought through the opening. It is important to identify the proximal and distal ends, and often a marking suture is used. The ileostomy is matured at the end after fascial and skin closure of the midline incision and placement of sterile dressing. The ileum is then incised transversely 1 cm above the skin on the distal limb of the loop. Next, the cut edges of the ileum are sewn to the skin with interrupted absorbable sutures, and the proximal limb can then be everted over the stoma rod. A diverting stoma does not protect against anastomotic leakage or prevent anastomotic complications, but it does diminish the morbidity resulting from leakage and reduce the likelihood of an emergency operation. The loop ileostomy is also easier to close than a diverting colostomy. Stoma formation is performed with a plastic ileostomy rod to prevent retraction during the initial postoperative period, and the rod is removed on postoperative day 5. A presacral sump drain is also placed and brought out through the skin opposite to the ileostomy.

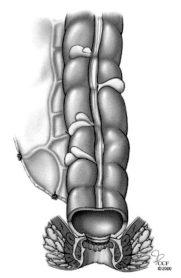

Figure 14-12. Anastomosis between descending colon and anus after complete resection of the rectum. The absence of the rectum often results in frequent, small bowel movements, a phenomenon known as "clustering" or "low anterior resection syndrome." (From Mantyh CR, Hull TL, Fazio VW: Coloplasty in low colorectal anastomosis: manometric and functional comparison with straight and colonic J-pouch anastomosis. Dis Colon Rectum 44:37–42, 2001, Fig 4. Reproduced with kind permission of Springer Science and Business Media.)

A hand-sewn, end-to-end colorectal anastomosis can be performed, if desired, in one or two layers with interrupted sutures. The sutures are all placed first, and then we parachute the proximal colon to the rectal cuff as the sutures are tied down. The knots are generally placed on the inside to invert the mucosa (see Fig. 14-12). Alternatively, a hand-sewn anastomosis can be performed transanally.

Coloanal Anastomosis

Patients with very low anastomoses often report urgency, frequency, seepage, and incontinence. To decrease these symptoms, a colonic reservoir is frequently created.

Colonic J Pouch

The colonic J pouch is considered for low anastomoses, less than 5 cm from the dentate line. The J pouch was first described in 1986 to increase colonic reservoir and improve quality of life after coloanal anastomosis. The European Organisation for Research and Treatment of Cancer (EORTC) conducted a randomized, prospective trial comparing the quality of life after a straight coloanal anastomosis with a J-pouch coloanal anastomosis and showed improved functional outcome and quality of life after J-pouch anastomosis. The improvement seen with the J pouch is most apparent in the first year after surgery. The J pouch has no advantage in patients whose anastomoses are more proximal than 8 cm from the dentate line. The splenic flexure must have been mobilized to provide adequate bowel length. The distal descending colon is folded into a J configuration with the efferent limb of the J pouch being 5 to 6 cm. The linear stapler is inserted through a colotomy on the antimesenteric side of the inferior-most aspect of the J pouch, then closed and fired. Multiple firings of the stapler may be needed (Fig. 14-13). The staple line is checked for bleeding, and the anvil of the circular stapler is placed using a purse-string suture. Further steps in the anastomosis are as previously described. We routinely use a diverting loop ileostomy for patients with a J pouch.

Transverse Coloplasty

A colonic J pouch may not be possible in about 25% of patients because of a narrow pelvis or

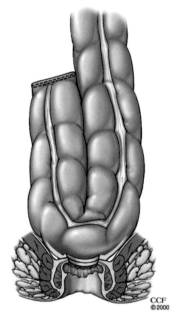

Figure 14-13. J pouch fashioned from descending colon to form proximal portion of coloanal anastomosis. This increases the "capacitance" to decrease the frequency of bowel movements. (From Mantyh CR, Hull TL, Fazio VW: Coloplasty in low colorectal anastomosis: manometric and functional comparison with straight and colonic J-pouch anastomosis. Dis Colon Rectum 44:37–42, 2001, Fig 3. Reproduced with kind permission of Springer Science and Business Media.)

inadequate reach of the proximal colon. In these patients, a transverse coloplasty is a suitable alternative, which was first described in 1997. A recent randomized trial demonstrated comparable functional results between transverse coloplasty and J-pouch coloanal reconstruction. A longitudinal colotomy is initiated, on the antimesenteric border, at a point 5 cm from the cut end of the descending colon and extended proximally for 8 to 10 cm (Figs. 14-14 and 14-15). The colotomy is then closed transversely in a manner similar to that of a Heineke-Mikulicz pyloroplasty with absorbable suture. An end-to-end anastomosis is next performed with the circular stapler in the usual manner, and a diverting ileostomy is made. However, the coloplasty has been thought to be associated with a higher leak rate ranging from 7% to 16% compared with J-pouch reconstruction and is reserved only for patients not amenable to a J-pouch reconstruction. The functional advantages of both coloplasty and colonic J pouches are best seen in the first 2 years after operation, including improve-

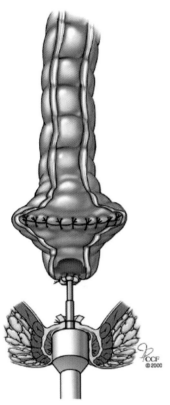

Figure 14-14. Coloplasty. A coloplasty is performed by making an 8- to 10-cm colotomy 4 to 6 cm from the cut end of the colon. The longitudinal colotomy is made between the taeniae on the antimesenteric side. It is closed transversely with absorbable sutures. An end-to-end stapled anastomosis then joins the colon to the distal rectum or anus. (From Mantyh CR, Hull TL, Fazio VW: Coloplasty in low colorectal anastomosis: manometric and functional comparison with straight and colonic J-pouch anastomosis. Dis Colon Rectum 44:37–42, 2001, Fig 1. Reproduced with kind permission of Springer Science and Business Media.)

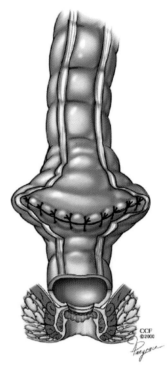

Figure 14-15. The completed stapled coloplasty with anastomosis. (From Mantyh CR, Hull TL, Fazio VW: Coloplasty in low colorectal anastomosis: manometric and functional comparison with straight and colonic J-pouch anastomosis. Dis Colon Rectum 44:37–42, 2001, Fig 2. Reproduced with kind permission of Springer Science and Business Media.)

ments in symptoms of urgency, frequency, nocturnal stooling, and continence.

Abdominoperineal Resection

Ernest Miles described the first APR operation in 1908. Currently, patients who are not amenable to sphincter salvage undergo APR resection, which involves the en bloc resection of the rectosigmoid, the rectum with the mesorectum, and the anus along with its surrounding mesentery and perianal soft tissues. There is increasing use of restorative procedures after radical surgery for rectal cancer, but APR is still performed in 30% to 55% of patients in the United States based on SEER (Surveillance, Epidemiology and End Results) registry data.

The abdominal portion of the operation is performed similarly to that of the sphincter salvage approach previously described with a total mesorectal excision. The total mesorectal excision should be carried down to the levator muscles inferiorly. Anteriorly, the dissection should be carried out to and beyond the level of the prostate in men and beyond the cervix in women. When the rectum is fully mobilized, the surgeon moves in between the legs to perform the perineal excision. A two-team approach may also be used to expedite the surgery.

The perineal dissection is done by making an elliptical incision around the anus. This incision should extend from the perineal body anteriorly to the coccyx posteriorly. Dissection is continued with electrocautery through the ischiorectal fat. A self-retaining retractor is very useful to facilitate deep dissection. We prefer to use the Lone Star Retractor, which has adjustable, flexible hooks that can be placed circumferentially to evert the tissues out. The dissection is carried outside the external sphincters toward the coccyx. The anococcygeal ligament is palpated posteriorly and is incised, creating an opening between the left and right levator muscles. At this point, it is helpful for the perineal surgeon to insert an index finger into the pelvis to guide the division of the posterolateral soft tissue with electrocautery by hooking the index finger under the levator muscles laterally on each side. A vessel-sealing device, such as the LigaSure (Covidien, Mansfield, MA), is useful during the deeper dissection. The anterior dissection should be done last. A narrow Deaver or appendectomy retractor may be used to improve the retraction during the deeper dissection.

When the perineal opening is wide enough, the proximal end of the specimen is passed from the abdominal portion through the perineum in the opening between the coccyx and the anus. The everted specimen is then used to help provide traction to develop the anterior dissection plane. In men, the anterior dissection requires careful attention to prevent injury to the urethra or the prostatic capsule, which may result in excessive bleeding. As the dissection proceeds, it is helpful to palpate the Foley catheter during anterior dissection to remain in the right plane. In women, a bulky anterior lesion may necessitate a posterior wall vaginectomy to ensure a negative margin.

Once the specimen is freed circumferentially, it is inspected and sent for pathologic evaluation. The pelvis is irrigated and hemostasis is obtained. The perineal incision (Fig. 14-16) is then closed in several layers with absorbable sutures to minimize the risk of perineal wound infection. A drain should be placed in this space below the peritoneal reflection and brought out either transabdominally or through the perineum. We prefer to also mobilize and place an omental pedicle in the pelvis to keep the small bowel out of the pelvis and decrease the risk of subsequent pelvic adhesions as well as to facilitate healing.

The end colostomy is created in a site marked preoperatively by the enterostomal therapist. The colostomy site opening is created, similar to the loop ileostomy just described, in the left lower quadrant. The mobilized colon is passed through this site, but it is not matured until the abdominal incision is closed and a dry sterile dressing has been applied. The colon is secured

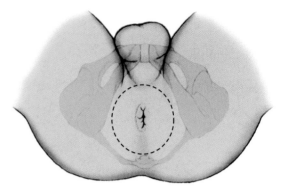

Figure 14-16. The topographic landmarks for the perineal dissection. (Adapted from Fazio VW [ed]: Current Therapy in Colon and Rectal Therapy. Ontario, BC Decker, 1990, pp 120–130.)

to the peritoneal cavity circumferentially as it exits the abdomen. The colostomy is generally matured to the skin with interrupted 3-0 absorbable sutures.

The mortality rate from radical rectal surgery is approximately 2%, with most deaths related to cardiopulmonary complications. The overall risk of anastomotic leak after rectal surgery is about 5%, but it can increase in patients who have a low coloanal anastomosis, who are immunosuppressed, and who have undergone neoadjuvant chemoradiation therapy. The risk of autonomic nerve dysfunction has declined from 60% to 85% down to less than 15% in most current series with TME dissection.[39,40]

Pelvic Exenteration and Sacrectomy

Pelvic exenteration involves resection of the anus, rectum, bladder, ureters, and pelvic reproductive organs. Sacrectomy is necessary when the rectal cancer is invading posteriorly but contraindicated when there is invasion of the upper sacral vertebrae. However, indications for pelvic exenteration are limited by the relatively high morbidity and mortality associated with the procedure. Wanebo and associates[41] have reported 5-year survival rates after pelvic exenteration for locally recurrent rectal cancer ranging from 20% to 30%. Curative exenteration cannot be performed when there is evidence of carcinomatosis, liver metastases, pelvic sidewall invasion, bilateral ureteral obstruction, or aortic node metastases. The surgeon should consider comfort care or additional adjuvant therapy (e.g., intraoperative radiation therapy, brachytherapy, and further chemoradiation) before performing palliative exenteration.

References

1. Weiser MR, Posner MC, et al: Adenocarcinoma of the colon and rectum. In Yeo CJ (ed): Shackelford's Surgery of the Alimentary Tract, 5th ed. Philadelphia: Elsevier, 2007.
2. Turnball RB Jr, Kyle K, Watson FR, et al: Cancer of the colon: the influence of the no-touch isolation technique on survival rates. Ann Surg 166(3):420–427, 1967.
3. Wiggers T, Jeekel J, Arends JW, et al: No-touch isolation technique in colon cancer: a controlled prospective trial. Br J Surg 75(5):409–415, 1988.
4. Hermanek P, Wiebelt H, Staimmer D, Riedl S: Prognostic factors of rectum carcinoma—experience of the German Multicenter Study SGCRC. German Study Group Colo-Rectal Carcinoima. Tumori 81(3):60–64, 1995.
5. Enker WE, Laffer UT, Block GE: Enhanced survival of patients with colon and rectal cancer is based upon wide anatomic resection. Ann Surg 190(3):350–356, 1979.
6. Hida JI, Okuno K, Yasutomi M, et al: Optimal ligation level of the primary feeding artery and bowel resection margin in colon cancer surgery. Dis Colon Rectum 48:2232–2237, 2005.
7. Nelson H, Petrelli N, Carlin A, et al: Guidelines 2000 for colon and rectal cancer surgery. J Natl Cancer Inst 93(8):583–596, 2001.
8. Chang GJ, Rodriguez-Bigas MA, Skibber JM, Moyer VA: Lymph node evaluation and survival after curative resection of colon cancer: a systemic review. J Natl Cancer Inst 99(6):433–442, 2007.
9. Baxter NN, Virnig DJ, Rothenberger DA, et al: Lymph node evaluation in colorectal patients: a population-based study. J Natl Cancer Inst 97(3):219–225, 2005.
10. Gabriel WB, Dukes C, Bussey HJ: Lymphatic spread in cancer of the rectum. Br J Surg 23:395–413, 1935.
11. Kim J, Huynh R, Abraham I, et al: Number of lymph nodes examined and its impact on colorectal cancer staging. Am Surg 72:902–905, 2006.
12. Tekkis PP, Smith JJ, Heriot AG, et al: A national study on lymph node retrieval in resectional surgery for colorectal cancer. Dis Colon Rectum 49:1673–1683, 2006.
13. Thomas KA, Lechner J, Shen P, et al: Use of sentinel node mapping for cancer of the colon: to map or not to map. Am Surg 72(7):606–611, 2006.
14. Stojadinovic A, Nissan A, Protic M, et al: Prospective randomized study comparing sentinel lymph node evaluation with standard pathologic evaluation for the staging of colon carcinoma: results from the United States Military Cancer Institute Clinical Trials Group Study GI-01. Ann Surg 245(96):846–857, 2007.
15. Grobmyer SR, Guillem JG: Colon cancer. In Cameron JL (ed): Current Surgical Therapy, 8th ed. Philadelphia: Elsevier, 2004, pp 211–215.
16. Sonoda T, Milson JW: Segmental colon resection, Chap. 34. In ACS Surgery: Principles and Practice. Chicago, IL: American College of Surgeons, 2006.
17. Britton J: Intestinal anastomosis. In Souba WV (ed): Online ACS Surgery: Principles and Practice. Chicago: American College of Surgeons, 2004.
18. Ota DM: Right hemicolectomy for cancer. In Fischer JE, Bland KI (eds): Mastery of Surgery. Boston: Little Brown, 1997, pp 1490–1507.
19. Bothwell WN, Bleicher RJ, Dent TL: Prophylactic ureteral catheterization in colon surgery. A five year review. Dis Colon Rectum 37(4):330–334, 1994.
20. Zollinger RM, Zollinger RM Sr: Left colon. In Zollinger's Atlas of Surgical Operations, 7th ed. New York: McGraw-Hill, 1993, pp 128–133.
21. Pilipshen SJ, Heilweil M, Quan SH, et al: Patterns of pelvic recurrence following definitive resections of rectal cancer. Cancer 53(6):1354–1362, 1984.
22. Nagtegaal ID, Majinen CA, Kranenbarg EK, et al: Circumferential margin involvement is still an important predictor of local recurrence in rectal carcinoma: not one millimeter but two millimeters is the limit. Am J Surg Pathol 26:350–357, 2002.
23. Tjandra JJ, Kilkenney JW, Buie WD, et al: Practice parameters for the management of rectal cancer. Dis Colon Rectum 48: 411–423, 2005.
24. Heald RJ, Husband EM, Ryall RD: The mesorectum in rectal cancer surgery: the clue to pelvic recurrence? Br J Surg 69: 613–616, 1982.
25. Heald RJ, Moran BJ: Embryology and anatomy of the rectum. Semin Surg Oncol 15(2):66–71, 1998.
26. Moynihan B: Surgical treatment of cancer of the sigmoid flexure and rectum. Surg Gynecol Obstet 6:463–466, 1908.
27. McAnena OJ, Heald RJ, Lockhart-Mummery HE: Operative and functional results of total mesorectal excision with ultra-low anterior resection in the management of carcinoma of the lower one-third of the rectum. Surg Gynecol Obstet 170:517–521, 1990.
28. MacFarlane JK, Ryall RD, Heald RJ: Mesorectal excision for rectal cancer. Lancet 341:457–460, 1993.
29. Enker WE, Thaler HT, Cranor ML, et al: Total mesorectal excision in the operative treatment of carcinoma of the rectum. J Am Coll Surg 181:335–346, 1995.
30. Zaheer S, Pemberton JH, Faroul R, et al: Surgical treatment of adenocarcinoma of the rectum. Ann Surg 227:800–811, 1998.
31. Heald RJ, Moran BJ, Ryall RD, et al: Rectal cancer: the Basingstoke experience of total mesorectal excision, 1978–1997. Arch Surg 133:894–898, 1998.
32. Havenga K, Enker WE, Norstein J, et al: Improved survival and local control after total mesorectal excision or D3 lymphadenectomy in the treatment of primary rectal cancer: an international analysis of 1411 patients. Eur J Surg Oncol 25:368–374, 1999.
33. Bolognese A, Cardi M, Muttillo IA, et al: Total mesorectal excision for surgical treatment of rectal cancer. J Surg Oncol 74: 21–23, 2000.
34. Martling AL, Holm T, Rutqvist LE, et al: Effect of a surgical training programme on outcome of rectal cancer in the County of Stockholm. Stockholm Colorectal Cancer Study Group, Basingstoke Bowel Cancer Research Project. Lancet 356:93–96, 2000.
35. Bissett IP, McKay GS, Parry BR, et al: Results of extrafascial excision and conventional surgery for rectal cancer at Auckland Hospital. Aust N Z J Surg 70:704–709, 2000.
36. Kapiteijn E, Marijnen CA, Nagtegaal ID, et al: Preoperative radiotherapy combined with total mesorectal excision for resectable rectal cancer. N Engl J Med 345:638–646, 2001.
37. Tocchi A, Mazzoni G, Lepre L, et al: Total mesorectal excision and low rectal anastomosis for the treatment of rectal cancer and prevention of pelvic recurrences. Arch Surg 136:216–220, 2001.
38. Wibe A, Rendedal PR, Svensson E, et al: Prognostic significance of the circumferential resection margin following total mesorectal excision for rectal cancer. Br J Surg 89:327–334, 2002.
39. Rothenberger DA, Ricciardi R: Procedures for rectal cancer. In Souba WV (ed): Online ACS Surgery: Principles and Practice, 2004.
40. Havenga K, Enker WE: Autonomic nerve preserving total mesorectal excision. Surg Clin North Am 82(5):1009–1018, 2002.
41. Wanebo HJ, Antoniuk P, Koness RJ, et al: Pelvic resection and recurrent rectal cancer. Dis Colon Rec 42(11):1438–1448, 1999.

15

Systemic Therapy for Colon Cancer

Khaled El-Shami,
Sujatha Nallapareddy,
and Wells Messersmith

KEY POINTS

- Systemic therapy for colorectal cancer is rapidly changing, with six new drugs introduced during the last decade.
- Several "targeted" drugs have shown benefit in advanced disease, but not in the postoperative adjuvant setting.
- *K-ras* mutational testing for epidermal growth factor receptor (EGFR)-targeting antibodies has ushered in an era of personalized therapy whereby genetic testing of colorectal tumors determines therapy.

Introduction

The fluoropyrimidine analog fluorouracil (5-FU) first developed by Heidelberger and coworkers[1] in 1957 was the only first-line chemotherapeutic option for patients with advanced colorectal cancer until the late 1990s. As such, 5-FU underwent extensive dose and schedule optimizations and combinations with different modulators to improve response and survival rates. Median survival beyond 12 months, however, was rarely attainable.[2-6]

Over the past 10 years, considerable investigational work has resulted in new drugs and more innovative combination strategies for treating colon cancer. The new landscape of systemic therapy for colon cancer has seen the addition of irinotecan, oxaliplatin, and capecitabine as cytotoxic agents. In addition, targeted therapies, such as the first monoclonal antibody against the vascular endothelial growth factor (VEGF), bevacizumab (Avastin), was approved in 2004 for first-line therapy for metastatic colorectal cancer. Two monoclonal antibodies against the epidermal growth factor receptor (EGFR), cetuximab and more recently panitumumab, have

been approved for chemotherapy-refractory colorectal cancer. *K-ras* codon 12/13 testing has revolutionized the way in which EGFR-targeting antibodies are used in the clinic. This chapter reviews the state of the art in systemic therapy of colon cancer, both in the metastatic and adjuvant setting, and explores future directions in this field.

Metastatic Colorectal Cancer

5-Fluorouracil and Leucovorin

The benefit of systemic therapy in the management of metastatic colorectal cancer was initially established in the 1980s and 1990s. Several phase III randomized trials showed improvement in the quality of life and overall responses despite low objective response rates (RR 10%–20%) with the use of 5-FU and leucovorin (LV).[7] According to a meta-analysis of 13 such trials, systemic chemotherapy significantly improved overall survival compared with best supportive care.[8] Fluorouracil forms the backbone of systemic therapy for advanced colorectal cancer, and the survival of these patients nearly doubled with the advent of new chemotherapeutic and targeted agents (Fig. 15-1).

Fluorouracil and leucovorin are administered intravenously in a variety of dosing schedules. In the loading bolus schedules, 5-FU and leucovorin are administered daily in bolus for 5 consecutive days and repeated every 28 days (Mayo Clinic Protocol)[9]; alternatively, in the weekly bolus schedule, 5-FU and leucovorin are given weekly for 6 of every 8 weeks (Roswell Park regimen).[10] For the infusional regimen, leucovorin and 5-FU are administered in bolus followed

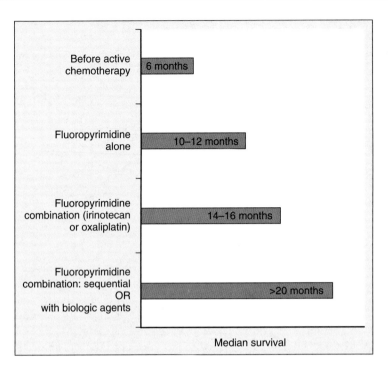

Figure 15-1. Median survival of patients with advanced colorectal cancer.

by 22 hours of 5-FU infusion through a central venous catheter on days 1 and 2 and repeated every 2 weeks (5-FU/LV2).[11]

These regimens differ in their toxicities, which may partly guide their use clinically. The bolus regimens tend to be associated with bone marrow suppression, mucostomatitis, and diarrhea; whereas palmar-plantar erythrodysesthesia (hand-foot syndrome) is more common in the infusional regimen. Central venous access is required for the infusional regimen. The difference in quality of life and cost between the infusional and bolus regimens is marginal, and the infusional method seems to be marginally more effective than the bolus approach.[12-16]

Irinotecan

The advent of a number of active agents allowed the use of combination chemotherapy (Box 15-1). The earliest combination regimens used irinotecan with various schedules of 5-FU/LV in first-line therapy of metastatic colorectal cancer.[17-19] Irinotecan (also known as CPT-11) is a semisynthetic derivative of the natural alkaloid camptotecin and exerts its cytotoxic effects by inhibiting topoisomerase I, which is necessary for the proper uncoiling of DNA for replication and transcription. The drug is hydrolyzed to its more potent active metabolite, SN38, by carbo-

xylesterase.[20] Irinotecan and its metabolites interact with DNA replication forks, leading to DNA fragmentation by stabilizing single-chain DNA breaks and subsequent cell death. When compared with infusional 5-FU or best supportive care, irinotecan showed single-agent activity in patients with advanced colorectal cancer who had previously received bolus 5-FU with improvement in median survival and quality of life.[21,22]

In first-line advanced colorectal cancer therapy, irinotecan improved median survival by about 2 months and almost doubled the response

---

Box 15-1. Selected Agents with Proven Efficacy in Metastatic Colorectal Cancer

Cytotoxic Agents

Fluoropyrimidines
  5-Fluorouracil (+ folinic acid/leucovorin modulation)
  Capecitabine
  Tegafur/uracil
  S-1
Irinotecan
Oxaliplatin

Biologic/Targeted Agents

Bevacizumab
Cetuximab
Panitumumab

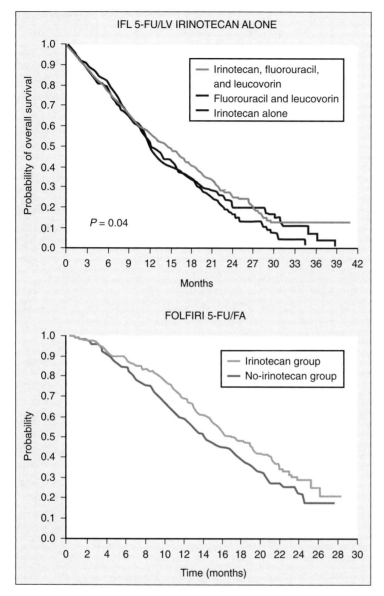

Figure 15-2. Kaplan-Meier estimates of overall survival for irinotecan-based regimens. FA, folinic acid. (**A,** Reprinted from Saltz LB, Cox JV, Blanke C, et al: Leucovorin and fluorouracil and leucovorin for metastatic colorectal cancer. Irinotecan Study Group. N Engl J Med 343: 905–914, 2000. **B,** Reprinted from Douillard JY, Cunningham D, Roth AD, et al: Irinotecan combined with fluorouracil compared with fluorouracil alone as first-line treatment for metastatic colorectal cancer: a multicentre randomized trial. Lancet 355:1041–1047, 2000.)

rate when combined with 5-FU and leucovorin in two randomized trials[16,19] (Fig. 15-2). In the North American trial, irinotecan added to weekly bolus schedule 5-FU (IFL) was compared with bolus 5-FU (Mayo regimen) and patients who received IFL had a longer median overall survival (14.8 versus 12.6 months; $P =$ .04) and a higher response rate (39% versus 21%; $P <$ .001). In the European trial, irinotecan combined with infusional 5-FU (FOLFIRI) was compared with infusional 5-FU regimens. Similar efficacy was found in patients who received the FOLFIRI with improvement of median overall survival from 14.1 to 17.4 months

($P <$ .001) and response rate from 22% to 35% ($P <$ .01).

The toxicity of irinotecan includes diarrhea, bone marrow suppression, nausea and vomiting, and alopecia. Certain toxicities, especially diarrhea and neutropenia, correlate with a polymorphism of uridine diphosphate glucuronosyltransferase isoform 1A1 (UGT1A1) in retrospective studies.[23,24] SN38, the active metabolite, is glucuronidated by UGT1A1 before elimination, so reduced UGT1A1 activity increases SN38. An (FDA)-approved clinical test for UGT1A1 polymorphism is available, and individualizing irinotecan dosage based on patients' pharmacogenomic profile may eventually be clinically feasible.[25] With no data from a prospective clinical trial, the usefulness of testing UGT1A1, and how to adjust dosages depending on the test results, are debatable.

Oxaliplatin

Oxaliplatin is a third-generation diaminocyclohexane-containing platinum compound that forms bulky DNA adducts and induces cellular apoptosis.[26] Unlike previous generations of platinum compounds, oxaliplatin showed promising activity against human colorectal cell lines in preclinical studies. In clinical studies, oxaliplatin had limited single-agent efficacy but was highly synergistic with fluoropyrimidines in first- and second-line therapy for metastatic colorectal cancers.[27-29] A possible mechanism was downregulation of thymidylate synthase by oxaliplatin.[30-32]

In April 2002, an interim analysis of a landmark trial ushered in oxaliplatin-based therapy to the first-line treatment of advanced colorectal cancer. The North Central Cancer Treatment Group/Intergroup Trial N9741 compared IFL with oxaliplatin/folinic acid/5-FU (FOLFOX4 regimen with oxaliplatin 85 mg/m^2 on day 1; LV 200 mg/m^2 for 2 hours; and bolus 5-FU, 400 mg/m^2 followed by 600 mg/m^2 continuous infusion for 22 hours on days 1 and 2) and a combination of irinotecan and oxaliplatin (IROX).[33] FOLFOX4 compared favorably with IFL, which was the standard of care at the time, in all efficacy parameters including response rate (45% versus 31%), time to progression (TTP, 8.7 months versus 6.9 months), and median overall survival (OS 19.5 months versus 15 months). In addition, toxicity analysis favored FOLFOX4. This trial eventually set the new standard of care in first-line therapy of colorectal cancer. Based on its results, FOLFOX has become the most widely used combination regimen in newly diagnosed advanced or metastatic colorectal cancer, particularly in the United States.

In the second-line setting, patients with metastatic colorectal cancer who received FOLFOX after IFL failure had a better outcome in median time to progression and response rate compared with those who received 5-FU and leucovorin.[34] In three first-line randomized trials, the oxaliplatin-containing regimens showed consistently better time to progression, response

rate, and overall survival than did 5-FU and leucovorin alone.[35,36]

When combined with 5-FU and leucovorin, oxaliplatin has side effects that are different from those of the other platinum compounds, namely, cisplatin and carboplatin. Nephrotoxicity, ototoxicity, and alopecia have been less common.[37-39] Approximately 15% of patients who received oxaliplatin-based regimens, however, have developed a unique neuropathy: an acute, reversible, transient, and cold-induced paresthesia of hands, feet, oral, or pharyngeal regions during or for a short period of time after infusion and a cumulative, dose-dependent, longer-lasting peripheral dysesthesia after months of treatment. The neuropathy is usually reversible when oxaliplatin is stopped and fortunately reverses in more than 99% of patients to a level not interfering with activities of daily living within 18 months after discontinuation.[40]

FOLFOX versus FOLFIRI

Despite the fact that FOLFOX showed significantly higher efficacy compared with irinotecan and bolus 5-FU (IFL), when administered in combination with infusional 5-FU and leucovorin, irinotecan (FOLFIRI), and oxaliplatin (FOLFOX) appear to be equally efficacious in patients with previously untreated metastatic colorectal cancer. The choice for first-line therapy is then often guided by the regimens' adverse effects and institutional practice. A phase III trial by Tournigand and associates[41] compared FOLFOX with FOLFIRI with crossover at progression. Response rates (56% versus 54%), progression-free survival ([PFS] 8.5 months versus 8.0 months), and median overall survival (21.5 versus 20.6 months) were almost identical. Comparable results were also reported by an Italian group.[42]

It is clear that the maximum impact on overall survival is related to exposure to all active drugs, with the actual sequence of this exposure playing a minor role or no role in changing the overall survival outcome. This observation was emphasized in a meta-analysis of seven phase III studies showing that the median overall survival correlates with the percentage of patients receiving all three active agents (5-FU, irinotecan, and oxaliplatin).[43] Regimens with all three drugs simultaneously (FOLFOXIRI) have also been tested with promising results.[44]

Oral Fluoropyrimidines

Capecitabine, a fluoropyrimidine carbamate, is an oral prodrug that undergoes enzymatic conversion in the liver to 5-FU.[45] The adverse-effect profile is similar to that of infusional 5-FU regimen, with hand-foot syndrome as the predominant toxicity. However, stomatitis, nausea, vomiting, bone marrow suppression, and diarrhea are observed as well. Capecitabine is superior to daily bolus Mayo regimen in terms of objective response rate (about 25% versus 16%, respectively) in two randomized controlled trials, but it did not confer significant survival advantage (median survival about 12.9 versus 12.8 months, respectively).[46–48]

Another oral fluoropyrimidine with similar response and survival rates compared with intravenous 5-FU was tegafur, a prodrug of 5-FU, plus uracil, an inhibitor of dihydropyrimidine dehydrogenase.[49,50] The combination is usually administered together with oral leucovorin and is approved by regulatory agencies outside of the United States. S-1 is another 5-FU-based oral combination drug, which has been developed mainly in Asia.[51–56]

The oral fluoropyrimidine that has been studied the most is capecitabine. Having been designed to recapitulate the pharmacokinetics of continuous infusion 5-FU via oral administration, capecitabine was compared with the Mayo Clinic regimen of bolus 5-FU/LV in a phase III trial. It was found to have superior response rates, equivalent PFS and overall survival, and a favorable toxicity profile.[48] These observations led to studies exploring capecitabine as an alternative to infusional 5-FU in combination with oxaliplatin or irinotecan. Two studies, TREE-1 and TREE-2, explored the best fluoropyrimidine in combination with oxaliplatin. Patients were randomized to FOLFOX6, bolus 5-FU/LV/oxaliplatin, or CAPOX (capecitabine + oxaliplatin).[57] Since the FDA approval of bevacizumab took place while the trials were ongoing, an amendment was made to add bevacizumab to various arms of the studies. Although bevacizumab appeared to enhance the efficacy of each individual regimen, the CAPOX regimen was comparable to its infusional counterpart FOLFOX6 as far as response rates, TTP (time to progression), and overall survival are concerned, with the regimen containing the bolus 5-FU/LV being the least effective.

Moreover, a large, randomized, international, phase III trial of 2035 advanced colorectal cancer patients, NO16966, compared first-line XELOX (capecitabine [Xeloda] + oxaliplatin) with FOLFOX4 (intravenous bolus and infusional 5-FU + oxaliplatin). After release of bevacizumab data in colorectal cancer in 2003, the protocol was amended to investigate, using a 2 by 2 factorial design, XELOX + placebo versus XELOX + bevacizumab (7.5 mg/kg every 3 weeks) versus FOLFOX4 + placebo versus FOLFOX4 + bevacizumab (5.0 mg/kg every 2 weeks). The primary objective of the study was to answer two questions: (1) whether the XELOX regimen is noninferior to FOLFOX and (2) whether the addition of bevacizumab to chemotherapy improved results compared with chemotherapy alone. The secondary endpoints included overall survival, overall response rates, time to and duration of response, and safety profile. The study showed that XELOX (capecitabine + oxaliplatin) is as effective as FOLFOX4 (infused 5-FU + oxaliplatin) in terms of PFS (hazard ratio [HR] 1.05; upper limit of the 95% confidence interval was below the noninferiority margin of 1.23). Adding bevacizumab to chemotherapy (FOLFOX4 and XELOX) significantly improved PFS compared with that with chemotherapy alone (HR 0.83), which meant that adding bevacizumab to chemotherapy combination with either 5-FU or capecitabine improves the chances of delaying progression of the disease by 20%.[58] In contrast, the combination of capecitabine and irinotecan (CAPIRI) is more controversial. CAPIRI was found to be inferior to its infusional counterpart (FOLFIRI) both in terms of PFS and tolerability in the phase III trial BICC-C,[59] but the difference in overall survival was not significant. Diarrhea appears to be a major hurdle in combining these agents, and care must be taken to prevent dehydration.

Epidermal Growth Factor Receptor (EGFR) Antibodies

The epidermal growth factor receptor (EGFR, or HER1) is a transmembrane receptor tyrosine kinase that belongs to the erbB, or HER, receptor family. Upon binding with a ligand such as epidermal growth factor (EGF) or transforming growth factor (TGF-α), EGFR pairs with another EGFR receptor (homodimerization) or another member of the erbB family (heterodi-

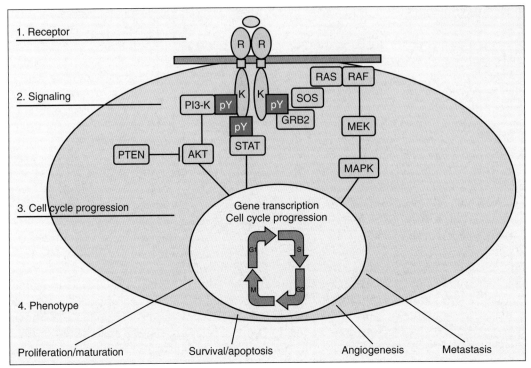

Figure 15-3. Epidermal growth factor signaling pathway. (Reprinted from Baselga J: Targeting the epidermal growth factor receptor: a clinical reality. J Clin Oncol 19:41S–44S, 2001.)

merization). Dimerization leads to receptor autophosphorylation and activation of intracellular signaling pathways that regulate cellular growth, survival, migration, adhesion, and differentiation (Fig. 15-3). The receptor was found to be abnormally activated in many epithelial malignancies including colorectal cancer.[60,61]

EGFR became a target of interest in colorectal cancer therapy when expression or upregulation of the EGFR gene was found in 60% to 80% of cases.[62–65] Overexpression of EGFR in colorectal cancer was also associated with poorer prognosis.[66,67] Inhibition of EGFR can be achieved by targeting the extracellular domain with monoclonal antibodies or the intracellular tyrosine kinase with small molecule inhibitors.[68]

Cetuximab is a chimeric murine/human IgG1 monoclonal antibody highly specific for EGFR and has a higher affinity than EGF and TGF-α, thereby blocking the ligand-dependent autophosphorylation of the receptor. Although preclinical studies showed primarily cytostatic single-agent activity, cetuximab plus irinotecan was highly synergistic in irinotecan-refractory colorectal cancer xenografts when tumor growth would have continued with respective agents

alone.[69–71] As an IgG1 subtype antibody, cetuximab can theoretically mediate immune functions and thus may have immunologic mechanisms as well.

Cetuximab was first of its class to be approved by the FDA in the United States for treatment of colorectal cancer in patients who had previous unsuccessful chemotherapy. The response rates for cetuximab alone and cetuximab plus irinotecan were 9% and 17%, respectively, in two nonrandomized trials involving colorectal cancer patients previously treated with an irinotecan-based regimen.[72,73] In a multi-institutional randomized study, 329 patients with metastatic colorectal cancer who progressed on irinotecan-based regimen were randomized to receive either cetuximab plus irinotecan or cetuximab monotherapy.[74] The patients receiving cetuximab plus irinotecan had a better response rate (22.9% versus 10.8%; $P = .007$) and median TTP (4.1 versus 1.5 months; $P < .001$) than cetuximab monotherapy, although median survival was not significantly different (8.6 versus 6.9 months; $P = .48$).

Cetuximab as monotherapy versus best supportive care (BSC) was investigated in the

NCIC CO.17 trial.[75] In this trial, 572 metastatic colorectal cancer patients who progressed after treatment with fluoropyrimidines, oxaliplatin, and irinotecan were randomized to cetuximab with BSC versus BSC alone without crossover. Cetuximab improved overall survival (HR for death 0.77; $P = .005$) from 4.6 months in the BSC-alone arm to 6.1 months in the cetuximab/BSC arm in unselected patients. The hazard ratio for PFS was 0.68; $P < .001$.

A more recent trial, CRYSTAL, evaluated cetuximab combined with the irinotecan-based chemotherapy regimen FOLFIRI versus FOLFIRI alone. Median PFS was slightly improved from 8.0 to 8.9 months ($P = .036$), but there was no significant difference in overall survival. The response rate was also improved by the addition of cetuximab (46.9% versus 38.7% in the FOLFIRI-only arm; $P = .0038$).[76] Furthermore, in a subgroup analysis of patients who had liver-limited disease, PFS was 11.4 months with cetuximab versus 9.2 months in the control arm. The number of complete resections of the metastases in the subgroup who had only liver metastases was more than double with cetuximab plus FOLFIRI compared with the control arm (9.8% versus 4.5%).

In addition, the combination of cetuximab plus the oxaliplatin-based regimen (FOLFOX) in irinotecan-refractory metastatic colorectal cancer appeared to be safe when examined in a multi-institutional randomized trial, the EXPLORE trial.[77] The OPUS trial, a phase II randomized study, further confirmed this result. In this trial, 337 patients were randomized to receive FOLFOX4 + cetuximab versus FOLFOX4. The best overall response rate was 45.6% in the FOLFOX/cetuximab arm versus 35.7% in the FOLFOX arm.[78]

The side effects of cetuximab are fairly well tolerated. About 75% of patients developed a mild acneiform rash. About 3% of patients developed hypersensitivity infusional reactions when receiving therapy. The development of rash to anti-EGFR therapy seemed to correlate with objective response, but this relationship needs to be better defined in a properly designed clinical study.[79]

Panitumumab is a fully human monoclonal antibody of the IgG2 type against EGFR with single-agent activity in chemotherapy-refractory colorectal cancer comparable to that of cetuximab.[80,81] Different dosing schedules have been proposed (weekly, every 2 weeks, or every 3 weeks).[82] Although more than 90% of patients experienced some degree of acneiform rash, only 3% were severe (grade 3 or 4). Based on the results of a phase III trial showing improved PFS compared with BSC in metastatic colon cancer, biweekly panitumumab has received FDA approval for use in chemotherapy-refractory advanced colorectal carcinoma.[83]

In previous cetuximab trials, only patients with EGFR expression by immunohistochemical stain were eligible, owing to preclinical evidence, which suggests the predictive value of EGFR expression for cetuximab efficacy. This led to the initial approval of cetuximab therapy for patients with EGFR-expressing colorectal cancer by FDA in the United States. Data from multiple EGFR antibody trials show that the degree of EGFR expression seems to be unrelated to response, and patients with EGFR-negative colorectal cancers have responded to cetuximab as well.[84,85] Hence, EGFR expression by the contemporary immunohistochemical analysis techniques did not seem to predict cetuximab response.

A revolution in the treatment of colorectal cancer patients with EGFR-targeting antibodies occurred with the discovery that patients with K-ras mutations do not benefit from EGFR-targeting antibodies. K-ras mutations are seen in 40% of colorectal tumors. Retrospective analyses of K-ras codon 12/13 mutational status in archived tumors from clinical trials involving cetuximab and panitumumab have shown that K-ras mutation is a negative predictive biomarker for the benefit of EGFR antibodies.

The predictive role of K-ras mutational status was retrospectively analyzed in the two trials in which cetuximab or panitumumab were compared with BSC in third-line setting.[86,87] In the NCIC CO.17 trial, in patients with wild-type K-ras, treatment with cetuximab compared with supportive care alone significantly improved overall survival (median 9.5 versus 4.8 months; HR for death, 0.55; $P < .001$) and PFS (median 3.7 months versus 1.9 months; HR for progression or death 0.40; $P < .001$).[86] Among patients with mutated K-ras tumors, there was no significant difference between those who were treated with cetuximab and those who received supportive care alone with respect to overall survival (HR 0.98; $P = .89$) or PFS (HR 0.99; $P = .96$).

The impact of *K-ras* status on response rate and PFS in the first-line treatment of patients with FOLFIRI or FOLFOX with or without cetuximab was also retrospectively investigated in the CRYSTAL, EVEREST, and OPUS trials. Data from all these trials suggest that the benefit from addition of cetuximab to standard treatment is higher in patients with wild-type *K-ras*. For patients with *K-ras* mutations, no benefit could be shown for adding cetuximab to FOLFOX or FOLFIRI. This led the FDA and the European Medicines Agency (EMEA) to change the labeling for cetuximab and panitumumab for patients with only wild-type *K-ras* colorectal cancer.

Other potential predictive biomarkers have been explored but are not ready for clinical implementation. Since colorectal cancer also has *BRAF* mutations, and *K-ras* and *BRAF* are mutually exclusive, the role of *BRAF* mutations as prognostic or predictive factors for response to cetuximab or panitumumab was analyzed in a retrospective analysis of 113 patients treated with either EGFR-targeting antibody. In this study, researchers confirmed that *K-ras* and *BRAF* mutations are mutually exclusive and that patients with *BRAF* mutations also did not respond to either cetuximab or panitumumab[88-90] (Table 15-1). Patients with *BRAF* mutations also had shorter PFS and overall survival, suggesting a role of *BRAF* as prognostic marker, but this result needs to be validated in large trials. Other predictive biomarkers such as high mRNA levels of the EGFR ligands epiregulin and amphiregulin as well as PTEN status are being investigated, with the hope of leading to better patient selection for these targeted therapies.[91,92]

Bevacizumab and Angiogenesis

Angiogenesis delivers essential nutrients and oxygen for the sustained growth and metastasis in tumors and presents a rational target in cancer therapy.[93] These tumor-induced blood vessels are often structurally and functionally abnormal, impairing the effective delivery of chemotherapeutic agents to the cancer.[94] The abnormal process is thought to be driven by an imbalance of pro- and antiangiogenic factors, and disrupting the process by neutralizing vascular endothelial growth factor, a key ligand for angiogenesis, has been a focus in colorectal cancer therapy.[95]

Bevacizumab is a humanized recombinant monoclonal antibody that binds vascular endothelial growth factor and inhibits ligand-dependent angiogenesis. The drug's efficacy was demonstrated in two randomized controlled trials, which led to FDA approval for use with any intravenous 5-FU-containing regimen in first- or second-line metastatic colorectal cancer therapy.[96] Several mechanisms have been speculated to explain the activity of bevacizumab and other antiangiogenic agents, including starving the tumor of essential nutrients and oxygen by inhibition of formation of tumor vasculature, and improving the delivery of chemotherapeutic agents by normalizing the tumor vasculature and decreasing interstitial pressures in tumors.

In a small randomized phase II trial, 104 patients were randomized to receive weekly bolus 5-FU and leucovorin (5-FU/LV) (control arm), bevacizumab 5 mg/kg or 10 mg/kg plus 5-FU/LV (low-dose and high-dose bevacizumab arms, respectively).[97] Compared with those in the control arm, patients in both bevacizumab

Table 15-1. Randomized Trial Results of EGFR Antibodies (Cetuximab and Panitumumab)

Study	Treatment	Patients	*K-ras* Mutant	*K-ras* Wild-Type
Amado (2008)[87]	Panitumumab* versus BSC (third line)	208	7.4 wk HR 0.99	12.3 wk HR 0.45
Karapetis (2005)[86]	Cetuximab* versus BSC	287	1.9 mo NR	3.7 mo HR 0.40
Van Cutsem (2009)[88]	FOLFIRI ± cetuximab (first line)	599	7.6 mo HR 1.07	9.9 mo HR 0.68
Bokemeyer (2009)[89]	FOLFOX ± cetuximab (first line)	169	5.5 mo HR 1.83	7.7 mo HR 0.57

*Median progression-free survival for the cetuximab- and panitumumab-containing arms.
BSC, best supportive care; EFGR, epidermal growth factor receptor; HR, hazard ratio; NR, not reported.

arms had better response rate (control 17%; low-dose 40%, high-dose 24%), longer median TTP (5.2, 9.0, and 7.2 months, respectively), and longer median survival (13.8, 21.5, and 16.1 months, respectively). It is interesting that the low-dose bevacizumab arm seemed to be superior to the high-dose arm and was partly attributed to some imbalance in randomization, resulting in more patients with poor prognostic factors in the latter group. The dose of 5 mg/kg for bevacizumab was thus chosen for the subsequent phase III trial. Bleeding (gastrointestinal and epistaxis), hypertension, thrombosis, and proteinuria were more common in the bevacizumab arms.

In the interim, irinotecan plus bolus 5-FU and leucovorin (IFL) became the standard first-line therapy for metastatic colorectal cancer in the United States (see earlier). As such, the subsequent phase III trial used IFL as the control regimen, and 813 patients with previously untreated metastatic colorectal cancer were randomized to IFL plus placebo, IFL plus bevacizumab 5 mg/kg, and 5-FU/LV plus bevacizumab 5 mg/kg.[98] The 5-FU/LV/bevacizumab arm was discontinued during a planned interim analysis when the data monitoring committee found that the addition of bevacizumab to IFL had an acceptable safety profile. The intention-to-treat analysis showed a superior median survival for the IFL plus bevacizumab arm compared with the control arm (20.3 versus 15.6

months; $P < .001$) (Fig. 15-4). The study arm also had a better response rate (44.8% versus 34.8%; $P = .004$) and median duration of response (10.4 versus 7.1 months; $P = .001$). Reversible hypertension and proteinuria were more frequent in the study arm. Other rare but serious adverse events included thrombotic events, gastrointestinal perforation (1.5% of the patients in the bevacizumab arm) and wound dehiscence.

The role of bevacizumab with oxaliplatin-based regimen for second-line therapy for patients with metastatic colorectal cancer was studied in a randomized phase III study (E3200).[99] In the study, previously treated patients were randomly assigned to FOLFOX4 alone or FOLFOX4 plus high-dose bevacizumab (10 mg/kg). Analysis of 829 patients showed superior median survival in the bevacizumab plus FOLFOX4 arm (12.9 versus 10.8 months; $P = .001$). Dose reduction of bevacizumab to 5 mg/kg was allowed in the study for hypertension, bleeding, thrombosis, proteinuria, and abnormal liver tests. About 56% of 240 patients in the FOLFOX4 plus bevacizumab had bevacizumab dose reduction, and the overall survival was not statistically different from the group without dose reduction.[100]

Despite the clear role of bevacizumab with intravenous 5-FU-based regimens in first- and second-line therapy for patients with metastatic colorectal cancer, more clinical questions still

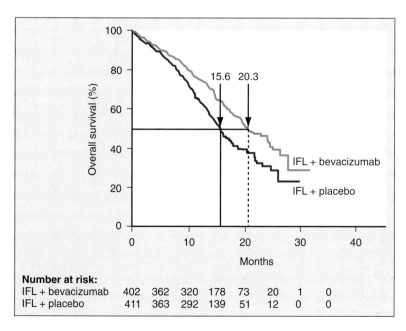

Figure 15-4. Kaplan-Meier estimates of survival with irinotecan, fluorouracil, and leucovorin (IFL) with or without bevacizumab. (Reprinted from Hurwitz H, Fehrenbacher L, Novotny W, et al: Bevacizumab plus irinotecan, fluorouracil, and leucovorin for metastatic colorectal cancer. N Engl J Med 350:2335–2342, 2004.)

need to be clarified, such as efficacy of continuing bevacizumab into second-line therapy and synergism with oral fluoropyrimidines. Studies addressing the combination of bevacizumab and cetuximab are ongoing. In the BOND (Bowel Oncology with Cetuximab Antibody)-2 trial,[101] patients with advanced colorectal cancer who had unsuccessful irinotecan-based therapy, more than 80% of whom had also been pretreated with oxaliplatin, were enrolled in a randomized phase II trial comparing cetuximab plus bevacizumab with cetuximab/bevacizumab plus irinotecan as salvage therapy. The primary objective of the trial was to document the feasibility of the dual-antibody combinations and to assess the response rate in both arms. In terms of the first objective, no unexpected adverse effects were encountered when cetuximab and bevacizumab were combined; the combination was feasible. Moreover, the addition of bevacizumab appeared to enhance the efficacy of cetuximab and cetuximab/irinotecan in terms of response rate, but more strikingly, in terms of time to tumor progression (TTP). This effect is even more noteworthy, since cetuximab monotherapy in BOND-1 was only associated with a rather disappointing median TTP of 1.5 months. Combining cetuximab with bevacizumab increased median TTP dramatically to 6.9 months. A similar effect was seen in the cetuximab + bevacizumab + irinotecan arm. Unfortunately, large clinical trials have indicated that "double biologic" strategies are harmful to patients.

With the latter data showing the feasibility of irinotecan with bevacizumab and cetuximab, several trials have investigated the combinations in first-line conventional chemotherapy and monoclonal antibodies.[102-104] In a randomized phase III trial of chemotherapy/bevacizumab with or without panitumumab (PACCE Study), median PFS in the experimental arm with both the biologics was 10 versus 11.4 months in the experimental versus control arms, respectively, and overall survival was 19.4 versus 24.5 months, also favoring the control arm.[102] The combination was inferior even in K-ras wild-type patients with more death rates and excess toxicity. The results are the same with another large study including cetuximab and bevacizumab (CAIRO 2 Study).[103] In this study, the combination of capecitabine/oxaliplatin/bevacizumab chemotherapy, with or without cetuximab, was tested

in 755 untreated metastatic colorectal cancer patients. The primary endpoint was PFS. The study demonstrated worsened PFS in the double biologic arm, 10.7 in the control arm, and 9.5 in the experimental arm (P = .01). The quality-of-life scores were worse and toxicities also more common in the experimental arm. In the subset analysis, even patients with wild-type K-ras also did not benefit.

Most double-biologic arms of ongoing studies were closed based on the latter results, and such combinations should not be used outside of a clinical trial. The CALGB/Southwest Oncology Group Intergroup 80405, a phase III intergroup trial comparing FOLFOX or FOLFIRI-based chemotherapy (investigators' choice) with bevacizumab, cetuximab or both was also evaluating the role of double biologics. This trial has been amended now to include patients with K-ras wild-type only.

Duration of Therapy

The prevailing dictum in systemic therapy of advanced or metastatic disease has been the continuation of therapy without interruption until tumor progression or substantial toxicity is observed. This concept has been challenged in the OPTIMOX-1 trial,[105] in which a stop-and-go approach for oxaliplatin was used. In this trial, FOLFOX regimen was given for a predetermined number of cycles followed by maintenance infusional 5-FU/LV for 6 months, which is followed by reintroduction of oxaliplatin. The OPTIMOX-1 trial included 620 patients and reported a modest decrease in oxaliplatin-induced neurotoxicity (grade 3, 13% versus 18%) without a significant decrease in efficacy. This novel concept was stretched even further in the OPTIMOX-2 trial,[106] which addressed the question of whether maintenance therapy was of any benefit. In this trial, PFS was significantly longer in patients who continued treatment compared to those who had treatment pauses (8.7 versus 6.9 months; P = .009), but overall "disease control" was similar. Of note, the OPTIMOX trials were conducted before the biologic agents such as bevacizumab and cetuximab became components of standard therapy. It remains to be seen whether maintenance therapy using these agents could provide comparable, or better, efficacy while limiting the toxicity of continuous treatment.

Adjuvant Systemic Therapy

Timely surgical resection offers the only chance for cure of colorectal cancer, and indeed advanced colorectal cancer that is not amenable to surgical resection is eventually lethal. In a remarkable recently reported observation, the majority of patients with colorectal cancer had evidence of circulating tumor cells in the peripheral blood when sensitive detection methods such as reverse transcriptase-polymerase chain reaction (RT-PCR) are used.[107] Therefore, disease recurrence is thought to derive from clinically occult micrometastases that are present at the time of apparently curative surgery. The goal of adjuvant systemic therapy has been to eradicate such micrometastases, thereby decreasing the likelihood of relapse and increasing the cure rate. The earliest studies in adjuvant systemic therapy of colorectal cancer used 5-FU monotherapy (i.e., without leucovorin modulation) without any improvement in 5-year survival.[108] These disappointing results led to a lull period in the field of adjuvant systemic therapy of colorectal cancer. The interest was revived, however, with the discovery of leucovorin modulation. As with advanced colorectal cancer, 5-FU/LV became the backbone of standard adjuvant therapy of colorectal cancer.

The Fluoropyrimidines

In 1995, the results of the IMPACT (International Multicentre Pooled Analysis of Colon Cancer Trials) study were published.[109] In this pivotal study, data were pooled from 1526 patients with resected Dukes' B and C colon cancer enrolled in three independent international trials. All the patients were randomized to either observation alone or 6 monthly cycles of 5-FU/LV. There was a significant 22% reduction in the risk of death in the 5-FU/LV arm with 3-year overall survival increasing by 5% (83% versus 78%) in the treated group. Subsequent subgroup analysis showed that the benefit was limited to patients with node-positive disease. Subsequently, a flurry of randomized studies trying to optimize this therapy was performed.[110–114] A number of important observations emerged from these trials. First, administering 5-FU/LV for 6 months was equally effective as it was for 12 months. Second, 5-FU administered with high-dose leucovorin

$(200–500 \text{ mg/m}^2)$ is equivalent to low-dose leucovorin (20 mg/m^2). Finally, no significant difference was found between the two most widely used regimens for administrating bolus 5-FU/LV, namely, the Mayo Clinic and the Roswell Park regimens. Furthermore, despite the significant survival advantage and lower hematologic toxicity with continuous infusion 5-FU over bolus regimens in advanced colorectal cancer, this observation did not pan out in the adjuvant setting. In at least three studies comparing continuous infusion to bolus 5-FU in adjuvant treatment of colon cancer, no statistically significant differences were observed in either disease-free survival or overall survival.[115–117]

The advent of the oral fluoropyrimidine, capecitabine, with its obvious convenience of administration, led to its being tested in the adjuvant setting. The Xeloda in Adjuvant Colon Cancer Therapy (X-ACT) trial was a large randomized study in which patients with stage III colon cancer were randomized after resection to receive either bolus 5-FU/LV or capecitabine at a dose of 1250 mg/m^2 twice daily.[118] This trial showed that capecitabine was at least equivalent (noninferior) to its intravenous counterpart 5-FU. Moreover, there was a nonstatistically significant trend toward a better clinical outcome. It is noteworthy, however, that the capecitabine dose used in the X-ACT trial appears to be more toxic when given to patients in the United States. This difference in the tolerance of capecitabine between patients on either side of the Atlantic remains largely a matter of conjecture. Capecitabine's activity as a single agent, together with its ease of administration, led to a number of studies evaluating the feasibility and efficacy of combining it with other active agents in the adjuvant setting (see text that follows).

Combination Adjuvant Chemotherapy (Oxaliplatin and Irinotecan)

The significant impact of oxaliplatin and irinotecan in metastatic colorectal cancer provided the rationale for their evaluation in the adjuvant setting. Two major trials evaluated the combination of 5-FU/LV with oxaliplatin. The MOSAIC trial[119] randomized 2200 patients, of whom 60% had stage III and 40% had stage II colon cancer, to either infusional 5-FU/LV or the same regimen combined with oxaliplatin (FOLFOX4). With a median follow-up of 3 years, there was a statistically significant 5% improvement in PFS for the oxaliplatin-containing regimen. The overall survival benefit reached statistical significance in only the stage III patients (68.3 vs. 72.9% probability of survival at 6 years), whereas there was no difference in overall survival for the stage II patients.[120] A second phase III randomized trial C-07, conducted in the United States by the National Surgical Adjuvant Breast and Bowel Project (NSABP),[121] included 2407 patients and showed almost identical observations.[122] Based on the results of these two trials, oxaliplatin, 5-FU, and leucovorin became the standard of care for stage III colon cancer patients.

In contrast to the results with oxaliplatin, benefit has not been shown for irinotecan in the adjuvant setting in three large trials that recruited over 3700 patients. The first trial randomly assigned 1264 patients with resected stage III colon cancer to weekly high-dose LV plus 5-FU with or without irinotecan.[123] In a preliminary report with a median 2.6-year follow-up, both failure-free survival and overall survival were similar. Moreover, IFL was associated with significantly higher rates of grade 3 or 4 neutropenia (42% versus 5%), febrile neutropenia (4% versus 1%) and treatment-related death (2.8 versus 1%).

The FOLFIRI regimen has been studied in the adjuvant setting in two trials, both of which have been reported in abstract form only. The multicenter PETACC-3 trial compared infusional 5-FU/LV with and without irinotecan (180 mg/m^2 over 90 minutes on day 1 every 14 days) in 3278 patients with resected colon cancer, of whom 2333 had stage III disease.[123] With a median 66.3-month follow-up, there was no significant difference in disease-free survival (DFS) from the addition of irinotecan to infusional 5-FU/LV in patients with stage III disease (5-year DFS 56.7% versus 54.3%, HR 0.90; $P =$ .94). Overall survival was also similar in the two arms. The similarly designed ACCORD trial randomly assigned 400 patients with high-risk features including node-positive or obstructed/perforated colon cancers to the same two treatment arms as in PETACC-3 trial.[124] In a preliminary report with median follow-up of 36 months, event-free survival was not significantly different in the groups. With over 3700 patients recruited into these three trials with no apparent benefit, further large-scale randomized controlled trials evaluating irinotecan as adjuvant treatment are unlikely to be performed. Therefore, adjuvant irinotecan-containing chemotherapy cannot be considered a standard approach for patients requiring adjuvant chemotherapy for resected colon cancer.

In the adjuvant trials incorporating monoclonal antibodies, results thus far have been disappointing. In the NSABP CO-8 study, 2672 patients with stages II and III colon cancer were randomized to mFOLFOX for 12 cycles (6 months) versus mFOLFOX (12 cycles) with bevacizumab (12 months total). Bevacizumab showed initial transient improvement in DFS in the first year, but the benefit diminished at 3 years.[125] The hazard ratio was 0.89 ($P =$ .15). The N0147 study, which randomized stage III colon cancer patients to FOLFOX ± cetuximab (6 months), was amended to include K-ras wild-type patients only. However, the study was closed in 2009 after a futility analysis was positive.

Adjuvant Systemic Therapy for Stage II Colon Cancer

Although the role of adjuvant treatment is well established in stage III disease, the comparatively lower rate of recurrence and better survival in stage II disease have rendered the benefit of adjuvant chemotherapy less clear-cut. A number of meta-analyses found no significant survival benefit for adjuvant therapy in stage II colorectal cancer. However, the largest randomized trial addressing this issue was recently reported. In the QUASAR study, 3239 patients were randomized between observation and 5-FU/LV.[126] Of note, 92% of enrolled patients had stage II disease. With a median follow-up of 4.6 years, adjuvant therapy was associated with significantly reduced risk of recurrence and with improved survival. The 5-year recurrence rates were 22.2% for the chemotherapy arm and 26.2% for the observation arm. In addition, the 5-year survival rates were 80.3% for the chemotherapy arm and 77.4% for the observation arm. The survival benefit in stage II patients treated with adjuvant chemotherapy was statistically significant ($P =$ .04). The American Society of Clinical Oncology (ASCO) guidelines state that the routine use of adjuvant therapy for stage II patients is not recommended.[127] However, ASCO guidelines suggested that several subsets of medically fit patients with high-risk stage II disease, including poorly differentiated histology, T4 lesions, bowel perforation, and inadequately sampled lymph nodes, could be considered for adjuvant therapy.

The recent focus on the role of molecular markers for risk stratification of colon cancer patients has created excitement and opened new opportunities for identifying patients who may benefit from systemic therapy. A number of markers have been looked at, including thymidylate synthase, cyclooxygenase 2, *ras* gene mutation, and circulating tumor cells, among others.[128] However, the two molecular markers that garnered the most attention are allelic loss of chromosome 18q and microsatellite instability. Stage II patients with loss of 18q have worse outcomes than those who maintained it.[129] Counterintuitively, however, the presence of microsatellite instability is associated with better prognosis,[130] although the benefit of chemotherapy in patients with microsatellite instability is debated.

Microsatellite instability in stage II and stage III colon cancer patients treated in PETACC-3 Trial was assessed retrospectively. Paraffin tissue blocks were analyzed for microsatellite instability status using the National Cancer Institute extended panel of 10 markers. Microsatellite instability is a strong prognostic factor for relapse-free survival (RFS) and overall survival in stage III and stage II disease, particularly in stage II colon cancer.[131]

These markers are being incorporated into a currently recruiting trial, E5202, in adjuvant therapy of stage II colorectal cancer (see following text).

Future Directions

The advent of monoclonal antibodies and their efficacy in metastatic colorectal cancer has paved the way for the next wave of adjuvant therapy trials. Large-scale phase III trials now underway evaluating cetuximab and bevacizumab in the adjuvant setting (Table 15-2) have thus far been negative. Further patient selection strategies may be necessary to successfully implement these agents successfully in the adjuvant setting.

In addition to the incorporation of antibodies in the adjuvant setting, the Eastern Cooperative Oncology Group (ECOG) E5202 will be the first clinical trial in colorectal cancer to make use of genetic markers for risk stratification and treatment arm allocation. In this trial, stage II patients will be stratified based on their genetic features into a low-risk group, those with microsatellite instability, and those with no 18q allelic loss for observation, whereas patients with genetic markers predictive of high risk will be randomized to either FOLFOX or FOLFOX plus bevacizumab.

There are currently a number of novel agents, particularly molecularly targeted therapies, that are in early stage of development (reference 132 and references therein). A good number of tyrosine kinase inhibitors as well as inhibitors of intracellular signaling, such as mTOR inhibitors, are being tested against colorectal cancer in early-phase clinical trials. Epigenetic-based therapies have also been the focus of interest.

Tumor immunotherapy has been extensively studied in the past in patients with colorectal cancer. The recent observation that the type and density of immune cells within colorectal tumor deposits are prognostic factors independent of and superior to the histopathologic methods currently used to stage colorectal cancer points to an important role of the adaptive immune system in the biology and natural history of colorectal cancers.[133,134] Whether the continued search for more effective vaccines and immuno-

Trial	Stage of Disease	Treatment Arm	No. Patients
		Table 15-2. Recent Adjuvant Therapy Trials	
NSABP C-08	II and III	FOLFOX vs FOLFOX + bevacizumab	2632
AVANT	II and III	FOLFOX vs FOLFOX + bevacizumab vs XELOX + bevacizumab	3450
Intergroup 0147	III	FOLFOX vs FOLFOX + cetuximab	2300
ECOG E5202	II	Molecular Testing and Stratification, then Observation vs FOLFOX vs FOLFOX + bevacizumab	3610

therapeutic interventions will bear fruit in the near future remains to be seen.

The achievement of milestones based on an increasing body of knowledge on the molecular basis of colorectal tumorigenesis has led to the recognition of specific targets for therapy and novel therapeutics. The predictive role of *K-ras* in patient selection for EGFR antibody therapy has paved a way of personalized medicine in colorectal cancer. The survival and quality of life of colorectal cancer patients have significantly improved as a result of immense effort in basic and clinical research. It is thus reasonable to predict that further improvement in molecular evaluation of tumors and the advent of more novel therapeutics will produce more tangible clinical benefit to patients with colorectal cancer.

References

1. Heidelberger C, Chaudhuri NK, Danneberg P, et al: Fluorinated pyrimidines: a new class of tumor-inhibitory compounds. Nature 179:663–666, 1957.
2. Efficacy of intravenous continuous infusion of fluorouracil compared with bolus administration in advanced colorectal cancer. Meta-analysis Group in Cancer. J Clin Oncol 16:301–308, 1999.
3. Meta-analysis of randomized trials testing the biochemical modulation of fluorouracil with methotrexate in metastatic colorectal cancer. Advanced Colorectal Cancer Meta-analysis Project. J Clin Oncol 12:960–969, 1994.
4. Randomized phase III study of high-dose fluorouracil given as a weekly 24-hour infusion with or without leucovorin versus bolus fluorouracil plus leucovorin in advanced colorectal cancer: European Organization of Research and Treatment of Cancer Gastrointestinal Group Study 40952. J Clin Oncol 21:3721–3728, 2003.
5. Piedbois P, Buye M: What can we learn from a meta-analysis of trials testing the modulation of 5-FU by leucovorin? Advanced Colorectal Meta-analysis Project. Ann Oncol 4(Suppl 2):15–19.
6. Modulation of fluorouracil by leucovorin in patients with advanced colorectal cancer: evidence in terms of response rate. Advanced Colorectal Cancer Meta-analysis Project. J Clin Oncol 10:896–903, 1992.
7. Simmonds PC: Palliative chemotherapy for advanced colorectal cancer: systematic review and meta-analysis. Colorectal Cancer Collaborative Group. BMJ 321:531–535, 2000.
8. Palliative chemotherapy for advanced or metastatic colorectal cancer. Colorectal Meta-analysis Collaboration. Cochrane Database Syst Rev 2(2):CD001545, 2000.
9. Poon MA, O'Connell MJ, Wieand HS, et al: Biochemical modulation of fluorouracil with leucovorin: confirmatory evidence of improved therapeutic efficacy in advanced colorectal cancer. J Clin Oncol 9(11):1967–1972, 1991.
10. Petrelli N, Herrera L, Rustum Y, et al: A prospective randomized trial of 5-fluorouracil versus 5-fluorouracil and high-dose leucovorin versus 5-fluorouracil and methotrexate in previously untreated patients with advanced colorectal carcinoma. J Clin Oncol 5(10):1559–1565, 1987.
11. de Gramont A, Bosset JF, Milan C, et al: Randomized trial comparing monthly low-dose leucovorin and fluorouracil bolus with bimonthly high-dose leucovorin and fluorouracil bolus plus continuous infusion for advanced colorectal cancer: a French intergroup study. J Clin Oncol 15:808–815, 1997.
12. Lokich JJ, Moore CL, Anderson NR: Comparison of costs for infusion versus bolus chemotherapy administration: analysis of five standard chemotherapy regimens in three common tumors—part one. Model projections for cost based on charges. Cancer 78:294–299, 1996.
13. Lokich JJ, Moore CL, Anderson NR: Comparison of costs for infusion versus bolus chemotherapy administration–part two. Use of charges versus reimbursement for cost basis. Cancer 78:300–303, 1996.
14. Kohne CH, Wils J, Lorenz M, et al: Randomized phase III study of high-dose fluorouracil given as a weekly 24-hour infusion with or without leucovorin versus bolus fluorouracil plus leucovorin in advanced colorectal cancer: European Organization of Research and Treatment of Cancer Gastrointestinal Group Study 40952. J Clin Oncol 21:3721–3728, 2003.
15. Efficacy of intravenous continuous infusion of fluorouracil compared with bolus administration in advanced colorectal cancer. Meta-analysis Group in Cancer. J Clin Oncol 16:301–308, 1998.
16. Meropol NJ: Turning point for colorectal cancer clinical trials. J Clin Oncol 24:3322–3324, 2006.
17. Douillard JY, Cunningham D, Roth AD, et al: Irinotecan combined with fluorouracil compared with fluorouracil alone as first-line treatment for metastatic colorectal cancer: a multicentre randomized trial. Lancet 355:1041–1047, 2000.
18. Kohne CH, van Cutsem E, Wils J, et al: Phase III study of weekly high-dose infusion fluorouracil plus folinic acid with or without irinotecan in patients with metastatic colorectal cancer: European Organization for Research and Treatment of Cancer Gastrointestinal Group Study 40986. J Clin Oncol 23:4856–4865, 2005.
19. Saltz LB, Cox JV, Blanke C, et al: Leucovorin and fluorouracil and leucovorin for metastatic colorectal cancer. Irinotecan Study Group. N Engl J Med 343:905–914, 2000.
20. Pizzolato JF, Saltz LB: The camptothecins. Lancet 361:2235–2242, 2003.
21. Cunningham D, Pyrhonen S, James RD, et al: Randomised trial of irinotecan plus supportive care versus supportive care alone after fluorouracil failure for patients with metastatic colorectal cancer. Lancet 352:1413–1418, 1998.
22. Rougier P, Van Cutsem E, Bajetta E, et al: Randomised trial of irinotecan versus fluorouracil by continuous infusion after fluorouracil failure in patients with metastatic colorectal cancer. Lancet 352:1407–1412, 1998.
23. Gupta E, Lestingi TM, Mick R, et al: Metabolic fate of irinotecan in humans: correlation of glucuronidation with diarrhea. Cancer Res 54:3723–3725, 1994.
24. Gupta E, Wang X, Ramirez J, et al: Modulation of glucuronidation of SN-38, the active metabolite of irinotecan, by valproic acid and phenobarbital. Cancer Chemother Pharmacol 39:440–444, 1997.
25. Innocenti F, Undevia SD, Iyer L, et al: Genetic variants in the UDP-glucuronosyltransferase 1A1 gene predict the risk of severe neutropenia of irinotecan. J Clin Oncol 22:1382–1388, 2004.
26. Raymond E, Faivre S, Chaney S, et al: Cellular and molecular pharmacology of oxaliplatin. Mol Cancer Ther 1:227–235, 2002.
27. Becouarn Y, Ychou M, Ducreux M, et al: Phase II trial of oxaliplatin as first-line chemotherapy in metastatic colorectal cancer patients. Digestive Group of French Federation of Cancer Centers. J Clin Oncol 16:2739–2744, 1998.
28. Diaz-Rubio E, Sastre J, Zaniboni A, et al: Oxaliplatin as single agent in previously untreated colorectal carcinoma patients: a phase II multicentric study. Ann Oncol 9:105–108, 1998.
29. Levi F, Perpoint B, Garufi C, et al: Oxaliplatin activity against metastatic colorectal cancer. A phase II study of 5-day continuous venous infusion at circadian rhythm modulated rate. Eur J Cancer 29A:1280–1284, 1993.
30. Plasencia C, Taron M, Martinez E, et al: Down-regulation of thymidylate synthase gene expression after oxaliplatin administration: implications for the synergistic activity of sequential oxaliplatin/5FU in sensitive and 5FU-resistant cell lines. [Abstract] Proc Am Assoc Cancer Res 42:508, 2001.
31. Fischel JL, Formento P, Ciccolini J, et al: Impact of the oxaliplatin-5 fluorouracil-folinic acid combination on respective intracellular determinants of drug activity. Br J Cancer 86:1162–1168, 2002.
32. Yeh KH, Cheng AL, Wan JP, et al: Down-regulation of thymidylate synthase expression and its steady-state mRNA by oxali-

platin in colon cancer cells. Anticancer Drugs 15:371–376, 2004.

33. Goldberg RM, Sargent DJ, Morton RF, et al: A randomized controlled trial of fluorouracil plus leucovorin, irinotecan, and oxaliplatin combinations in patients with previously untreated metastatic colorectal cancer. J Clin Oncol 22:23–30, 2004.

34. Rothenberg ML, Oza AM, Bigelow RH, et al: Superiority of oxaliplatin and fluorouracil-leucovorin compared with either therapy alone in patients with progressive colorectal cancer after irinotecan and fluorouracil-leucovorin: interim results of a phase III trial. J Clin Oncol 21:2059–2069, 2003.

35. Giacchetti S, Perpoint B, Zidani R, et al: Phase III multicenter randomized trial of oxaliplatin added to chronomodulated fluorouracil-leucovorin as first-line treatment of metastatic colorectal cancer. J Clin Oncol 18:136–147, 2000.

36. Grothey A, Deschler B, Kroening H, et al: Phase III study of bolus 5-fluorouracil (5-FU)/folinic acid (FA) (Mayo) vs weekly high-dose 24h 5-FU infusion/FA + oxaliplatin (OXA) (FUFOX) in advanced colorectal cancer (ACRC). [Abstract 512] Proc Am Soc Clin Oncol 21:129a, 2002.

37. Raymond E, Faivre S, Woynarowski JM, et al: Oxaliplatin: mechanism of action and antineoplastic activity. Semin Oncol 25(2 Suppl 5):4–12, 1998.

38. Raymond E, Chaney SG, Taamma A, et al: Oxaliplatin: a review of preclinical and clinical studies. Ann Oncol 9(10): 1053–1071, 1998.

39. Grothey A: Oxaliplatin-safety profile: neurotoxicity. Semin Oncol 30(4 Suppl 15):5–13, 2003.

40. de Gramont A, Boni C, Navarro M, et al: Oxaliplatin/5FU/LV in the adjuvant treatment of stage II and stage III colon cancer: efficacy results with a median follow-up of 4 years. 2005 ASCO Annual Meeting Proceedings. Part I of II. [Abstract] J Clin Oncol 23(16S):3501, 2005.

41. Tournigand C, Andre T, Achille E, et al: FOLFIRI followed by FOLFOX6 or the reverse sequence in advanced colorectal cancer: a randomized GERCOR study. J Clin Oncol 22: 229–237, 2004.

42. Colucci G, Gebbia V, Paoletti G, et al: Phase III randomized trial of FOLFIRI versus FOLFOX4 in the treatment of advanced colorectal cancer: a multicenter study of the Gruppo Oncologico dell'Italia Meridionale. J Clin Oncol 23:4866–4875, 2005.

43. Grothey A, Sargent D, Goldberg RM, et al: Survival of patients with advanced colorectal cancer improves with the availability of fluorouracil-leucovorin, irinotecan, and oxaliplatin in the course of treatment. J Clin Oncol 22:1209–1214, 2004.

44. Falcone A, Ricci S, Brunetti I, et al: Phase III trial of infusional fluorouracil, leucovorin, oxaliplatin, and irinotecan (FOLFOX-IRI) compared with infusional fluorouracil, leucovorin, and irinotecan (FOLFIRI) as first-line treatment for metastatic colorectal cancer: The Gruppo Oncologico Nord Ovest. J Clin Oncol 25:1670–1676, 2007.

45. Pentheroudakis G, Twelves C: The rational development of capecitabine from the laboratory to the clinic. Anticancer Res 22:3589–3596, 2002.

46. Van Cutsem E, Twelves C, Cassidy J, et al: Oral capecitabine compared with intravenous fluorouracil plus leucovorin in patients with metastatic colorectal cancer: results of a large phase III study. J Clin Oncol 19:4097–4106, 2001.

47. Hoff PM, Ansari R, Batist G, et al: Comparison of oral capecitabine versus intravenous fluorouracil plus leucovorin as first-line treatment in 605 patients with metastatic colorectal cancer: results of a randomized phase III study. J Clin Oncol 19:2282–2292, 2001.

48. Van Cutsem E, Hoff PM, Harper P, et al: Oral capecitabine vs intravenous 5-fluorouracil and leucovorin: integrated efficacy data and novel analyses from two large, randomised, phase III trials. Br J Cancer 90:1190–1197, 2004.

49. Douillard JY, Hoff PM, Skillings JR, et al: Multicenter phase III study of uracil/tegafur and oral leucovorin versus fluorouracil and leucovorin in patients with previously untreated metastatic colorectal cancer. J Clin Oncol 20:3605–3616, 2002.

50. Carmichael J, Popiela T, Radstone D, et al: Randomized comparative study of tegafur/uracil and oral leucovorin versus parenteral fluorouracil and leucovorin in patients with previously untreated metastatic colorectal cancer. J Clin Oncol 20:3617–3627, 2002.

51. Tsunoda A, Shibusawa M, Tsunoda Y, et al: Antitumor effect of S-1 on DMH induced colon cancer in rats. Anticancer Res 18:1137–1141, 1998.

52. Konno H, Tanaka T, Baba M, et al: Therapeutic effect of 1 M tegafur-0.4 M 5-chloro-2,4-dihydroxypyridine-1 M potassium oxonate (S-1) on liver metastasis of xenotransplanted human colon carcinoma. Jpn J Cancer Res 90: 448–453, 1999.

53. Maehara Y, Sugimachi K, Kurihara M, et al: Clinical evaluation of S-1, a new anticancer agent, in patients with advanced gastrointestinal cancer. S-1 Cooperative Gastrointestinal Study Group. Gan To Kagaku Ryoho 26:476–485, 1999.

54. Takemoto H, Fukunaga M, Ooshiro R, et al: A case of peritoneal dissemination disappeared by CPT-11 + TS-1 combination chemotherapy. Gan To Kagaku Ryoho 32:1768–1770, 2005.

55. Nakao K, Tsunoda A, Amagasa H, et al: A case report of poorly-differentiated adenocarcinoma in sigmoid colon cancer with liver and pulmonary metastasis responding to TS-1 and CPT-11. Gan To Kagaku Ryoho 33:109–112, 2006.

56. Kanazawa S, Seo A, Tokura N, et al: Liver metastasis from sigmoid colon cancer with peritoneal dissemination showed a complete response to TS-1. Gan To Kagaku Ryoho 33: 113–117, 2006.

57. Hochster HS, Hart LL, Ramanathan RK, et al: Safety and efficacy of oxaliplatin/fluoropyrimidine regimens with or without bevacizumab as first line treatment for metastatic colorectal cancer (mCRC): final analysis of the TREE study. [Abstract of Meeting] J Clin Oncol 24:3510, 2006.

58. Saltz L, Clarke E, Diaz-Rubio W, et al: Bevacizumab in combination with XELOX or FOLFOX4: updated efficacy results from XELOX-1/NO16966, a randomized phase III trial in first-line metastatic colorectal cancer. [Abstract of Meeting] J Clin Oncol 25:4028, 2007.

59. Fuchs CS, Marshall J, Mitchell E, et al: Randomized, controlled trial of irinotecan plus infusional, bolus, or infusional fluoropyrimidines in first-line treatment of metastatic colorectal cancer: results from the BICC-C study. J Clin Oncol 25(30): 4779–4786, 2007.

60. Carpenter G, Cohen S: Epidermal growth factor. J Biol Chem 265:7709–7712, 1990.

61. Real FX, Rettig WJ, Chesa PG, et al: Expression of epidermal growth factor receptor in human cultured cells and tissues: relationship to cell lineage and stage of differentiation. Cancer Res 46:4726–4731, 1986.

62. Yasui W, Sumiyoshi H, Hata J, et al: Expression of epidermal growth factor receptor in human gastric and colonic carcinomas. Cancer Res 48:137–141, 1988.

63. Messa C, Russo F, Caruso MG, et al: EGF, TGF-alpha, and EGF-R in human colorectal adenocarcinoma. Acta Oncol 37:285–289, 1998.

64. Porebska I, Harlozinska A, Bojarowski T: Expression of the tyrosine kinase activity growth factor receptors (EGFR, ERB B2, ERB B3) in colorectal adenocarcinomas and adenomas. Tumour Biol 21:105–115, 2000.

65. Salomon DS, Brandt R, Ciardiello F, et al: Epidermal growth factor-related peptides and their receptors in human malignancies. Crit Rev Oncol Hematol 19:183–232, 1995.

66. Mayer A, Takimoto M, Fritz E, et al: The prognostic significance of proliferating cell nuclear antigen, epidermal growth factor receptor, and mdr gene expression in colorectal cancer. Cancer 71:2454–2460, 1993.

67. Hemming AW, Davis NL, Kluftinger A, et al: Prognostic markers of colorectal cancer: an evaluation of DNA content, epidermal growth factor receptor, and ki-67. J Surg Oncol 51:147–152, 1992.

68. Baselga J: Why the epidermal growth factor receptor? The rationale for cancer therapy. Oncologist 4:2–8, 2002.

69. Fan Z, Baselga J, Masui H, et al: Antitumor effect of anti-epidermal growth factor receptor monoclonal antibodies plus cis-diamminedichloroplatinum on well established A431 cell xenografts. Cancer Res 53:4637–4642, 1993.

70. Goldstein NI, Prewett M, Zuklys K, et al: Biological efficacy of a chimeric antibody to the epidermal growth factor receptor in a human tumor xenograft model. Clin Cancer Res 1: 1311–1318, 1995.

71. Prewett MC, Hooper AT, Bassi R, et al: Enhanced antitumor activity of anti-epidermal growth factor receptor monoclonal antibody IMC-C225 in combination with irinotecan (CPT-11) against human colorectal tumor xenografts. Clin Cancer Res 8:994–1003, 2002.

72. Saltz LB, Meropol NJ, Loehrer PJS, et al: Phase II trial of cetuximab in patients with refractory colorectal cancer that

expresses the epidermal growth factor receptor. J Clin Oncol 22:1201–1208, 2004.

73. Saltz L, Rubin MS, Hochster HS: Cetuximab (IMC-C225) plus irinotecan (CPT-11) is active in CPT-11-refractory colorectal cancer (CRC) that expresses epidermal growth factor receptor (EGFR). [Abstract 7] Proc Am Soc Clin Oncol 20:3a, 2001.

74. Cunningham D, Humblet Y, Siena S, et al: Cetuximab monotherapy and cetuximab plus irinotecan in irinotecan-refractory metastatic colorectal cancer. N Engl J Med 351:337–345, 2004.

75. Jonker DJ, O'Callaghan CJ, Karapetis CS, et al: Cetuximab for the treatment of colorectal cancer. N Engl J Med 357: 2040–2048, 2007.

76. Van Cutsem E, Nowacki M, Lang S, et al: Randomized phase III study of irinotecan and 5-FU/FA with or without cetuximab in the first-line treatment of patients with metastatic colorectal cancer (mCRC): the CRYSTAL trial. J Clin Oncol 25:4000, 2007.

77. Badarinath S, Mitchell EO, Hennis CD, et al: Cetuximab plus FOLFOX for colorectal cancer (EXPLORE): preliminary safety analysis of a randomized phase III trial. 2004 ASCO Annual Meeting Proceedings Post-Meeting Edition. [Abstract] J Clin Oncol 22(14S):3531, 2004.

78. Bokemeyer C, Bondarenko I, Hartmann JT, et al: Fluorouracil, leucovorin, and oxaliplatin with and without cetuximab in the first-line treatment of metastatic colorectal cancer. The Opus Experience. J Clin Oncol 27:663–671, 2009.

79. Perez-Soler R, Saltz L: Cutaneous adverse effects with HER1/EGFR-targeted agents: is there a silver lining? J Clin Oncol 23:5235–5246, 2005.

80. Malik S, Hecht J, Patanaik A: Safety and efficacy of panitumumab monotherapy in patients with metastatic colorectal cancer (mCRC). [Abstract of Meeting] J Clin Oncol 23:3520, 2005.

81. Berlin J, Neubauer M, Swanson P, et al: Panitumumab antitumor activity in patients with metastatic colorectal cancer (mCRC) expressing ≥10% epidermal growth factor receptor (EGFR). [Abstracts of Meeting] J Clin Oncol 24:3548, 2006.

82. Arends R, Yang BB, Schwab G, et al: Flexible dosing schedules of panitumumab (ABX-EGF) in cancer patients. [Abstracts of Meeting] J Clin Oncol 23:3089, 2005.

83. Wainberg Z, Hechts JR: A phase III randomized, open label, controlled trial of chemotherapy and bevacizumab with or without panitumumab in the first line treatment of patients with metastatic colorectal cancer. Clin Colorectal Cancer 5:363–367, 2006.

84. Lenz H, Mayer RJ, Gold PJ: Activity of cetuximab in patients with colorectal cancer refractory to both irinotecan and oxaliplatin. 2004 ASCO Annual Meeting Proceedings Post-Meeting Edition. [Abstract] J Clin Oncol 22(14S, July 15 Suppl):3510, 2004.

85. Chung KY, Shia J, Kemeny NE, et al: Cetuximab shows activity in colorectal cancer patients with tumors that do not express the epidermal growth factor receptor by immunohistochemistry. J Clin Oncol 23:1803–1810, 2005.

86. Karapetis CS, Khambata-Ford S, Jonker DJ, et al: KRAS mutations and benefit from cetuximab in advanced colorectal cancer. N Engl J Med 359:1757–1765, 2008.

87. Amado RG, Wolf M, Peeters M, et al: Wild-type KRAS is required for panitumumab efficacy in patients with metastatic colorectal cancer. J Clin Oncol 26:1626–1634, 2008.

88. Van Cutsem E, Kohne CH, Hitre E, et al: Cetuximab and chemotherapy as initial treatment for metastatic colorectal cancer. N Engl J Med 360:1408–1417, 2009.

89. Bokemeyer C, Bondarenko I, Makhson A, et al: Fluorouracil, leucovorin, and oxaliplatin with and without cetuximab in the first-line treatment of metastatic colorectal cancer. J Clin Oncol 27(5):663–671, 2009.

90. Di Nicolantonio F, Martín M, Molinari F, et al: Wild-type BRAF is required for response to panitumumab or cetuximab in metastatic colorectal cancer. J Clin Oncol 26(35): 5705–5712, 2008.

91. Khambata-Ford S, Garrett CR, Meropol NJ, et al: Expression of epiregulin and amphiregulin and K-ras mutation status predict disease control in metastatic colorectal cancer patients treated with cetuximab. J Clin Oncol 25:3230–3237, 2007.

92. Tejpar S, De Roock W, Piessevaux H, et al: Amphiregulin and epiregulin mRNA expression in primary tumors predicts

outcome in metastatic colorectal cancer treated with cetuximab. J Clin Oncol 27(30):5068–5074, 2009.

93. Folkman J: Seminars in medicine of the Beth Israel Hospital, Boston. Clinical applications of research on angiogenesis. N Engl J Med 333:1757–1763, 1995.

94. Jain RK: Normalizing tumor vasculature with anti-angiogenic therapy: a new paradigm for combination therapy. Nat Med 7:987–989, 2001.

95. Ferrara N, Gerber HP, LeCouter J: The biology of VEGF and its receptors. Nat Med 9:669–676, 2003.

96. Ferrara N, Hillan KJ, Novotny W: Bevacizumab (Avastin), a humanized anti-VEGF monoclonal antibody for cancer therapy. Biochem Biophys Res Commun 333:328–335, 2005.

97. Kabbinavar F, Hurwitz HI, Fehrenbacher L, et al: Phase II, randomized trial comparing bevacizumab plus fluorouracil (FU)/leucovorin (LV) with FU/LV alone in patients with metastatic colorectal cancer. J Clin Oncol 21:60–65, 2003.

98. Hurwitz H, Fehrenbacher L, Novotny W, et al: Bevacizumab plus irinotecan, fluorouracil, and leucovorin for metastatic colorectal cancer. N Engl J Med 350:2335–2342, 2004.

99. Giantonio BJ, Catalano PJ, Meropol NJ, et al: Bevacizumab in combination with oxaliplatin, fluorouracil, and leucovorin (FOLFOX4) for previously treated metastatic colorectal cancer: results from the eastern cooperative oncology group (ECOG) study E3200. J Clin Oncol 25:1539–1544, 2007.

100. Giantonio BJ, Catalano PJ, O'Dwyer PJ, et al: Impact of bevacizumab dose reduction on clinical outcomes for patients treated on the Eastern Cooperative Oncology Group's study E3200 trial. 2006 ASCO Annual Meeting Proceedings Part I. [Abstract] J Clin Oncol 24:3538, 2006.

101. Saltz LB, Lenz HJ, Hoechster H, et al: Randomized phase II trial of cetuximab/bevacizumab/irinotecan (CBI) versus cetuximab/bevacizumab (CB) in irinotecan-refractory colorectal cancer. [Abstracts of Meeting] J Clin Oncol 23:3508, 2005.

102. Hecht JR, Mitchell E, Chidiac T, et al: Randomized phase IIIB trial of chemotherapy, bevacizumab, and panitumumab compared with chemotherapy and bevacizumab alone for metastatic colorectal cancer. J Clin Oncol 27:672–680, 2009.

103. Tol J, Koopman M, Cats A, et al: Chemotherapy, bevacizumab, and cetuximab in metastatic colorectal cancer. N Engl J Med 360:563–572, 2009.

104. Punt CJ, Tol J, Rodenburg CJ, et al: Randomized phase III study of capecitabine, oxaliplatin, and bevacizumab with or without cetuximab in advanced colorectal cancer: the CAIRO2 Study of the Dutch Colorectal Cancer Group. [Abstract LBA 4011] J Clin Oncol 26(Suppl):180s, 2008.

105. Tournigand C, Cervantes A, Figer A, et al: OPTIMOX-1: a randomized study of FOLFOX4 or FOLFOX7 with oxaliplatin in a stop-and-go fashion in advanced colorectal cancer—a GERCOR study. J Clin Oncol 24:394–400, 2006.

106. Maindrault-Goebel F, Lledo G, Chibaudel B, et al: OPTIMOX2, a large randomized phase II study of maintenance therapy or chemotherapy-free intervals (CFI) after FOLFOX in patients with metastatic colorectal cancer (MRC). A GERCOR study. [Abstracts of Meeting] J Clin Oncol 24:3504, 2006.

107. Wang JY, Wu CH, Lu CY, et al: Molecular detection of circulating tumor cells in the peripheral blood of patients with colorectal cancer using RT-PCR: significance of the prediction of postoperative metastasis. World J Surg 6:1007–1013, 2006.

108. Buyse M, Zeleniuch-Jacquote A, Chalmers TC: Adjuvant therapy of colorectal cancer. Why we still don't know. JAMA 259:3571, 1988.

109. Efficacy of adjuvant fluorouracil and folinic acid in colon cancer. International Multicentre Pooled Analysis of Colon Cancer Trials (IMPACT) investigators. Lancet 345:939–944, 1995.

110. Di Constanzo F, Sobero A, Gasperoni S, et al: Adjuvant chemotherapy in the treatment of colon cancer: randomized multicenter trial of the Italian National Intergroup of Adjuvant Chemotherapy in Colon Cancer (INTACC). Ann Oncol 14:1365–1372, 2003.

111. Link KH, Kornmann M, Saib L, et al: Increase in survival benefit in advanced resectable colon cancer by extent of adjuvant treatment: results of randomized trial comparing modulation of 5-FU + levamisole with folinic acid or with interferon-alpha. Ann Surg 242:178–187, 2005.

112. Porschen R, Bermann A, Loffler T, et al: Fluorouracil plus leucovorin as effective adjuvant therapy in curatively resected

stage III colon cancer: results of trial adjCCA-01. J Clin Oncol 19:1787–1794, 2001.

113. QUASAR Collaborative Group: Comparison of fluorouracil with additional levamisole, higher dose folinic acid, or both, as adjuvant chemotherapy for colorectal cancer: a randomized trial. Lancet 355:1588–1596, 2000.

114. Schippinger W, Jagoditch M, Sorre C, et al: A prospective randomised trial to study the role of levamisole and interferon-alpha in an adjuvant therapy with 5-FU for stage III colon cancer. Br J Cancer 92:24–29, 2005.

115. Andre T, Colin P, Louvet C, et al: Semimonthly versus monthly regimen of fluorouracil and leucovorin for 24 or 36 weeks as adjuvant therapy in stage II and III colon cancer: results of a randomized trial. J Clin Oncol 21:2896–2903, 2003.

116. Chau I, Norman AR, Cunningham D, et al: A randomized comparison between 6 months of bolus fluorouracil/leucovorin and 12 weeks of protracted venous infusion fluorouracil as adjuvant treatment in colorectal cancer. Ann Oncol 16: 549–557, 2005.

117. Poplin EA, Benedetti JK, Estes NC, et al: Phase III Southwest Oncology Group 9415/Intergroup 0153 randomized trial of fluorouracil, leucovorin, and levamisole versus continuous infusion and levamisole for adjuvant treatment of stage III and high risk stage II colon cancer. J Clin Oncol 23:1819–1825, 2005.

118. Scheithauer W, McKendrick J, Begbie S, et al: Oral capecitabine as an alternative to i.v. 5-fluorouracil-based adjuvant therapy for colon cancer: safety results of a randomized, phase III trial. Ann Oncol 14:1735–1743, 2003.

119. Andre T, Boni C, Mounedji-Boudiaf L, et al: Multicenter International Study of oxaliplatin/5-fluorouracil/leucovorin in the Adjuvant Treatment of Colon Cancer (MOSAIC) investigators. Oxaliplatin, fluorouracil, and leucovorin as adjuvant treatment for colon cancer. N Engl J Med 350:2343–2351, 2004.

120. de Gramont A, Boni C, Navarro M, et al: Oxaliplatin/5FU/LV in adjuvant colon cancer: updated efficacy results of the MOSAIC trial, including survival, with a median follow-up of six years. J Clin Oncol 25:4007, 2007.

121. Kuebler JP, Wieand HS, O'Connell MJ, et al: Oxaliplatin combined with weekly bolus fluorouracil and leucovorin as surgical adjuvant chemotherapy for stage II and III colon cancer: results from NSABP C-07. J Clin Oncol 16:2198–2204, 2007.

122. Saltz LB, Niedzwicki D, Hoillis D, et al: Irinotecan fluorouracil plus leucovorin is not superior to fluorouracil plus leucovorin alone as adjuvant treatment for stage III colon cancer: results of CALGB 89803. J Clin Oncol 25:3456–3461, 2007.

123. Van Cutsem E, Labianca R, Hossfeld D, et al: Randomized phase III trial comparing biweekly infusional fluorouracil/leucovorin alone or with irinotecan in the adjuvant treatment of stage III colon cancer: PETACC-3. J Clin Oncol 27: 3117–3125, 2009.

124. Ychou M, Raoul JL, Douillard JY, et al: A phase III randomized trial of LV5FU2 + CPT-11 versus LV5FU2 alone in adjuvant high risk colon cancer (FNCLCC Accord02/FFCD9802 trial). [Abstract] J Clin Oncol 23:246s, 2005.

125. Wolmark N, Yothers G, O'Connell MJ, et al: A phase III trial comparing mFOLFOX6 to mFOLFOX6 plus bevacizumab in stage II or III carcinoma of the colon: results of NSABP Protocol C-08.N. [Abstract LBA4] J Clin Oncol 27(Suppl):18s, 2009.

126. Gray RG, Barnwell J, Hills R, et al: QUASAR: a randomized study of adjuvant chemotherapy (CT) vs observation including 3238 colorectal cancer patients. [Abstracts of Meeting] J Clin Oncol 22:3501, 2004.

127. Benson AB, Schrag D, Somerfield MR, et al: American Society of Clinical Oncology recommendations for adjuvant therapy for stage II colon cancer. J Clin Oncol 22:3408–3419, 2004.

128. Westra JL, Plukker JT, Buys CH, et al: Genetic alterations in locally advanced stage II/III colon cancer: a search for prognostic markers. Clin Colorectal Cancer 4:252–259, 2004.

129. Jen J, Kim H, Piantadosi S, et al: Allelic loss of chromosome 18q and prognosis in colorectal cancer. N Engl J Med 331: 213–221, 1994.

130. Kohonen-Corish MR, Daniel JJ, Chan C, et al: Low microsatellite instability is associated with poor prognosis in stage C colon cancer. J Clin Oncol 23:2318–2324, 2005.

131. Tejpar S, Bosman F, Delorenzi M, et al: Microsatellite instability (MSI) in stage II and III colon cancer treated with 5FU-LV or 5FU-LV and irinotecan (PETACC 3-EORTC 40993-SAKK 60/00 trial). [Abstract 4001] J Clin Oncol 27(Suppl):15s, 2009.

132. Baranda J, Williamson S: The new paradigm in the treatment of colorectal cancer: are we hitting the target?. Expert Opin Investig Drugs 16:311–324, 2007.

133. Pages F, Berger A, Camus M, et al: Effector memory T cells, early metastasis, and survival in colorectal cancer. N Engl J Med 353:2654–2666, 2005.

134. Galon J, Costes A, Sanchez-Cabo F, et al: Type, density, and location of immune cells within human colorectal tumors predict clinical outcome. Science 313:1960–1964, 2006.

16 Radiation Therapy for Colorectal Adenocarcinoma: External Beam and Intraoperative Radiation Therapy

Joseph M. Herman and Timothy M. Pawlik

KEY POINTS

- Despite aggressive surgical management, up to 40% of patients with rectal cancer and 30% of patients with colon cancer will experience locoregional failure.
- External beam radiation therapy (EBRT) combined with chemotherapy is a well-established method of enhancing locoregional control in patients with rectal cancer; it is preferentially given before surgery.
- Intraoperative radiation therapy is a method of delivering high doses of radiation to the operative field at the time of surgery. The method of delivery can be either EBRT or brachytherapy. EBRT has been associated with greater toxicity owing to dose overlap. Brachytherapy can be administered continually in the postoperative setting or intraoperatively using high-dose rate brachytherapy, which is administered robotically through a multichanneled applicator.
- Intraoperative radiation therapy is most beneficial in the setting of resection of all gross disease (R0 or R1).
- All patients with recurrent rectal cancer would benefit from a multidisciplinary team approach.

Background

In 2009, an estimated 40,870 new cases of rectal cancer and 106,100 cases of colon cancer were diagnosed in the United States.[1] Despite aggressive surgical management, 5% to 40% of rectal cancer patients and 30% of advanced colon cancer (T4) patients will experience locoregional relapse.[2-4] Radiation has been shown to decrease the risk of local recurrence after blunt and mesorectal excisions.[5,6] The German rectal cancer trial demonstrated that preoperative chemoradiation (CRT) improves local control and sphincter preservation and results in less treatment-related toxicity compared with postoperative CRT.[7] Relapse rates for rectal cancer are especially high when tumors are adherent to or invading adjacent structures (T4). In these cases, even aggressive management with neoadjuvant CRT and total mesorectal excision (TME) can often result in margin-positive resections. In turn, a positive surgical resection margin is associated with an increased risk of local recurrence. Without treatment, patients with pelvic recurrences may experience severe pain and in general have a median survival of about 8 months.[8] Palliative surgery alone improves survival up to a median of 11 months.[2] Although radiation therapy or chemotherapy plus radiation can successfully palliate pain, 5-year survival rates for either therapy when used alone are less than 5%.[9,10] When colorectal cancers recur, a multimodality approach is required.

After decades of treating locally advanced colorectal cancer (CRC) with 5-fluorouracil (5-FU) and radiation, newer cytotoxic and biologic agents are now available. Combinations of cytotoxic agents (e.g., irinotecan and oxaliplatin) and targeted therapies (e.g., cetuximab and bevacizumab) have led to increases in disease-free and overall survival in patients with colorectal cancer.[11-15] With the advances in adjuvant systemic treatment, patients with colorectal cancer are now living longer. As such, durable control of the primary tumor site has renewed importance. In addition to appropriate aggressive surgical management (e.g., mesorectal excision, en bloc resection of involved organs, and so on), there has been a renewed interest in intraoperative radiation therapy (IORT) for locally advanced or locally recurrent pelvic adenocarcinoma. Specifically, some clinicians have advocated that preoperative CRT followed by IORT and adjuvant chemotherapy may lead to improved outcomes for patients.

IORT has the advantage of escalating the radiation dose at the tumor bed after resection of all gross disease. By allowing higher doses of radiation to be administered to specific anatomic sites, IORT can limit the dose of radiation to adjacent normal structures, thereby reducing potential toxicity. IORT has historically been associated with an improvement in local control; however, the effect of IORT on overall survival is more controversial. The role, as well as the efficacy, of IORT continues to evolve. In this chapter, we review the relative indications, feasibility, and efficacy of EBRT and IORT. In addition, we attempt to highlight which patients are most likely to benefit from IORT in the treatment of locally advanced or locally recurrent colorectal adenocarcinoma. We also briefly discuss the role of adjuvant radiation therapy and IORT for T4 colon cancer.

External Beam Radiation Therapy for Rectal Cancer

Sauer and colleagues[7] conducted a randomized clinical trial that established preoperative CRT and surgery followed by maintenance chemotherapy as the standard of care for clinical stage T3, T4, or node-positive rectal cancer. Early studies evaluating preoperative therapy used hypofractionated radiation alone. Specifically, the Swedish rectal trial demonstrated a statistically significant improvement in local control and survival with the addition of radiation alone (25 Gy in five fractions) to the pelvis before a non–TME.[6] This trial showed that local therapy alone can improve survival after surgical resection. The Dutch rectal trial evaluated whether radiation therapy (25 Gy) was still necessary after a TME.[16] Although local control was improved with TME, there remained a statistically significant improvement in local control with the addition of radiation, but no improvement was seen in overall survival.

In the United States, conventionally fractionated preoperative irradiation alone is supported by several single-institutional studies.[17] Three more recent randomized clinical trials from Europe have investigated the role of preoperative irradiation with or without chemotherapy. Two of these studies (EORTC 22921 and FFCD 9203) demonstrated a significant improvement in local control when 5-FU-based chemotherapy was added to radiation (45 Gy) in the neoadjuvant setting.[5,18] As expected, acute toxicity was increased with the addition of chemotherapy, as had been noted in the French trial (FFCD 9203).[5] A third trial from Poland compared a short-course (25 Gy) with a standard-course radiation therapy regimen (45 Gy). No statistically significant difference was found with regard to local control, survival, or late toxicity between the two arms, although the trial had several flaws including inconsistencies with maintenance chemotherapy after surgery.[19]

Although local control has been improved with neoadjuvant CRT, many patients still succumb to metastatic disease. Therefore, several studies have explored adding a second chemotherapeutic agent concurrent with 5-FU. Oxaliplatin has been shown to be efficacious in the metastatic setting and now appears to be reasonably well tolerated when added to 5-FU and radiation therapy.[14,20,21] Targeted therapies such as erlotinib (epidermal growth factor tyrosine kinase inhibitor) and bevacizumab have also been evaluated in the neoadjuvant setting and may result in further improvements in local control and survival.[14,15]

Radiation Therapy Treatment Planning

Generally, patients are treated prone on a belly board with three fields of radiation (one posterior and two laterals). Patients undergo computed tomography simulation, and the primary tumor (tumor bed if adjuvant) and iliac vessels (representing lymph node areas at risk) are delineated. Standard borders include L4/L5 vertebral bodies superiorly and the bottom of the ischial tuberosity inferiorly. Lateral borders correspond to the lateral aspect of the iliac lymph nodes or approximately 1.5 cm lateral to the pelvic brim. To limit the dose to normal structures, many centers have begun using intensity-modulated radiation therapy (IMRT) for localized rectal cancer in the neoadjuvant setting.[22]

Adjuvant Radiation Therapy With or Without Chemotherapy

Several classic trials have examined the use of adjuvant radiation alone or in combination with chemotherapy. Several studies demonstrated that chemotherapy and radiation improved local control and survival.[23-25] The method of administration of chemotherapy appears to be important for obtaining optimal results. Infusional 5-FU was found to be superior to bolus 5-FU. The toxicity between the regimens also differed, with infusional 5-FU causing more diarrhea and bolus 5-FU resulting in pancytopenias.[26-28] The timing of chemotherapy may also be important according to a recent randomized study. Starting radiation therapy with the first cycle of chemotherapy led to a better outcome compared with the traditional "sandwich" approach (chemotherapy alone, combined CRT, chemotherapy alone), which was used in most trials.[29] Thus, infusional 5-FU with radiation therapy can be considered a standard adjuvant therapy, and it may be reasonable to begin radiation with the first cycle of chemotherapy. Capecitabine, an orally active prodrug of 5-FU has been shown to be equally efficacious in the adjuvant and neoadjuvant setting.[30]

Intraoperative Radiation Therapy: Overview

Intraoperative radiation therapy (IORT) refers to the delivery of high doses of radiation to the tumor bed at the time of surgical resection. IORT has been advocated as an adjunct to external beam radiation therapy (EBRT) to escalate the dose of radiation at the site of resection. IORT can be delivered using electrons (intraoperative electron beam radiation therapy [IOERT]) or with brachytherapy catheters.[31,32] Both methods involve retraction of mobile normal structures, most notably bowel. Structures that cannot be retracted out of the treatment field (e.g., blood vessels, ureters, and peripheral nerves) are shielded using lead.

IOERT is administered using a standard or mobile linear accelerator (Mobetron, IntraOp Medical Corporation, Sunnyvale, California; Linac Systems, LLC, Albuquerque, New Mexico), which can deliver various electron beam energies (i.e., doses) to prespecified tissue depths[33] (Fig. 16-1). With IOERT, various cone shapes and sizes can be used to adapt to diverse tumor bed volumes. One limitation of IOERT is that it may require several overlapping IOERT

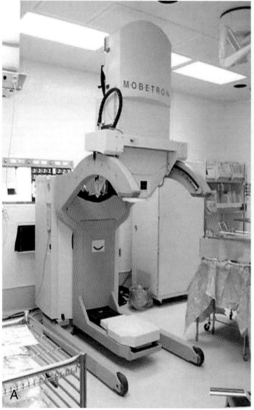
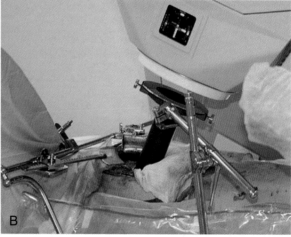

Figure 16-1. **A,** Intraoperative electron beam radiation therapy (IOERT) is administered using a mobile linear accelerator (Mobetron). **B,** Cone used to deliver focused IOERT to the tumor bed. (Courtesy of L.L. Gunderson, Mayo Clinic, Rochester, Minnesota.)

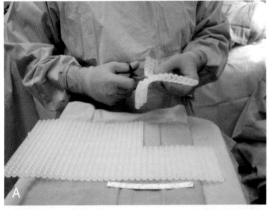

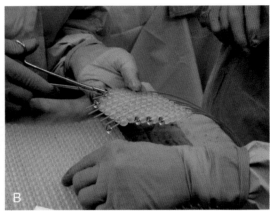

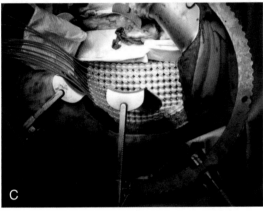

Figure 16-2. High-dose rate brachytherapy involves placement of catheters in the tumor bed after en bloc resection of the rectal cancer. The catheters are often placed into a silicone flap that can be cut to conform to the tumor bed (**A**). After adjusting the wires to the appropriate length (**B**), the flap is placed into the operative field with the appropriate shielding (**C**). A wire with a single iridium source (Ir-192) at the end then passes through the catheters embedded in the flap at evenly spaced 1-cm intervals to deliver the radiation.

cones to adequately cover the area of interest. Overlapping cones may result in radiation "hot spots" that may increase toxicity, especially peripheral neuropathy.[34] To decrease these hot spots, some institutions (e.g., Mayo Clinic, Rochester, Minnesota) use rectangular or ellipsoid applicators while eliminating the need for overlapping circular fields. In contrast, the University of Heidelberg Department of Radiation Oncology uses horseshoe-shaped applicators that simplify abutting two smaller fields.[35] For the Mobetron, square and rectangular applicators are being developed that allow for field sizes of up to 8 cm × 20 cm as a single field size (personal communication, Mobetron).

Brachytherapy involves placement of catheters in the tumor bed after en bloc resection of the tumor. The catheters are placed individually or into a silicone flap (Freiburg Flap, Nucletron, Veenendaal, The Netherlands, or Harrison-Anderson-Mick [HAM] applicator, Mick-Radio Nuclear Instruments, Inc., Mount Vernon, New York), which can be cut to conform to the tumor bed (Fig. 16-2A–C). IORT brachytherapy can be administered using either low-dose rate

IORT (LDR-IORT) or high-dose rate IORT (HDR-IORT).

LDR-IORT involves the placement of brachytherapy catheters into the operative bed after surgical resection. With LDR-IORT, the catheters are manually loaded with individual brachytherapy sources (e.g., iridium) after surgery. The loaded catheters are then left in place for a specified period of time based on the depth and dose prescribed.

In contrast, with HDR-IORT the complete dose of IORT is administered at the time of surgery. Specifically, HDR-IORT is administered through a wire with a single iridium source (Ir-192) at the end, which passes through catheters embedded in a silicon flap at evenly spaced 1-cm intervals. A robot guides the brachytherapy wire through the catheters and stops at "dwell" positions that have been designated by the radiation treatment plan. These dwell positions and times can be used to manipulate the dose at various points along the flap. With HDR-IORT, the tumor bed can be covered by a single flap, in contrast to IOERT, which may require several overlapping IOERT cones. In addition,

Table 16-1. Potential Differences Between IOERT and HDR-IORT

	IOERT	HDR-IORT
Treatment time	2–4 minutes	5–30 minutes
Procedure time	30–45 minutes	45–120 minutes
Treatment sites	Accessible locations	Depth at risk ≤0.5–1.0 cm from surface
Surface dose	Lower (75–93%)	Higher (200%)
Dosimetric homogeneity	≤10% variation	≥100 variation
Dose at depth (2 cm)	Higher (70–100%)	Lower (30%)

HDR-IORT, high-dose rate intraoperative radiation therapy; IOERT, intraoperative electron beam radiation therapy.

HDR-IORT results in a higher surface dose (HDR 200% of prescribed dose versus IOERT 75%–95% of prescribed dose) with a lower dose at 2 cm (HDR 30% versus IOERT 70%–100%) compared with IOERT.[33] Unlike LDR-IORT, with HDR-IORT the flap and catheters are removed immediately after treatment has been delivered, thereby limiting radiation exposure to physicians and surgical staff. However, compared with IOERT, HDR/LDR brachytherapy treatment and procedure times are typically longer and depend on the source strength at the time of the procedure (Table 16-1).

In general, the biologic effectiveness of single-dose IORT is thought to be equivalent to 1.5 to 2.5 times the same total dose of fractionated EBRT.[36] Therefore, adding 15 Gy of IORT to 45 Gy of EBRT is equivalent to an EBRT dose of 75 to 87.5 Gy—the dose range believed to be most effective at controlling microscopic residual disease.

Patient Selection for Intraoperative Radiation Therapy

Whenever possible, patients should be presented at a multidisciplinary conference with surgeons, medical oncologists, and radiation oncologists where imaging and pathology can be reviewed. Patients who are most likely to benefit from IORT are those with locally advanced or locally recurrent colorectal tumors that are deemed amenable to surgical resection. Determinations of resectability require close collaboration with the surgeon. IORT has no established role for treating gross residual pelvic disease after an R2 resection (e.g., macroscopically positive/debulking operation). As such, a multimodality approach involving IORT requires that the surgeon anticipate an R0 (microscopically negative) or R1 (microscopically positive) resection.

A good history and physical examination and adequate cross-sectional imaging are required to determine whether a colorectal lesion is resectable. Patients with advanced pelvic tumors can present with a wide range of symptoms. Tumor involvement of surrounding pelvic structures can lead to symptoms such as pain, constipation, tenesmus, recurrent urinary tract infections, vaginal or rectal bleeding, hematuria, and pneumaturia. A digital rectal examination, bimanual examination (in females), proctoscopy, as well as endoscopic rectal ultrasound provide critical information for planning the operative approach and need to be performed before the operation. The distance of the rectal mass from the anal verge, the orientation of the tumor and its association with adjacent bony structures, and whether the mass is mobile or fixed should be ascertained. Accurate assessment of the pelvic mass on physical examination can be difficult, especially in patients with recurrent tumor and in those previously treated with radiation therapy.

All patients being considered for pelvic exenteration should undergo preoperative computed tomography (CT) or magnetic resonance imaging (MRI) to evaluate the extent of local disease and to exclude extrapelvic metastasis. Fluorodeoxyglucose-positron emission tomography (FDG-PET) can be used as an adjunct to CT to better identify metastatic disease. The accuracy of CT in the preoperative assessment of rectal cancer has been reported to range from 55% to 72%.[37,38] MRI has been reported to be superior to CT in accurately predicting tumor invasion through the bowel wall. In addition, MRI has been reported to be more accurate than CT in the identification of sacral bone and piriform muscle involvement.[39] However, even with MRI it can be difficult to reliably distinguish radiation changes from tumor involvement in patients with pelvic sidewall abnormalities.[40]

Most studies indicate that 24% to 64% of patients with locally recurrent rectal cancer can have resection with negative margins.[41–48] In patients with locally advanced disease, extirpation of structures such as the bladder, reproductive organs (e.g., vagina, uterus), or bony structures including the sacrum-coccyx may be necessary. Although sphincter preservation is a goal of resection, oncologic principles and adequate margins should not be compromised to maintain sphincter function. In patients with metastatic disease who have synchronous locally advanced or locally recurrent disease, IORT should be considered in conjunction with local extirpation of the pelvic tumor—usually after a course of chemotherapy to ensure that the systemic burden of disease is stable or responsive.[49]

Review of Literature on IORT

Early studies investigating advanced and recurrent rectal cancer have demonstrated that local control and survival are stage- and margin-dependent.[43,50–54] For locally advanced disease, the 5-year local recurrence and survival rates range between 5% to 37% and 46% to 70%, respectively. These studies also show that the rate of local control and survival for primary locally advanced rectal cancer is clearly superior to that for recurrent disease (recurrent locoregional disease: local recurrence 21%–74%, overall survival 16%–41%) (Tables 16-2 and 16-3).

The Radiation Therapy Oncology Group (RTOG) reported a phase I/II study that evaluated patients with advanced, unresectable, or recurrent carcinoma of the rectum.[55] Of the 86 evaluable patients, 42 patients received either IORT alone ($n = 15$) or in combination with EBRT ($n = 27$). The investigators reported that local control rates were dependent on the amount of residual disease after surgical resection before IOERT. Specifically, patients who had grossly negative surgical margins (e.g., either R0 or R1 resection) had a significantly better 2-year actuarial local control rate and overall survival rate compared with patients who had gross residual disease (e.g., R2 resection) at the IOERT site (local control 88% versus 77%, $P = .001$; overall survival 48% versus 10%, $P = .006$; R0/R1 versus R2, respectively). These findings have been corroborated by Willett and colleagues,[56] who similarly reported a 5-year disease-free survival rate of only 6% for patients with locally advanced rectal cancer who underwent IORT after an R2 resection compared with 54% when the margins were grossly negative. Data from a recent update of this study confirm the long-term implications of margin status before IOERT therapy (5-year overall survival rate, no gross residual disease 40% versus gross residual disease 13%; $P = .0001$).[48]

Table 16-2. Studies Evaluating HDR-IORT or IOERT in Patients with Locally Advanced/Unresectable Primary Rectal Cancer

Study	n	%LR	%OS	Gy IORT/EBRT/Chemo?	Toxicity
HDR-IORT					
Huber et al (1996)[63]	38	2-yr, 27	NA	15/50/yes	2 US, poor sacral healing
Nuyttens et al (2004)[65]	18	3-yr, 19	3-yr, 61	10/50/no	3 late (diarrhea/pain)*
Harrison et al (1998)[47]	22	2-yr, 37	2-yr, 69	10–20/45–50/yes	11 WH (all)
IOERT					
Gunderson et al[3]	61	5-yr, 16	5-yr, 46	10–20/45–55/yes	32% PN, 23% BO, 16% WH
Calvo et al[80]	100	4-yr, 6	4-yr, 65	12.5/45–50/yes	30 patients w/morbidity
Willett et al[56]	20	5-yr, 23	5-yr, 54 (DFS)	15/50.4/yes	1 US, 3 BO
Krempien et al[61]	210	5-yr, 7	5-yr, 69	10/41.4/yes*	Acute 17%, late 13%

*CRT delivered preoperatively or postoperatively.
BO, bowel obstruction; CRT, chemoradiation; DFS, disease-free survival; EBRT, external beam radiation therapy; HDR-IORT, high-dose rate intraoperative radiation therapy; IOERT, intraoperative electron beam radiation therapy; IORT, intraoperative radiation therapy; LR, local recurrence; n, number; NA, not applicable; OS, overall survival; PN, peripheral neuropathy; US, ureteral stenosis; WH, wound healing.

Table 16-3. Studies Evaluating HDR-IORT or IOERT in Patients with Locally Recurrent Rectal Cancer

Study	n	%LR	%OS	No. IORT	Toxicity
HDR-IORT					
Alektiar et al (2000)[46]	74	5-yr, 61	5-yr, 23	All	16%PN, 23%US, 24% WH
Harrison et al (1998)[47]	46	2-yr, 37	2-yr, 47	All	11 WH (all)*
Nuyttens et al (2004)[65]	19	3-yr, 52	2-yr, 35	All	46% WH, 14% PN
IOERT					
Valentini et al (1999)[45]	47	5-yr, 68	5-yr, 22	11	1 US, 1 WH
Rutten et al (2001)[81]	62	5-yr, 37	5-yr, 33	All	16% PN
Lindel et al (2001)[48]	69	5-yr, 65	5-yr, 27	46	3 BO, 4 WH, 4 PN
Wiig et al (2002)[67]	107	5-yr, 50	5-yr, 30	59	NA
Shoup et al (2002)[42]	100	5-yr, 38	5-yr, 33	All	23% US, 16% PN
Eble et al (1998)[60]	31	2-yr, 29	4-yr, 58	All	17 WH, 2 US, 0 PN
Suzuki et al (1995)[69]	106	5-yr, 40	5-yr, 19	42	6 BO, 3 US
Wallace et al (1995)[51]	41	5-yr, 70	5-yr, 16 (DFS)	All	4 PN, 3 BO, 4 WH
Abuchaibe et al (1993)[54]	27	2-yr, 74	2-yr, 47	All	37% enteritis, 52% PN

*Not clarified if toxicity in primary or recurrent.
BO, bowel obstruction; DFS, disease-free survival; HDR-IORT, high-dose rate-intraoperative radiation therapy/IOERT, intraoperative electron beam radiation therapy; IORT, intraoperative radiation therapy; LR, local recurrence; n, number; NA, not applicable; OS, overall survival; PN, peripheral neuropathy; US, ureteral stenosis; WH, wound healing.

To see whether IORT might improve outcomes after state-of-the-art rectal surgery alone, Pacelli and colleagues[57] compared preoperative radiation therapy (no chemotherapy) plus IORT after rectal resection with TME versus TME alone for patients with middle and lower T3 rectal cancer. From 1991 to 1997, 113 patients received either preoperative radiation therapy (38 Gy) plus IORT (10 Gy; n = 69) or TME alone (n = 44). Postoperative complications were comparable in the two groups. Patients who received preoperative radiation therapy followed by TME and IORT tended to have a longer 5-year disease-specific survival rate (81%) compared with patients who underwent TME alone (58%) (P = .052). The differences in local control, however, were more dramatic. Specifically, local recurrence at 5 years was more than three times more common in the TME-alone group (23.2%) compared with the combined-modality group (6.6%) (P = .017). The data from this study demonstrated the superiority of a combined-modality approach that includes preoperative radiation therapy, TME, and IOERT over TME alone in patients with T3 rectal cancer. This study, however, was not able to address the relative benefit of IORT itself (e.g., preoperative radiation therapy, TME, and

IOERT versus preoperative radiation therapy, TME, without IOERT).

In aggregate, data from these studies show a local control benefit for IOERT in patients with locally advanced/recurrent rectal pelvic tumors. The benefit of IOERT appears to be confined to patients undergoing resection of all gross disease (e.g., either R0 or R1 resection). When surgery is unable to extirpate all gross disease, local control can be anticipated to be poor even if IOERT is used.

Preoperative Chemoradiation Followed by Surgery and IOERT

With the introduction and widespread acceptance of TME, the incidence of positive margins and the rate of local recurrence for patients with rectal cancer have decreased. After the German rectal trial, neoadjuvant CRT became the standard of care for patients with either T3 or node-positive tumors.[7] Because many patients are now being treated with preoperative radiation, the role of IORT for locally advanced rectal cancer has been questioned. Several studies have specifically addressed this clinical question. Sanfilippo and colleagues[58] examined patients with rectal cancers treated with preoperative 5-

FU-based CRT (median dose 45 Gy) followed by resection and IORT. Patients with T4 rectal cancer who were treated with preoperative combined CRT followed by multivisceral resection had a local recurrence rate of 20% at 31 months. Similar to other studies, positive margin status predicted worse local control and long-term survival. Although the addition of IORT was not associated with an improved local control rate, the study was underpowered to examine this endpoint, since only a few patients received IORT.

In a separate study, Kim and colleagues[59] combined IOERT (orthovoltage radiation median dose 12.5 Gy) with 5-FU-based preoperative EBRT (50.4 Gy) and surgical resection in 40 patients with locally advanced, unresectable rectal carcinoma. Twenty-seven patients had primary tumors, and 13 had recurrent disease. The crude local control rate for locally advanced primary rectal cancer was 73% compared with 27% in patients with recurrent cancer. All patients ($n = 4$) with gross residual disease had recurrence. In contrast, the 5-year actuarial local control and overall survival rates for patients undergoing complete gross resection (e.g., R0 or R1) along with IORT were 75% and 64%, respectively. Whereas preoperative CRT followed by orthovoltage IORT failed to control gross residual disease, this therapeutic approach was successful in the setting of minimal residual disease.

Eble and colleagues[60] evaluated 63 patients with locally advanced stage II or III rectal cancer who received neoadjuvant radiation (with or without 5-FU chemotherapy) followed by resection and IOERT. The median EBRT dose was 41.4 Gy for those receiving preoperative CRT, with 45 (71.4%) of these patients receiving concomitant 5-FU chemotherapy. At the time of surgery, 54 (86%) patients had a microscopically negative resection (R0). The mean IOERT dose was 11.3 Gy. At a median follow-up of 30.6 months, patients who received neoadjuvant CRT, resection, and IOERT had a higher 4-year actuarial recurrence-free survival rate (82% and 17.6%, respectively) and were less likely to develop distant metastases, compared with those who underwent neoadjuvant radiation (no 5-FU) resection and IOERT (59% and 38.8%, respectively). This study demonstrates the importance of adding 5-FU to neoadjuvant radiation before IOERT.

Krempien and associates[61] investigated 210 patients who were treated with TME, IOERT (12 Gy for R1, and 15 Gy for R2), and either pre- ($n = 88$) or postoperative ($n = 122$) concurrent CRT (41.4 Gy). The 5-year actuarial disease-free and overall survival rate for the entire cohort was 69% and 66%, respectively; the 5-year actuarial local control rate was 93%. Tumor stage and surgical resection margin status (R0, R1, versus R2) each were associated with disease-free, overall, and local recurrence-free survival. Resection margin status was the strongest predictor of local control, with history of R2 resection being strongly associated with the highest risk of local recurrence. The study was unique in that patients who received IOERT were allowed to have a 20% dose reduction in EBRT (41.4 Gy); yet this did not seem to compromise long-term control rates. In fact, control results were similar to those reported by Sauer and colleagues[7] despite having more patients with T4 disease (22% versus 4%). In addition, the authors reported a perioperative complication rate (9%) that was comparable to that with TME alone and neoadjuvant CRT followed by TME. At a median follow-up of 61 months, there was no reported neuropathy and only a 2% incidence of ureteral obstruction.

Diaz-Gonzalez and associates[62] evaluated 115 patients with stage T3/T4 rectal tumors or node-positive disease who were treated with preoperative 5-FU-based CRT, surgery, and IOERT. With a median follow-up of 36.9 months (range 6–83.4), the median disease-free and overall survival had not been reached. Both the 3-year disease-free and overall survival rate was 74%, whereas the pelvic control rate was 94%. Seven (6%) patients developed pelvic recurrence (three isolated and four with synchronous metastatic disease), and 24 (21%) patients had recurrences with distant metastases alone. Two recurrences were localized to the presacral area—the area previously boosted with IOERT. The median time to local relapse was 23 months (range 10–55). Patients with microscopic residual disease had fewer local relapses compared with patients who had gross residual disease (2% versus 9%, respectively; $P = .136$). The overall relapse rate and incidence of systemic metastasis were significantly lower in the microscopic residual subgroup compared with the macroscopic residual group (8% versus 37% and 6% versus 32%, respectively; both $P = .001$). On multivariate analysis, male gender and persistence of macroscopic disease were associated with a shorter disease-free survival. The authors hypothesized that the shape of the female pelvis may allow for a larger IORT field, thus decreasing the risk of local recurrence compared with that of the male pelvis. Using male gender and residual macroscopic disease as risk factors, the investigators reported a progressively worse disease-free survival rate associated with none (100%), one (81%), or two (53%) of these risk factors.

HDR-IORT for Locally Advanced Rectal Cancer

In patients with locally advanced rectal cancer, the results with high-dose rate-intraoperative radiation therapy (HDR-IORT) appear to be similar to results with IOERT. Harrison and colleagues[47] reported on 22 patients with primary unresectable rectal cancer who received preoperative EBRT (45–50.5 Gy) with 5-FU followed by surgery plus HDR-IORT (10–20 Gy). Similar to other studies, local control and disease-free survival rates were markedly better in patients undergoing a resection with negative margins compared with those with positive margins (local control: margin-negative 92% versus margin-positive 38%; $P = .002$; disease-free survival: margin-negative 77% versus margin-positive 38%, $P = .03$).

Huber and associates[63] evaluated HDR-IORT combined with preoperative or postoperative 5-FU-based CRT. Median IORT dose was 15 Gy. From 1989 to 1993, 38 patients were included in this study. The tumors of 19 patients were staged as T3 tumors by preoperative endosonography (group I) and tumors of another 19 were staged as T4 tumors (group II). Patients in group I underwent resection (16 abdominoperineal resections [APR]; 3 low anterior resections [LAR]) and IORT, followed by postoperative CRT (50 Gy/5-FU), whereas patients in group II received preoperative CRT (40 Gy/5-FU) followed by resection (18 APR; 1 LAR) and IORT. Mean follow-up was 25.5 months. In groups I/II, most patients had an R0 resection ($n = 13$, $n = 14$ respectively). No perioperative mortality occurred in group I, 10.5% ($n = 2$) in group II. Postoperative morbidity was 53% ($n = 10$) in group I and 84% ($n = 16$) in group II. Delayed sacral wound healing was the predominant toxicity. Ureteral stenosis occurred in two

patients (group II). Late or persistent therapy-related complications were seen in two patients in group I and in six patients in group II. Local recurrence developed in three patients in group I (16%) and in two patients in group II (11%). Patients receiving preoperative CRT had a nonsignificant trend in survival compared with the adjuvant group. When compared with a matched historical control group of patients undergoing resection only, this cohort had a significant improvement in survival.

In another study by Ferenschild and colleagues,[64] the investigators prospectively evaluated 123 patients between 1987 and 2002 with initially unresectable locally advanced rectal cancer. All patients received preoperative radiation therapy (50 Gy). After 1997, patients ($n = 27$) received HDR-IORT (10 Gy) if the surgical margins were believed to be microscopically positive or were 2 mm. These patients had improved 5-year local control (58% versus 0%) and overall survival (38% versus 0%) compared with patients who did not receive HDR-IORT (pre-1997). Of note, some patients with R1/R2 resections did not receive IORT because of prior high radiation therapy (cervical cancer) or poor performance status or because IORT was not available.

HDR-IORT is a relatively new modality compared with IOERT; therefore, it is difficult to make a direct comparison of the two. In addition, improvements in IOERT treatment planning allow for better tumor bed coverage, which should result in less morbidity. Studies by Ferenschild[64] and Nuyttens and colleagues[65] suggest favorable outcomes with HDR-IORT in patients with positive margins (2 mm). This has not been reported with IOERT. However, Harrison and colleagues[47] reported inferior outcomes with R1/R2 resections despite the use of HDR-IORT. Both studies used neoadjuvant 5-FU-based CRT, and therefore the reason for the divergent outcomes is unclear. For both HDR-IORT and IOERT, these studies suggest improved local control and less morbidity when EBRT is delivered neoadjuvantly rather than adjuvantly. The addition of 5-FU appears to improve local control and survival of patients in some studies, but it is also associated with increased morbidity compared with EBRT alone. In patients with locally advanced (T3/T4) tumors, the addition of IORT to neoadjuvant CRT results in improved local control compared with neoadjuvant CRT alone. However, additional studies are needed to determine whether this trend persists.

Factors Associated With Outcome After IORT for Locally Advanced Rectal Cancer

Virtually all studies have demonstrated inferior outcomes with IORT after an incomplete surgical resection. To maximize the benefit of IORT, an oncologically appropriate resection is mandatory. IORT does not compensate for inadequate surgery that unnecessarily leaves residual tumor. As such, surgical resection to achieve negative margins is critical and is warranted even if an R0 resection requires extirpation of adjacent structures (e.g., ureter) or pelvic organs (e.g., bladder, reproductive organs).

Response to preoperative CRT may also help identify patients who are more likely to respond to or benefit from IORT. In two separate studies, Valentini and colleagues[45] and Stipa and colleagues[66] demonstrated improved local control, disease-free survival, and overall survival in patients who were downstaged with preoperative CRT followed by treatment with IORT. Others have identified specific factors associated with response to IORT. Diaz-Gonzalez and colleagues[62] evaluated 115 patients who were treated with either oral 5-FU or tegafur in combination with preoperative radiation therapy followed by surgery and IOERT. Patients treated with tegafur had a higher rate of complete pathologic response than those treated with 5-FU. Other factors associated with worse local control and disease-free survival following IORT include male gender,[62] pain, and positive lymph nodes at resection.[64] Tumor fixation has also been shown to adversely influence both local control and overall survival even in patients treated with IORT.[4,41,67]

Locally Recurrent Rectal Cancer

Many institutional reports on IORT have traditionally combined patients with locally advanced primary rectal lesions and those with recurrent rectal cancer. The combination of these patients can make it difficult to ascertain the relative benefit of IORT, especially in patients with recurrent rectal tumors. Patients with recurrent rectal cancer have often received previous che-

motherapy and radiation, therefore increasing the risk of treatment-related toxicity with IORT.

In general, most studies have demonstrated worse local control and survival rates for patients treated with IORT for recurrent pelvic lesions compared with primary locally advanced rectal lesions (see Table 16-3). For recurrent rectal cancer, Martinez-Monge and associates[68] suggest that the availability of IOERT, high-dose rate brachytherapy, and iodine-125 permanent seed implants can allow for optimal dosimetry. Most patients with locally recurrent rectal cancer have already received radiation; additional radiation and resection can therefore increase the likelihood of morbidity. In these cases, it may be beneficial to use HDR-IORT to limit the dose to the superficial surface of the resection bed, thus decreasing the risk of neuropathy. Another potential benefit of HDR-IORT is improved local control, as seen in some reports after margin-positive (2-mm) resections.[65] Additional studies, however, are needed to validate these findings.

Importance of Multimodality Therapy in Treatment of Locally Recurrent Rectal Cancer

Suzuki and colleagues[69] reported on 106 patients with locally recurrent rectal cancer who were treated with resection plus IORT (15–20 Gy) or resection plus EBRT (45 Gy). The investigators reported that margin status (33% microscopic residual disease versus 9% gross disease) and no history of IORT (IORT, 19% vs. no IORT, 7%) were associated with a worse 5-year overall survival (both $P < .05$). Other factors associated with a worse overall survival in patients with a recurrent rectal tumor were pelvic symptoms, tumor fixation, and performance status.

Eble and colleagues[70] reported on 31 consecutive patients with recurrent rectal carcinomas treated with IOERT and adjuvant EBRT after complete (R0, $n = 14$) or incomplete (R1, $n = 9$; R2, $n = 8$) resection. The mean IOERT dose was 13.7 Gy (range 12–20) supplemented with an EBRT dose of 41.4 Gy. Twenty-two patients had preoperative EBRT only, and 22 patients had concomitant CRT (5-FU and leucovorin). After a median follow-up of 28 months, 16 patients had re-recurrent disease, and 11 patients had died. Nine patients had failure only locally (four in-field, four marginal, and one anastomotic re-recurrence), and three patients had recurrence with both local and distant metastasis. The overall and IOERT in-field local control rates were 71% and 87%, respectively. The 4-year overall and relapse-free survival rates were 58% and 48%, respectively. After incomplete resection, the local failure rate increased (R0 21% versus R1/R2 35%), whereas the 4-year relapse-free survival rate significantly decreased (29% versus 71%). Of note, in addition to having higher local recurrence rates, patients who underwent an R1/R2 resection also had an increased rate of distant metastasis (R0 7% versus R1/R2 53%).

Treatment with IOERT was not associated with an increase in either acute or late toxicities. In aggregate, the data from these studies suggest that IOERT in combination with EBRT is a safe and efficacious multimodality treatment approach for patients with locally recurrent disease.

Harrison and colleagues[47] evaluated 46 patients with recurrent rectal cancer who underwent surgical resection followed by HDR-IORT (10–20 Gy). As expected, the 2-year local control and disease-free survival rates were better for patients undergoing resection with negative compared with positive margins (local control: 82% versus 19%, $P = .02$; disease-free survival: 71% versus 0%, $P = .04$, respectively).

Similar to primary rectal tumors, outcome after management of recurrent pelvic tumors depends on surgical margin status. A recent study by Nuyttens and colleagues[65] evaluated 37 patients (recurrent rectal cancer, $n = 19$) who were treated with EBRT, surgery, and HDR-IORT. HDR-IORT was administered only when the resection margins were 2 mm. A dose of 10 Gy was prescribed at a 1-cm depth from the template surface. At a median follow-up of 3 years, there were five in-field recurrences. The 3-year local failure rate was 19% for patients with primary rectal cancer compared with 52% for patients with recurrent tumors ($P = .0042$). These results suggest that when positive margins are suspected, HDR-IORT may be superior to IOERT. However, additional studies are needed.

In a series of 100 patients reported by Shoup and colleagues,[42] factors associated with survival in patients with recurrent rectal cancer included surgical margin status and vascular invasion in the resected specimen. In a separate study of 394 patients reported by Hahnloser and colleagues[43] EBRT was delivered perioperatively to 80% of patients, and IORT was delivered to 43% of patients. Overall survival was significantly decreased in patients with symptomatic pain or tumor fixation. Extended resection of adjacent organs, however, was not associated with a difference in local control or overall survival as long as all gross disease was extirpated. If, however, there was gross residual disease after extensive resection, patients remained at high risk for recurrence despite the use of IORT.

In general, patients with recurrent pelvic disease should be considered for IORT. Patients with locally recurrent rectal cancer should be considered for IORT when the pelvic disease is amenable to surgical resection (e.g., no evidence of unresectable extrapelvic disease, bilateral ureteric obstruction, or circumferential involvement of the pelvic wall). Even patients with extensive recurrent pelvic disease can achieve overall 5-year survival rates of about 20% using a combination of resection, EBRT, and IORT.

Re-irradiation

Recurrent disease in previously irradiated patients is a challenging situation in which treatment components should be balanced in an individualized fashion. The Mayo Clinic reported long-term local control rates of 60% in patients treated with moderate doses of re-irradiation with IORT.[52] Toxicity was moderate with a 32% incidence of neuropathy. A trend toward improved local control was observed in patients receiving more than 30 Gy (EBRT) of re-irradiation (81% versus 54%). In view of the high systemic failure rates in patients with recurrent rectal cancer, maintenance chemotherapy should become standard, and more aggressive systemic therapy regimens should be evaluated before, during, and after re-irradiation.

IORT Toxicity

The acute and long-term effects of IORT are often difficult to discern from surgical complications and tumor recurrence. Therefore, it is crucial to rule out tumor recurrence before attributing the symptoms to the side effects of treatment. Local relapses should also be distinguished from second malignancies.[71] In general, IORT most often correlates with late toxicity secondary to the radiobiology of a single high dose of radiation. It is difficult for normal tissues to repair damage from single high doses of radiation in contrast to fractionated low-dose radiation. Acute toxicity for HDR-IORT and IOERT are often associated with impaired wound healing. The dosimetric characteristics of HDR-IORT and IOERT are different (see Table 16-1) and therefore may have variant toxicity profiles. For example, to cover a large tumor bed with IOERT, multiple overlapping fields are necessary, thus increasing the likelihood of delivering higher doses to deep normal structures such as peripheral nerves. However, the newer methods described previously may result in less toxicity. Conversely, large fields can be easily treated with HDR-IORT, but it may be more difficult to avoid specific structures within the tumor bed such as the ureters and vessels.

Extensive animal studies have evaluated the acute and chronic adverse effects of IOERT. These experiments suggest that 10 to 20 Gy of IOERT plus EBRT (40–50 Gy) do not compromise the outcome of adult dogs.[33] In addition to treatment dose, the volume of tissue treated with IOERT is also critical (large vessels and ureters). Peripheral neuropathy is the dominant IOERT-related late normal tissue complication observed in patients after 5 years (8%).

The risk of ureteral obstruction or stenosis often depends on whether the tumor involved the ureter and whether the ureter was able to be removed from the IORT field or sufficiently blocked with lead. In addition, doses higher than 12.5 Gy increase the likelihood of ureteral damage and obstruction.[72] Another report demonstrated that lower doses of IOERT (median 10.4 Gy) and EBRT (41.4 Gy), as well as efforts to avoid or block the ureter, resulted in low rates of ureteral obstruction (2%).[61]

Secondary malignancies have not been directly attributed to radiation from IORT. Some studies, however, have demonstrated a possible correlation between IORT and second malignancies when used in conjunction with CRT.[71]

Functional Outcome and Quality of Life

Kienle and colleagues[73] compared functional outcome in 100 patients treated with no radiation, IORT (10–15 Gy), or IORT plus adjuvant EBRT (39.3–45 Gy). Anorectal function and rectal volume manometry were worse in the combined IORT/adjuvant EBRT arm. Specifically, rectal frequency, urgency, and number of pads needed were increased in patients treated with both IORT and EBRT. Although this study was concerning because it suggested worse functional outcome for patients treated with IORT plus EBRT, EBRT was administered in the postoperative rather than the preoperative setting, which may have contributed to worse functional outcomes. Since this was a retrospective study, patients who received combined IORT plus chemotherapy and radiation may also have had more advanced disease, which is frequently associated with more extensive surgery and increased morbidity.[73] Nevertheless, these data serve to emphasize that neoadjuvant CRT should be focused to limit the dose to the sphincter so that rectal function and quality of life may be preserved. Future studies will need to use standardized methods to prospectively evaluate quality of life in patients with rectal cancer treated with IORT.

Role of Adjuvant EBRT in Locally Advanced Colon Cancer

The standard of care for T3/T4 or node-positive rectal cancer is neoadjuvant 5-FU-based CRT.[7] Pathologic T3/T4 or node-positive resections require 5-FU-based CRT. The role of radiation in colon cancer is less clearly defined. If colon cancer patients undergo upfront surgical resection and have a pathologic T1/T2N0 resection, adjuvant radiation is unnecessary. Patients with pathologic T3/T4N+ colon cancer have an increased risk of local recurrence and may benefit from adjuvant therapy. The ascending colon and descending colon are considered anatomically immobile, and their close proximity to the retroperitoneal tissues often limits a wide surgical resection.[74] Incomplete resection results in residual disease and consequently increased local failure. When colon cancer tumors adhere to or invade adjacent structures, local failure rates exceed 30% with surgery alone.[75,76] Five-year survival rate with surgery alone drops to approximately 35% after a T4N+ resection. As with rectal cancer, adjuvant therapy has been used in colon cancer to improve local control, which may translate to a survival benefit.

Single-institution studies have demonstrated improved local control with adjuvant radiation therapy.[77] In a Massachusetts General Hospital series, patients with T4N0/N+ and T3N0 lesions with margins of less than 1 cm who received adjuvant radiation therapy were compared with historical controls who underwent surgery alone. Patients ($n = 171$) were treated with adjuvant radiation which was administered to the tumor plus a 3- to 5-cm margin to a total dose to 45 Gy with a boost to 50.4 Gy. 5-FU-based chemotherapy was delivered concomitantly with radiation in 63 patients. Five-year local control was improved when adjuvant radiation was implemented for T4N0 lesions (93% versus 69%) and T4N+ lesions (72% versus 47%). A smaller nonsignificant benefit was seen for T3 lesions. Patients receiving 5-FU had a trend toward improved local control and also a higher rate of acute enteritis (16% versus 4%), but no increase in late bowel toxicity. As with rectal cancer patients, patients with margin- and node-negative resections had improved 10-year local control and relapse-free survival rates.[75]

The Mayo Clinic reported a series of 103 patients treated with mostly 5-FU-based CRT with 11 patients receiving an IORT boost of 10 to 20 Gy. Patients with margin-negative resections had a 5-year local control rate of 90% compared with those with margin-positive resections (46% microscopic). It is surprising that patients who received IORT for residual disease fared better than those who did not (5-year local control 89% versus 18%). IORT also resulted in improved 5-year survival rate (76% versus 26%). A University of Florida series also reported improved local control rates with adjuvant radiation (88%) and found a dose-response relation to local control 96% (50–55 Gy) versus 76% (less than 50 Gy).

The only randomized trial to evaluate the efficacy of adjuvant radiation therapy for colon cancer was the US Gastrointestinal Intergroup phase III trial, which randomized patients to receive adjuvant radiation plus 5-FU and levamisole versus 5-FU and levamisole alone. Enrolled patients had to have margin-negative resections with adherence or invasion into surrounding structures (T4N0 or N+) or T3N+ lesions arising in the ascending or descending colon. The recommended total dose was 45 Gy with an optional 4.5-Gy boost. In 1996, the trial was closed because of poor accrual (189 evaluable

patients), and so there was not enough power to detect any differences between the groups. This study was flawed because many patients did not have clips placed at the time of surgery or preoperative imaging to clearly delineate the tumor bed. The study showed no difference in local control but showed increased toxicity with the addition of adjuvant CRT. Despite these limitations and insufficient power, this study has questioned the efficacy of adjuvant radiation in patients with resected colon cancer.

It is unlikely that additional randomized trials will be conducted to address the efficacy of adjuvant radiation in patients with resected colon cancer. However, newer chemotherapeutic agents have resulted in improved survival; therefore, local control can influence long-term survival. Treatment recommendations should be made on a case-by-case basis and should be discussed in a multidisciplinary setting with surgeons, radiation oncologists, and medical oncologists. In essence, adjuvant chemotherapy and radiation should be used in situations of invasion into adjacent structures and margin-positive resections and in situations in which the tumor bed can be clearly identified to enable focused radiation to be delivered while limiting the radiation dose to normal bowel.

IORT should be considered after a margin-positive resection or when the tumor is fixed to adjacent structures. All patients who receive adjuvant CRT should be considered for additional maintenance chemotherapy. As in rectal cancer, if a tumor is fixed based on preoperative imaging, the patient should receive neoadjuvant 5-FU-based CRT followed by IORT and maintenance chemotherapy.

Conclusions and Future Directions

Multiple single-institution studies have demonstrated improved local control, as well as survival, when IORT is combined with preoperative CRT and surgical resection to treat patients with locally advanced or recurrent rectal cancer.[2,4] Patient selection is crucial and should be determined in a multidisciplinary setting. Not only are the timing and choice of CRT critical, but a complete extirpation of all pelvic disease (e.g., an R0 or R1 resection) is mandatory if IORT is to be successful.

Recently, EORTC 22921 and FFCD 9203 demonstrated improved local control and complete response rates with the addition of 5-FU to preoperative radiation in patients with T2/N+ rectal cancer.[5,18] The addition of newer chemotherapeutic agents (e.g., oxaliplatin, irinotecan, bevacizumab) has resulted in improved response rates and longer survival for patients with locally advanced or metastatic disease. As such, integration of newer systemic agents into current treatment strategies should result in improved long-term survival in patients with locally advanced and recurrent rectal cancer.[4,78] With the improved survival associated with these novel chemotherapeutic and targeted therapies, use of IORT for long-term local control will become increasingly important.

Advances in MRI and functional imaging technology will not only improve patient selection, but also allow the radiation oncologist to optimize the IORT treatment field and the site of specific dose escalation and to better spare adjacent normal tissues. Use of specific sensitizers at the time of IORT may further improve local control, especially in patients with residual microscopic or macroscopic disease. In addition, tissue protectors such as amifostine may allow for better protection of normal structures.[79]

The role of adjuvant therapy in patients with locally advanced or node-positive colon cancer is unclear. Several institutions have demonstrated improved local control and even improved survival when adjuvant radiation (with or without chemotherapy) is used in patients with T4N0N1 or margin-positive resections. The only randomized trial showed no benefit in the addition of CRT for colon cancer patients with margin-negative T3/T4 resections, although there was limited power to detect a difference between the treatment arms. IORT appears to improve local control and possibly survival in single-institutional series, although data are limited. Therefore, the role of adjuvant CRT and IORT for patients with colon cancer should be discussed on a case-by-case basis in a multidisciplinary setting.

References

1. Jemal A, Siegel R, Ward E, et al: Cancer statistics, 2009. CA Cancer J Clin 59:225–249.
2. Hahnloser D, Haddock MG, Nelson H: Intraoperative radiotherapy in the multimodality approach to colorectal cancer. Surg Oncol Clin North Am 12(4):993–1013, ix, 2003.
3. Gunderson LL, Nelson H, Martenson JA, et al: Locally advanced primary colorectal cancer: intraoperative electron and external beam irradiation +/– 5-FU. Int J Radiat Oncol Biol Phys 37(3):601–614, 1997.
4. Willett CG, Czito BG, Tyler DS: Intraoperative radiation therapy. J Clin Oncol 25(8):971–977, 2007.
5. Gerard JP, Conroy T, Bonnetain F, et al: Preoperative radiotherapy with or without concurrent fluorouracil and leucovorin in T3–4 rectal cancers: results of FFCD 9203. J Clin Oncol 24(28):4620–4625, 2006.
6. Improved survival with preoperative radiotherapy in resectable rectal cancer. Swedish Rectal Cancer Trial. N Engl J Med 336(14):980–987, 1997.
7. Sauer R, Becker H, Hohenberger W, et al, and German Rectal Cancer Study Group. Preoperative versus postoperative chemoradiotherapy for rectal cancer. N Engl J Med 351(17):1731–1740, 2004.
8. Willett CG, Shellito PC, Tepper JE, et al: Intraoperative electron beam radiation therapy for recurrent locally advanced rectal or rectosigmoid carcinoma. Cancer 67(6):1504–1508, 1991.
9. Sofo L, Ratto C, Valentini V, et al: IORT in integrated treatment of high-risk rectal cancers. Front Radiat Ther Oncol 31:209–212, 1997.
10. Morganti AG, Santoni R, Osti MF: Radiotherapy in pelvic recurrences of rectal cancer. Ann Ital Chir 72(5):585–594, 2001.
11. Hurwitz H: Integrating the anti-VEGF-A humanized monoclonal antibody bevacizumab with chemotherapy in advanced colorectal cancer. Clin Colorectal Cancer 4(Suppl 2):S62–S68, 2004.
12. Goldberg RM, Venook AP, Schilsky RL: Cetuximab in the treatment of colorectal cancer. Clin Adv Hematol Oncol 2(11):1–10; quiz 11–12, 2004.
13. Cunningham D, Humblet Y, Siena S, et al: Cetuximab monotherapy and cetuximab plus irinotecan in irinotecan-refractory metastatic colorectal cancer. N Engl J Med 351(4):337–345, 2004.
14. Czito BG, Bendell JC, Willett CG, et al:. Bevacizumab, oxaliplatin, and capecitabine with radiation therapy in rectal cancer: phase I trial results. Int J Radiat Oncol Biol Phys 68(2):472–478, 2007.
15. Willett CG, Duda DG, Czito BG, et al: Targeted therapy in rectal cancer. Oncology 21(9):1055–1065; discussion 1065, 1070, 1075 passim, 2007.
16. Kapiteijn E, Marijnen CA, Nagtegaal ID, et al, and Dutch Colorectal Cancer Group: Preoperative radiotherapy combined with total mesorectal excision for resectable rectal cancer. N Engl J Med 345(9):638–646, 2001.
17. Mendenhall WM, Bland KI, Copeland EM III, et al: Does preoperative radiation therapy enhance the probability of local control and survival in high-risk distal rectal cancer? Ann Surg 215(6):696–705; discussion 705–706, 1992.
18. Bosset JF, Collette L, Calais G, et al, and EORTC Radiotherapy Group Trial 22921: Chemotherapy with preoperative radiotherapy in rectal cancer. N Engl J Med 355(11):1114–1123, 2006.
19. Bujko K, Nowacki MP, Nasierowska-Guttmejer A, et al: Long-term results of a randomized trial comparing preoperative short-course radiotherapy with preoperative conventionally fractionated chemoradiation for rectal cancer. Br J Surg 93(10):1215–1223, 2006.
20. Diaz-Rubio E, Tabernero J, Gomez-Espana A, et al, and Spanish Cooperative Group for the Treatment of Digestive Tumors Trial 2007: Phase III study of capecitabine plus oxaliplatin compared with continuous-infusion fluorouracil plus oxaliplatin as first-line therapy in metastatic colorectal cancer: final report of the Spanish Cooperative Group for the Treatment of Digestive Tumors Trial. J Clin Oncol 25(27):4224–4230, 2007.
21. Gerard JP, Chapet O, Nemoz C, et al: Preoperative concurrent chemoradiotherapy in locally advanced rectal cancer with high-dose radiation and oxaliplatin-containing regimen: the Lyon R0–04 phase II trial. J Clin Oncol 21(6):1119–1124, 2003.
22. Meyer JJ, Czito BG, Willett CG: Intensity-modulated radiation therapy for gastrointestinal tumors. Curr Oncol Rep 10(3):206–211, 2008.
23. Krook JE, Moertel CG, Gunderson LL, et al: Effective surgical adjuvant therapy for high-risk rectal carcinoma. N Engl J Med 324(11):709–715, 1991.
24. Thomas PR, Lindblad AS: Adjuvant postoperative radiotherapy and chemotherapy in rectal carcinoma: a review of the Gastrointestinal Tumor Study Group experience. Radiother Oncol 13(4):245–252, 1988.
25. Tveit KM, Guldvog I, Hagen S, et al: Randomized controlled trial of postoperative radiotherapy and short-term time-

scheduled 5-fluorouracil against surgery alone in the treatment of Dukes B and C rectal cancer. Norwegian Adjuvant Rectal Cancer Project Group. Br J Surg 84(8):1130–1135, 1997.
26. O'Connell MJ, Martenson JA, Wieand HS, et al: Improving adjuvant therapy for rectal cancer by combining protracted-infusion fluorouracil with radiation therapy after curative surgery. N Engl J Med 331(8):502–507, 1994.
27. Smalley SR, Benedetti JK, Williamson SK, et al: Phase III trial of fluorouracil-based chemotherapy regimens plus radiotherapy in postoperative adjuvant rectal cancer: GI INT 0144. J Clin Oncol 24(22):3542–3547, 2006.
28. Tepper JE, O'Connell MJ, Petroni GR, et al: Adjuvant postoperative fluorouracil-modulated chemotherapy combined with pelvic radiation therapy for rectal cancer: initial results of intergroup 0114. J Clin Oncol 15(5):2030–2039, 1997.
29. Lee JH, Lee JH, Ahn JH, et al: Randomized trial of postoperative adjuvant therapy in stage II and III rectal cancer to define the optimal sequence of chemotherapy and radiotherapy: a preliminary report. J Clin Oncol 20(7):1751–1758, 2002.
30. Liauw SL, Minsky BD: The use of capecitabine in the combined-modality therapy for rectal cancer. Clin Colorectal Cancer 7(2):99–104, 2008.
31. Calvo FA, Meirino RM, Orecchia R: Intraoperative radiation therapy part 2. Clinical results. Crit Rev Oncol Hematol 59(2):116–127, 2006.
32. Merrick HW III, Gunderson LL, Calvo FA: Future directions in intraoperative radiation therapy. Surg Oncol Clin North Am 12(4):1099–1105, 2003.
33. Calvo FA, Meirino RM, Orecchia R: Intraoperative radiation therapy part 1: rationale and techniques. Crit Rev Oncol Hematol 59(2):106–115, 2006.
34. Sindelar WF, Kinsella TJ: Normal tissue tolerance to intraoperative radiotherapy. Surg Oncol Clin North Am 12(4):925–942, 2003.
35. Eble MJ, Lehnert T, Herfarth C, Wannenmacher M: IORT as adjuvant treatment in primary rectal carcinomas: multi-modality treatment. Front Radiat Ther Oncol 31:200–203, 1997.
36. Gunderson LL, Shipley WU, Suit HD, et al: Intraoperative irradiation: a pilot study combining external beam photons with "boost" dose intraoperative electrons. Cancer 49(11):2259–2266, 1982.
37. Cance WG, Cohen AM, Enker WE, Sigurdson ER: Predictive value of a negative computed tomographic scan in 100 patients with rectal carcinoma. Dis Colon Rectum 34(9):748–751, 1991.
38. Vining DJ: Rectal imaging and cancer. Semin Surg Oncol 15(2):72–77, 1998.
39. Beets-Tan RG, Beets GL, Borstlap AC, et al: Preoperative assessment of local tumor extent in advanced rectal cancer: CT or high-resolution MRI? Abdom Imaging 25(5):533–541, 2000.
40. Popovich MJ, Hricak H, Sugimura K, Stern JL: The role of MR imaging in determining surgical eligibility for pelvic exenteration. AJR Am J Roentgenol 160(3):525–531, 1993.
41. Mannaerts GH, Rutten HJ, Martijn H, et al: Effects on functional outcome after IORT-containing multimodality treatment for locally advanced primary and locally recurrent rectal cancer. Int J Radiat Oncol Biol Phys 54(4):1082–1088, 2002.
42. Shoup M, Guillem JG, Alektiar KM, et al: Predictors of survival in recurrent rectal cancer after resection and intraoperative radiotherapy. Dis Colon Rectum 45(5):585–592, 2002.
43. Hahnloser D, Nelson H, Gunderson LL, et al: Curative potential of multimodality therapy for locally recurrent rectal cancer. Ann Surg 237(4):502–508, 2003.
44. Lopez-Kostner F, Fazio VW, Vignali A, et al: Locally recurrent rectal cancer: predictors and success of salvage surgery. Dis Colon Rectum 44(2):173–178, 2001.
45. Valentini V, Morganti AG, De Franco A, et al: Chemoradiation with or without intraoperative radiation therapy in patients with locally recurrent rectal carcinoma: prognostic factors and long term outcome. Cancer 86(12):2612–2624, 1999.
46. Alektiar KM, Zelefsky MJ, Paty PB, et al: High-dose-rate intraoperative brachytherapy for recurrent colorectal cancer. Int J Radiat Oncol Biol Phys 48(1):219–226, 2000.
47. Harrison LB, Minsky BD, Enker WE, et al: High dose rate intraoperative radiation therapy (HDR-IORT) as part of the management strategy for locally advanced primary and recurrent rectal cancer. Int J Radiat Oncol Biol Phys 42(2):325–330, 1998.
48. Lindel K, Willett CG, Shellito PC, et al: Intraoperative radiation therapy for locally advanced recurrent rectal or rectosigmoid cancer. Radiother Oncol 58(1):83–87, 2001.
49. Assumpcao L, Choti MA, Gleisner AL, et al: Patterns of recurrence following liver resection for colorectal metastases: effect of primary rectal tumor site. Arch Surg 143(8):743–749; discussion 749–750, 2008.
50. Willett CG: Intraoperative radiation therapy. Int J Clin Oncol 6(5):209–214, 2001.
51. Wallace HJ III, Willett CG, Shellito PC, et al: Intraoperative radiation therapy for locally advanced recurrent rectal or rectosigmoid cancer. J Surg Oncol 60(2):122–127, 1995.
52. Haddock MG, Gunderson LL, Nelson H, et al: Intraoperative irradiation for locally recurrent colorectal cancer in previously irradiated patients. Int J Radiat Oncol Biol Phys 49(5):1267–1274, 2001.
53. Gunderson LL, Martin JK, Beart RW, et al: Intraoperative and external beam irradiation for locally advanced colorectal cancer. Ann Surg 207(1):52–60, 1988.
54. Abuchaibe O, Calvo FA, Azinovic I, et al: Intraoperative radiotherapy in locally advanced recurrent colorectal cancer. Int J Radiat Oncol Biol Phys 26(5):859–867, 1993.
55. Lanciano RM, Calkins AR, Wolkov HB, et al: A phase I/II study of intraoperative radiotherapy in advanced unresectable or recurrent carcinoma of the rectum: a Radiation Therapy Oncology Group (RTOG) study. J Surg Oncol 53(1):20–29, 1993.
56. Willett CG, Shellito PC, Tepper JE, et al: Intraoperative electron beam radiation therapy for primary locally advanced rectal and rectosigmoid carcinoma. J Clin Oncol 9(5):843–849, 1991.
57. Pacelli F, Di Giorgio A, Papa V, et al: Preoperative radiotherapy combined with intraoperative radiotherapy improve results of total mesorectal excision in patients with T3 rectal cancer. Dis Colon Rectum 47(2):170–179, 2004.
58. Sanfilippo NJ, Crane CH, Skibber J, et al: T4 rectal cancer treated with preoperative chemoradiation to the posterior pelvis followed by multivisceral resection: patterns of failure and limitations of treatment. Int J Radiat Oncol Biol Phys 51(1):176–183, 2001.
59. Kim HK, Jessup JM, Beard CJ, et al: Locally advanced rectal carcinoma: pelvic control and morbidity following preoperative radiation therapy, resection, and intraoperative radiation therapy. Int J Radiat Oncol Biol Phys 38(4):777–783, 1997.
60. Eble MJ, Lehnert T, Treiber M, et al: Moderate dose intraoperative and external beam radiotherapy for locally recurrent rectal carcinoma. Radiother Oncol 49(2):169–174, 1998.
61. Krempien R, Roeder F, Oertel S, et al: Intraoperative electron-beam therapy for primary and recurrent retroperitoneal soft-tissue sarcoma. Int J Radiat Oncol Biol Phys 65(3):773–779, 2006.
62. Diaz-Gonzalez JA, Calvo FA, Cortes J, et al: Prognostic factors for disease-free survival in patients with T3–4 or N+ rectal cancer treated with preoperative chemoradiation therapy, surgery, and intraoperative irradiation. Int J Radiat Oncol Biol Phys 64(4):1122–1128, 2006.
63. Huber FT, Stepan R, Zimmermann F, et al: Locally advanced rectal cancer: resection and intraoperative radiotherapy using the flab method combined with preoperative or postoperative radiochemotherapy. Dis Colon Rectum 39(7):774–779, 1996.
64. Ferenschild FT, Vermaas M, Nuyttens JJ, et al: Value of intraoperative radiotherapy in locally advanced rectal cancer. Dis Colon Rectum 49(9):1257–1265, 2006.
65. Nuyttens JJ, Kolkman-Deurloo IK, Vermaas M, et al: High-dose-rate intraoperative radiotherapy for close or positive margins in patients with locally advanced or recurrent rectal cancer. Int J Radiat Oncol Biol Phys 58(1):106–112, 2004.
66. Stipa F, Chessin DB, Shia J, et al: A pathologic complete response of rectal cancer to preoperative combined-modality therapy results in improved oncological outcome compared with those who achieve no downstaging on the basis of preoperative endorectal ultrasonography. Ann Surg Oncol 13(8):1047–1053, 2006.
67. Wiig JN, Tveit KM, Poulsen JP, et al: Preoperative irradiation and surgery for recurrent rectal cancer: will intraoperative radiotherapy (IORT) be of additional benefit? A prospective study. Radiother Oncol 62(2):207–213, 2002.
68. Martinez-Monge R, Nag S, Martin EW: Three different intraoperative radiation modalities (electron beam, high-dose-rate brachytherapy, and iodine-125 brachytherapy) in the adjuvant treatment of patients with recurrent colorectal adenocarcinoma. Cancer 86(2):236–247, 1999.

69. Suzuki K, Gunderson LL, Devine RM, et al: Intraoperative irradiation after palliative surgery for locally recurrent rectal cancer. Cancer 75(4):939–952, 1995.
70. Eble MJ, Lehnert T, Herfarth C, Wannenmacher M: Intraoperative radiotherapy as adjuvant treatment for stage II/III rectal carcinoma. Recent results in cancer research. Fortschr Krebsforschung 146:152–160, 1998.
71. Azinovic I, Calvo FA, Puebla F, et al: Long-term normal tissue effects of intraoperative electron radiation therapy (IOERT): late sequelae, tumor recurrence, and second malignancies. Int J Radiat Oncol Biol Phys 49(2):597–604, 2001.
72. Miller RC, Haddock MG, Petersen IA, et al: Intraoperative electron-beam radiotherapy and ureteral obstruction. Int J Radiat Oncol Biol Phys 64(3):792–798, 2006.
73. Kienle P, Abend F, Dueck M, et al: Influence of intraoperative and postoperative radiotherapy on functional outcome in patients undergoing standard and deep anterior resection for rectal cancer. Dis Colon Rectum 49(5):557–567, 2006.
74. Gunderson LL, Tepper JE (eds): Clinical Radiation Oncology, 2nd ed. Philadelphia: Churchill Livingstone, 2000.
75. Willett CG, Goldberg S, Shellito PC, et al: Does postoperative irradiation play a role in the adjuvant therapy of stage T4 colon cancer? The Cancer Journal from Scientific American 5(4): 242–247, 1999.
76. Gunderson LL, Russell AH, Llewellyn HJ, et al: Treatment planning for colorectal cancer: radiation and surgical techniques and value of small-bowel films. Int J Radiat Oncol Biol Phys 11(7):1379–1393, 1985.
77. Willett CG, Fung CY, Kaufman DS, et al: Postoperative radiation therapy for high-risk colon carcinoma. J Clin Oncol 11(6):1112–1117, 1993.
78. Gambacorta MA, Valentini V, Coco C, et al: Sphincter preservation in four consecutive phase II studies of preoperative chemoradiation: analysis of 247 T3 rectal cancer patients. Tumori 93(2):160–169, 2007.
79. Myerson R, Zobeiri I, Birnbaum E, et al: Early results from a phase I/II radiation dose-escalation study with concurrent amifostine and infusional 5-fluorouracil chemotherapy for preoperative treatment of unresectable or locally recurrent rectal carcinoma. Semin Oncol 29(6 Suppl 19):29–33, 2002.
80. Calvo FA, Gómez-Espí M, Díaz-González JA, et al: Intraoperative presacral electron boost following preoperative chemoradiation in T3-4Nx rectal cancer: initial local effects and clinical outcome analysis. Radiother Oncol 62(2):201–206, 2002.
81. Rutten HJ, Mannaerts GH, Martijn H, Wiggers T: Intraoperative radiotherapy for locally recurrent rectal cancer in The Netherlands. Eur J Surg Oncol 26(Suppl A):S16–S20, 2000.

Surveillance and Follow-up

17 *Matthew T. Hueman and Nita Ahuja*

KEY POINTS

- The majority of colorectal recurrences occur within the first 2 to 3 years after diagnosis, and 90% occur within the first 5 years; as such, surveillance is recommended for all patients.
- The goal of surveillance is to detect recurrences earlier in order to improve overall survival and chance for long-term cure.
- At least 50% of colon cancer patients will develop a recurrence in the liver. Patients with isolated liver metastases are candidates for curative surgical resection, with 5-year survival rates now ranging from 35% to 58% in most series.
- There is controversy over the exact combination and frequency within the different major oncology organizations at which testing should be performed. However, all of the societies recommend frequent surveillance for 5 years following the diagnosis of colon cancer and include frequent physical examinations and endoscopic evaluation for local and metachronous recurrence. CT evaluations for distant recurrence as well as blood tests including CEA are often also included.
- Prospective randomized studies have not shown a conclusive benefit of improved survival, but these studies have multiple confounders, including varying surveillance strategies, small number, and so on. Meta-analyses, however, show a sustained survival benefit with increased surveillance.
- No definitive evidence exists to determine the optimal frequency and duration of follow-up after curative resection of colon cancer. However, existing data suggest a regimen of quarterly follow-up for the first 2 years and a gradual decrease in frequency of follow-up through a total of at least 5 years.

Introduction

In the United States, approximately 146,970 new cases of colorectal cancer are estimated to occur in 2009, which will account for more than 49,900 (49,920 to be exact) cancer-related deaths.[1] Up to 30% to 50% of patients with stage II or III colon cancer are estimated to develop locoregional recurrence, distant metastasis, and/or metachronous colon cancers after 5 years of follow-up.[2-5] Most of these recurrences occur in the first 2 (60%) to 3 (80%) years.[6] Given the high percentage of patients who have a recurrence within 2 to 3 years after curative intent therapy, surveillance performed after treatment for colon cancer is aimed at improving overall survival and the chances for long-term cure. Surveillance improves outcomes by maximizing the efficacy of and potential for curative intent re-resection by (1) identifying locoregional or distant metastasis (liver, lung) recurrence as early as possible and (2) detecting metachronous primary tumors at the earliest stage.

The most common site of recurrence after curative resection of colon cancer is the liver; in fact, at least 50% of patients with colon cancer develop liver metastases during the course of their disease.[7] In up to 30% of patients with liver metastases, the liver is the only site of metastatic disease.[8] Although historically an estimated 8% to 10% of patients who have undergone curative intent therapy for colorectal cancer develop isolated liver metastases,[3,9,10] improvements in imaging, notably helical spiral computed tomography (CT), have increased the ability to detect such recurrence, presumably before additional evidence of spread. Patients with isolated liver metastases are potential candidates for curative intent surgical resection, with the possibility of long-term survival. Several series report overall 5-year survival rates of 35% to 58% after curative intent hepatic resection.[11-13] Surveillance regimens that aim to detect metachronous metastatic colon cancer

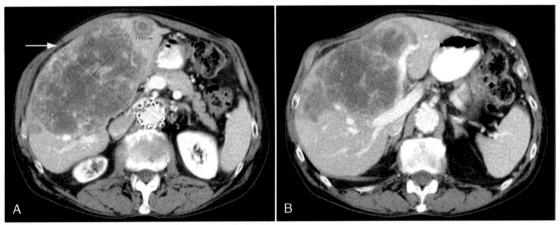

Figure 17-1. A 65-year-old man was diagnosed with T3N2 sigmoid colon cancer in 2004 and underwent adjuvant FOLFOX chemotherapy.   He was lost to follow-up until 2008, at which point he presented with abdominal discomfort and a palpable large abdominal mass. He also had a very high serum carcinoembryonic antigen (CEA) level. CT scan revealed multiple bilobar liver metastases but no extrahepatic disease. He had a centrally located dominant mass (**A**) (*white arrow*) measuring 15 by 10 cm, which straddles the right and left portal pedicles (**B**), precluding resectability. Presumably, if the man had undergone serial follow-up with CEA testing and CT, his liver-only recurrence might have been discovered when it was asymptomatic and still resectable.

liver metastases with such methods as measurement of serum carcinoembryonic antigen (CEA) and liver imaging (CT, ultrasound) may therefore be the most successful strategy for achieving the ultimate goal of improving overall survival (Fig. 17-1).

Although the rate of metachronous, or second, neoplasms is relatively low (7%–8%),[14] the early detection of presumably early-stage new primary lesions—and subsequent adequate surgical treatment—may provide the most efficacious target for surveillance. Although the rate of second neoplasms is relatively low compared with the rates of true recurrence, patients with diagnosed colon cancer are clearly at much higher risk and might benefit from the identification of lesions more likely to be amenable to cure than true recurrences. The population of patients with the best prognosis with respect to their colon cancer is most likely to benefit from such a strategy. The identification of metachronous new primary colonic neoplasms is clearly best accomplished through endoscopy, although fecal occult blood testing has also been promoted for detecting such new tumors.

The rate of local recurrence in colon cancer is decidedly low and is at least half the rate of distant recurrence. For colon cancer, about 15% of patients are estimated to develop locoregional recurrence.[15,16] In a recent prospective randomized controlled trial of patients with stage II and III resected colorectal cancer, the rate of local

recurrence was surprisingly high (approximately 30%) but still about half the rate of distant recurrences (almost 60%). These recurrences, including metachronous tumors, occurred in a background of a total recurrence rate of about 27%.[17] The authors themselves were surprised at the high rate of local recurrences seen in their study. They concluded that it was possible, even likely, that some intramural relapses were misdiagnosed and were in fact metachronous new primaries (which would also explain the higher than expected resectability rate).[17]

Although the endoscopic identification of both local recurrences and metachronous tumors may offer the greatest chance for discovering recurrences that can be both resected and cured, several studies have shown that the rate of intraluminal recurrences and metachronous tumors is very low.[15,18,19] This low rate has caused some investigators to state that the intensification of efforts to identify these lesions is of little benefit.[20] Therefore, the contribution of the identification of these lesions, primarily through endoscopy, to the overall efficacy of the strategy of surveillance remains controversial.[21]

Ultimately, the goal of post-treatment surveillance of patients who have undergone curative resection of colon cancer is to improve overall survival and chances for long-term cure. By identifying recurrences as early as possible, the oncology community aims to maximize the efficacy of and potential for curative

Table 17-1. Comparison of Follow-up Guidelines

	ASCO	NCCN	ESMO
Physical examination	Every 3–6 mo for 3 yr, then every 6 mo up to 5 yr	Every 3 mo for 2 yr, then every 6 mo up to 5 yr	Every 3–6 mo for 3 yr, then every 6–12 mo up to 5 yr
CEA routine	Every 3 mo for at least 3 yr (stage II or III)	Every 3 mo for 2 yr, then every 6 mo up to 5 yr (T2 or greater)	No
Liver sonography	No	No	Every 6 mo for 3 yr, then annually for 2 yr
Colonoscopy	3 yr after surgery, then every 5 yr	After 1 yr if polypectomy, then every 2–3 yr	After 1 yr, then every 3 yr (colon) Every 5 yr (rectal cancer)
Proctosigmoidoscopy (rectal cancer)	Every 6 mo for 5 yr if not pelvic radiation	—	Every 6 mo for 2 yr (with endosonography)
Abdominal CT	Annually for 3 yr (high risk of recurrence)	Annually for 3 yr (high risk of recurrence)	With suspicion
Chest CT	Annually for 3 yr (high risk of recurrence)	Annually for 3 yr (high risk of recurrence)	With suspicion
Chest x-ray	No	—	Every yr for 5 yr

ASCO, American Society of Clinical Oncology; CEA, carcinoembryonic antigen; CT, computed tomography; ESMO, European Society of Medical Oncology; NCCN, National Comprehensive Cancer Network.
From Li Destri G, Di Cataldo A, Puleo S: Colorectal cancer follow-up: useful or useless? Surg Oncol 15(1):1–12, 2006.

intent resection. Several overlapping, yet distinct, goals of surveillance regimens include the following:

1. To facilitate the earlier diagnosis of inevitable local and/or distant recurrences (to remove while still locally resectable)
2. To assist in identifying a greater number of local recurrences before evidence of distant disease (to remove before distant spread of locally recurrent disease)
3. To aid in discovering recurrences while they are still asymptomatic (to remove local or distant disease before becoming symptomatic, when presumably a larger proportion of recurrences have advanced to the point of unresectability).

All these goals are to improve the ability to provide curative intent, margin-negative (R0) resection. An often unstated and less optimal but important goal in post–curative intent resection of colorectal cancer is to identify incurable disease while it can still be reasonably palliated and before it becomes so advanced as to preclude even effective palliation. An additional goal is to provide a proven survival advantage—though not a cure—for patients with unresectable metastatic disease by initiating earlier systemic therapy.[22]

The optimal frequency and specific strategies of surveillance have not been defined; however, the overall interpretation of several prospective randomized controlled trials and meta-analyses indicates that rates of resectable tumor recurrence and overall survival are increased in intermediate-risk patients who undergo high-intensity rather than low-intensity programs of surveillance.[15,19,20,23,24] Controversy remains over the right combination of tests and the optimal frequency of evaluations, as evidenced by the different (although similar) surveillance guidelines from three major oncology organizations (Table 17-1). Although there may be disagreements about the optimal and most cost-effective strategy, general consensus exists that surveillance of patients with colon cancer who have undergone curative intent therapy improves overall survival.

Overview of Prospective Evidence

To date, eight prospective randomized controlled trials have been performed studying the possible benefit of colon cancer surveillance after apparent cure[17,21,25-30] (Table 17-2); only half of these trials[17,21,25,29,30] have been categorized as being of good quality.[20] Most of these prospective studies have compared low-intensity with high-intensity surveillance programs. The low-intensity surveillance was truly minimal in two studies,[25,29] whereas only one trial compared a schedule of surveillance with that with essentially no follow-up.[27] Only three

Table 17-2. Comparison of All Randomized Controlled Trials Performed to Evaluate the Efficacy of More Intensive versus Less Intensive Surveillance After Curative Resection of Colorectal Cancer

Randomized Trials of More versus Less Intensive Surveillance	Study Period	Comparison (Main Difference Between More and Less Intensive Arms)	Frequency of Follow-up Visit in Higher-Intensity Arm	CT in Higher Intensity Arm*	Liver Ultrasound in Higher-Intensity Arm*	Endoscopy in Higher-Intensity Arm*	CEA
Makela et al (1995)[26]	1988–1990	More tests versus less tests (same frequency of follow-up)	q 3 mo Y1-2; q 6 mo Y3-5	Yearly	q 6 mo	Yearly	CEA at each visit; no difference between arms
Ohlsson et al (1995)[27]	1983–1986	Surveillance arm versus no follow-up	q 3 mo Y1-2; q 6 mo Y3-4; q 1 year Y5	CT pelvis post APR at 3, 6, 12, 18, and 24 mo postop	None	3, 15, 30, and 60 months postop	CEA at each visit
Kjeldsen et al (1997)[25]	1987–1990	Same tests in each arm but only q 5-year evaluations in minimal follow-up arm	q 6 mo Y1-3; q 1 year Y4-5	None	None	q 6 mo Y1-3; q 1 yr Y4-5; Less intensive arm at 60, 120, and 150 mo	No CEA testing
Pietra et al (1998)[28]	1983–1984	In less intensive arm, less frequent follow-up and no CT scan	q 3 mo Y1-2; q 6 mo Y3; q 1 year Y4-	Yearly	q 3 mo Y1-2; q 6 mo Y3; q 1 year Y4-; Less intensive arm underwent ultrasound: q 6 mo Y1; q 1 year Y2-	Yearly; Less intensive arm: Yearly	CEA at each visit
Schoemaker et al (1998)[21]	1984–1990	More tests versus less tests (same frequency of follow-up)	q 3 mo Y1-2; q 6 mo Y3-7	Yearly	None	Yearly	CEA at each visit
Secco et al (2002)[29]	1988–1996	Surveillance arms (high risk high intensity, low risk intermediate intensity) versus minimal follow-up	High Risk: q 3 mo Y1-2; q 4 mo Y3; q 6 mo Y4-5; Low Risk: q 6 mo Y1-2; q 1 year Y3-5	None	High risk: q 6 mo Y1-3; q 1 yr Y4-5; Low risk: q 6 mo Y1-2	None	CEA at each visit
Rodriguez-Moranta et al (2006)[17]	1999–2001	More tests versus less tests (same frequency of follow-up)	q 3 mo Y1-2; q 6 mo Y3-5	q 6 mo Y1-2; q 1 yr Y3-	q 6 mo Y1-2; q 1 year Y3-	Yearly; Less intensive arm at 12 and 36 mo	CEA at each visit; no difference between arms
Wattchow et al (2006)[30]	1998–2001	Surgeon versus general practitioner follow-up	q 3 mo Y1-2; q 6 mo Y3-5	None	None	Every 3 years, including less intensive arm	None

*Unless otherwise stated, patients in the less intensive arm did not undergo this test.

APR, abdominoperineal resection; CEA, carcinoembryonic antigen; CT, computed tomography. mo, month; Y, year.

trials—one overall[28] and two in subset analysis only[17,29]—were able to demonstrate a survival benefit of more intensive surveillance. Pietra and associates[28] found that the overall survival advantage was attributed to earlier detection of asymptomatic local recurrence (primarily by CEA). However, these results were confounded by the fact that 30% of the patients had rectal cancer and more than half of the local recurrences in both the intensive and conventional follow-up groups were in patients with a history of rectal cancer.[28] To date, no single prospective randomized controlled trial provides definitive evidence of improved survival compared with surveillance, or with intensifying surveillance.

Without a gold standard multi-institutional study to provide guidance, at least five meta-analyses have coalesced the results of these prospective single-institution reports. Each meta-analysis independently revealed a survival benefit to high- versus low-intensity surveillance.[15,19,20,23,24] It is interesting and perhaps obvious to note in hindsight that the intensification of surveillance did not result in an increase or decrease in the rate of recurrence, presumably because it is inevitable. It is hoped that such an effort at least changes the type, if not the pattern, of recurrence, perhaps identifying it earlier before the progression or spread of locally recurrent lesions or before the local progression of distant hepatic or pulmonary metastases. Contrary to expectations, in a study by Secco and associates,[29] high-risk patients randomized to the minimal follow-up arm were found to have a shorter disease-free survival compared with the intensive surveillance arm. More intensive surveillance should result in finding recurrences sooner (and thus the patients will artificially have "shorter" disease-free intervals). Therefore, the expectation is that high-risk patients in the minimal follow-up arm would have longer disease-free intervals because the recurrence would be found later. The paradoxical finding in Secco and associates[29] that high-risk patients in the minimal follow-up arm had a shorter disease-free interval implies that more intensive surveillance does not identify recurrence earlier.

Despite this anomaly in a single study,[29] the meta-analyses provide support that intensifying follow-up significantly reduces the time to diagnosis of such inevitable recurrence. In doing so, intensive surveillance presumably aids in identifying a greater proportion of recurrences amenable to curative intent therapy. This reduction in time has been estimated to be as long as 8.5 months (95% confidence interval [CI], 7.6–9.4).[19] Many studies corroborate that under intensive surveillance, recurrences are more often discovered while asymptomatic, are uncovered at routine visits, and/or are amenable to curative intent therapy.[17,25,26,29] Perhaps because there are fewer patients in some of these reports, this benefit does not necessarily result in a measurable survival benefit,[17,25,29] or only in subset analysis.[29] Even in several of the meta-analyses, the overall survival benefit of more intensive surveillance (estimated to be about 10%) is disproportionately greater than the survival advantage obtained from detecting more recurrences amenable to curative intent therapy (estimated between 2% and 5%).[24] This conclusion has led some to speculate that the increased intensity of surveillance has other, less tangible, benefits such as improved sense of well-being, decreased anxiety, or enhanced global care of unrelated but coincident medical disease, which contribute to the reduction in mortality rate related to the intensive surveillance of colon cancer.[24]

The interpretation of these studies is hampered by the broad span of time in which they were performed (1983–2002), by the inclusion of both colon and rectal cancers, by the wide variation in surveillance strategies, and by the single-institutional nature of and small numbers of patients included in many of these reports. The inclusion of rectal cancers in the surveillance regimens complicates the interpretation of the results because of the much higher rate of locoregional recurrence in rectal cancer, as well as the relative ease of identifying endoscopic evidence of recurrence in left-sided or rectal cancers compared with right-sided lesions. Because of the broad span of time of these reports, many of these studies were performed before the more efficacious and better-tolerated chemotherapy of today, before the much higher-quality and sensitive CT scans of the current era, and before the much more aggressive, efficacious, and safer major liver resections seen in the last decade. Perhaps most significantly, the combination of improved CT imaging and of more aggressive and simultaneously safer major liver resection expands the ability to provide curative intent therapy to patients with metachronous colon cancer liver metastases. These relatively recent changes thus increase the chances that the earlier discovery of asymptomatic colon cancer liver metastases may provide a survival benefit.

In the background of these limitations and uncertainties, the heterogeneity of surveillance strategies studied to date prevents definitive determinations of the frequency or type of tests and prevents an estimation of the harms or costs of such tests. Given these lingering uncertainties, we eagerly await the final or preliminary results of three large-scale prospective randomized controlled trials: the GILDA study in Italy,[31] the Follow-up After Colorectal Surgery (FACS) study in the United Kingdom,[32] and the multicenter COLOFOL study in Denmark, Sweden, Poland, Ireland, and Uruguay.[33] All three large-scale studies are said to be adequately powered to independently support different aspects of the question of whether more intensive surveillance improves outcomes, including whether increased frequency of colonoscopy and liver ultrasound (GILDA), hospital-/imaging-based follow-up over primary care/CEA (FACS), or more versus fewer clinic visits (COLOFOL) improves outcomes.

Frequency and Duration

Two thirds of patients with colon cancer undergo curative intent therapy, including adjuvant therapy.[1] Up to 50% of these patients develop recurrent disease,[34] and most recurrences are within the first 2 years (60%).[6] Although the pace of recurrence decreases at this point, a significant number of patients continue to have recurrence within the next few years, with 80% of recurrences happening within the first 3 years and 90% within the first 5 years.[6,14,15,34] No definitive evidence exists to support the optimal frequency and duration of surveillance to detect these recurrences. Given the heterogeneity of follow-up strategies, the suggestion in several studies that more intense follow-up allows detection of a greater number of resectable recurrences, and the conclusion of several meta-analyses that more intense surveillance provides a survival benefit, several societies have designed a rationale design for follow-up based on the timing of recurrence (see Table 17-1). This rationale is based on scattered strategies of the several studies previously discussed; however, ultimately a cogent plan can still be distilled

from these attempts at defining the optimal surveillance strategy.

Considering the wide variety of strategies and combination of tests, it is difficult to analyze the meta-analyses and make a conclusion about the optimal frequency and duration of follow-up (see Tables 17-1 and 17-2). The review of a single randomized prospective trial demonstrating a survival benefit associated with intensive or conventional follow-up compared with minimal or no follow-up, in the background of a similar intensity and combination of tests in each arm, may provide some foundation for this determination. Unfortunately, only one of the randomized prospective studies (Pietra and associates[28]) revealed an overall survival benefit to more intensive surveillance in the background of a similar combination of tests in each arm. Interpretation of this study in the more broad application of determining the optimal frequency and duration of evaluations is complicated by the inclusion of patients with rectal cancer (whose earlier detection of local recurrence in the more intensive follow-up arm provided a substantial portion of the overall measured survival benefit seen in the study). Nonetheless, patients with a high risk for recurrence fared better in the more intensive follow-up arm, in which patients underwent evaluation every 3 months for the first 2 years and then every 6 months for the next 3 years. This frequency of testing is in comparison to the minimal follow-up arm, in which patients underwent evaluations every 6 months for the first year and then annually.[28]

In both groups, clinical examination, ultrasound, and serum CEA measurements were performed at each visit, and chest radiography and colonoscopy were performed annually. In the more intensive arm, patients also underwent annual CT scans, but these scans detected recurrence in only 1 of 104 asymptomatic patients when not previously detected by another method.[28] Given a similar combination of tests in study arms of differing frequency of follow-up, the survival benefit attributed to the arm with more frequent evaluations should give some credence to this particular schedule. Unfortunately, the study can be criticized on several other fronts. The survival benefit, attributed mostly to an asymptomatic CEA-directed detection of recurrence, is solely ascribed to local, not distant, recurrence. Both CT and CEA should be useful primarily for detecting asymptomatic resectable recurrences in the liver and lung; this should provide the bulk of the measurable survival benefit of detecting recurrent disease.[35] The identification of the less common event of local recurrence in colon cancer should contribute less to the survival benefit of surveillance, and it should certainly not be the sole contributor to such a benefit. It is likely that not just the incorporation of a significant portion of patients with rectal cancer (who have higher rates of local recurrence) but the performance of the study in the age before high-quality CT scans and before expanded criteria for resection of pulmonary and hepatic metastases contributed to the skewed findings. Nonetheless, it provides the only evidence of a survival benefit attributed to a particular frequency and schedule of follow-up seen in a single trial, and this particular frequency of follow-up has been independently adopted by many of the other studies. As such, it provides a rational schedule of follow-up.

Although the meta-analyses all support a survival benefit associated with more intense surveillance, the frequency of surveillance varied widely among studies; the intense and more frequent surveillance arm of one study could be interpreted to equate with the minimal and less frequent arm in another study. With this caveat, six of the eight prospective randomized controlled trials had a similar frequency of early follow-up in the higher-intensity arm of surveillance, with every-3-month evaluations in the first 2 years of follow-up and every-6-month evaluations through year 5.[17,21,26–28,30] In one of the remaining two studies, Secco and associates[29] attempted to risk-stratify frequency of follow-up and is therefore not neatly included in these six studies. In comparison, Secco and associates provided a similar level of frequency of follow-up only to the highest-risk patients who were randomized to the more intense follow-up strategy; the remainder of the study participants—including the low-risk patients randomized to the more intensive strategy and both the high-risk and low-risk patients randomized to the less intensive arm—did not undergo such frequent follow-up in the first 2 years.[29] This variation of strategies is further complicated by the fact that three studies varied the combination and performance of tests, but not the frequency or duration of follow-up, to provide an intensive arm and a minimal arm of surveillance.[17,21,26]

In all three studies, patients in both the intensive and less intensive arms of surveillance were clinically assessed every 3 months (years 1 and 2) and then every 6 months (years 3 through 5). Therefore, in essence, many of the studies do not allow a fair comparison of frequency and schedule of follow-up because the schedule is either the same in the two arms or both the schedule and combination of tests differ.

When comparing the higher-intensity surveillance arm in these trials, only four of the studies continued with every-6-month evaluations through the 5-year follow-up point without regard to risk of recurrence.[17,21,26,30] In one of these studies, Wattchow and associates[30] randomized follow-up for patients between general practitioners and surgeons; the researchers only *suggested* surveillance guidelines, including frequency of evaluations, which by study design were not enforced. Other studies provided less frequent follow-up in their higher-intensity surveillance arm in different combinations. The majority of differences in the schedule were seen after year 3. After this time point, at either year 4 or year 5, some investigators progressed from every-6-month visits to annual evaluations. Despite this significant variation, a specific frequency and schedule (every 3 months for the first 2 years and every 6 months through year 5) clearly dominates the studies analyzed, though without a valid comparison to other schedules. In meta-analysis, when combined with the more intensive tests, this schedule appears to provide a survival benefit.

No definitive evidence exists to determine the optimal frequency and duration of follow-up after curative intent therapy for colon cancer; however, the early clustering of recurrences juxtaposed with the survival benefit associated with more intensive surveillance provides a strong evidence-based rationale for quarterly follow-up for the first 2 years and a gradual decrease in frequency of follow-up through a total of at least 5 years.

History and Physical Examination

Several of the meta-analyses and some of the single prospective trials have attempted to isolate the contribution of the several methods of follow-up that may contribute to detection of recurrence. In large part, this analysis is motivated by identifying the most effective—and ineffective—method of detection, given the considerable cost of performing serial laboratory, imaging, and endoscopic examinations for a large population. The clinical examination is largely felt to be a minimal standard of follow-up and an accepted, almost forgotten, cost, although at least a couple of studies can be analyzed to attempt to demonstrate its worth. Although no specific analysis is able to demonstrate the contribution of the clinical examination, given the emphasis on the costly adjunctive methods of detection, it is certain that the busy clinician would agree that the clinical examination (the history and physical exam) can be the first to uncover evidence of recurrence.

Many relapses are first uncovered by new symptoms.[27,28,36] A randomized prospective study comparing bolus fluorouracil/leucovorin or protracted venous infusion fluorouracil helps to illustrate that despite close follow-up and sophisticated testing, a significant number of recurrences (42%) are still uncovered by symptoms alone.[35] In this trial, stage II and stage III resected colorectal cancer patients underwent serial CEA scanning at each clinic visit through 5 years of follow-up as well as CT scan of the thorax, abdomen, and pelvis at 12 and 24 months of follow-up. Twenty-nine percent of patients had recurrence.[35] In addition to these tests, the surveillance schedule consisted of clinical examination with trained oncologists every 3 months for the first year, every 6 months for the second year, and annually thereafter. In the first 2 years of follow-up, despite CT scans performed at 1 and 2 years and several CEA measurements, clinical examination uncovered 30% of all of the recurrences that occurred in the first 2 years.[35] Although only 21% of patients who had recurrences were able to undergo curative intent re-operation, 27% of these recurrences were uncovered by symptoms alone—as many as uncovered by CEA (27%) but not as many as by CT (45%).[35] Beyond the ability of the history and physical examination to detect recurrence, however, is the often unspoken role of the follow-up physician to advise and reassure, and many patients view follow-up as important even if it does not result in earlier detection of recurrence.[37]

An indirect way of analyzing the contribution of the clinical examination to the detection of

recurrence and to the promotion of survival is to examine the studies that compared clinic visits with no clinic visits (i.e., no follow-up). Two studies—one for reduction in mortality (Ohlsson and associates[27]) and two for reduction in incurable recurrence (Ohlsson and colleagues[27] and Secco and associates[29])—were analyzed in a recently updated meta-analysis.[23] This meta-analysis included all of the eight prospective randomized controlled trials cited and described in this chapter (see Table 17-2). Though statistically not significant, both examinations seemed to favor clinic visits in reducing mortality (odds ratio [OR] 0.57, [95% confidence interval (CI), 0.26–1.29], $P = .18$) and in reducing incurable recurrence (OR 0.85 [95% CI, 0.58–1.25], $P = .42$).[23] In Kjeldsen and associates[25] and Pietra and associates,[28] the investigators attempted to discern a survival benefit associated with more clinic visits compared with that with fewer clinic visits. These two studies were also analyzed together in the same meta-analysis,[23] which reveals a statistically insignificant trend favoring more clinic visits for both overall survival (OR 0.78 [95% CI, 0.58–1.05], $P = .098$) and reduction in incurable recurrence (OR 0.93 [95% CI, 0.69–1.26], $P = .64$).

Ultimately, as a running theme in this chapter, the overall heterogeneity of the eight prospective trials limits the ability to coalesce their results into an overall analysis. This theme is underlined by the findings in the Cochrane review and meta-analysis that the use of more tests versus fewer tests (the focus of five of the eight studies in this meta-analysis)[17,21,26–28] seems to improve overall survival (OR 0.64 [95% CI, 0.49–0.85], $P = .0018$), but that the use of CEA, the preeminent test of most surveillance strategies, does not statistically significantly improve survival (mortality, OR 0.57 [95% CI, 0.26–1.29], $P = .18$).[23] These findings reveal the emphasis of the several groups of investigators on the use of tests over clinical examination and highlight the significant limitations imposed by attempting to coalesce results of heterogeneous studies in a meta-analysis.

Carcinoembryonic Antigen Testing

Despite many well-known limitations, the American Society of Clinical Oncology (ASCO) panel of experts had determined by the 2000 Guidelines that enough evidence existed to recommend the addition of serial CEA measurement to periodic clinical evaluations (see Table 17-1). This addition was included as part of a comprehensive strategy of surveillance for patients with colorectal cancer who have undergone apparent curative therapy. The National Comprehensive Cancer Network (NCCN) also recommends CEA as the primary test to be uniformly added to clinical examination. Despite this expert consensus, the literature is rife with disparate results in the evaluation of the usefulness of serial serum CEA measurements. No definitive evidence exists to support postoperative CEA measurement in improving overall survival, but several evidence-based conclusions can be made to support the rationale for its use.

The primary rationale for CEA measurement is its ability to detect asymptomatic recurrences (primarily hepatic metastases, but also locoregional recurrence) (Figs. 17-2 and 17-3). CT scan must be used to anatomically define the presence of such a recurrence (see Figs. 17-2 and 17-3), but CEA can help select the patients who require additional imaging. With the caveat that one authority has recently concluded that no useful data on cost-effectiveness can be obtained from a review of the pertinent studies,[23] at least one study has shown that the use of CEA in an intensive surveillance program is cost-effective,[38] in part because CEA measurement may be more cost-effective than radiologic imaging in the detection of potentially curable recurrence.[39]

As described in the previous section, the challenge imposed by the limitations of meta-analysis help describe, in part, the contrasting outcomes observed in the literature. In the Cochrane review, five of the studies were available to be analyzed for the comparison of more tests versus fewer tests, but only the studies of Ohlsson and colleagues[27] and Secco and associates[29] were felt to be able to be analyzed regarding the effect of CEA versus no CEA testing.[23] The fact that no significant difference could be found in favor of CEA testing in a surveillance strategy is emblematic of the challenge in coalescing results of heterogeneous trials.

Though somewhat controversial, CEA has been found in a separate meta-analysis of the same prospective studies to be the test that has been most convincingly associated with a significant reduction in mortality, an increased detection of asymptomatic tumor recurrence, and an improvement in finding recurrences amenable to curative intent therapy.[20] In this separate meta-analysis, the researchers combined not only the Ohlsson[27] and Secco[29] studies, as in the Cochrane review,[23] but also the study of Pietra and associates.[28] The Pietra study compared more with less CEA testing, rather than CEA testing versus no CEA testing, as seen in the other two studies. Although no individual study was able to make a definitive conclusion, the analysts combined all three studies to make the conclusion that CEA testing did indeed have a positive effect on survival.[20]

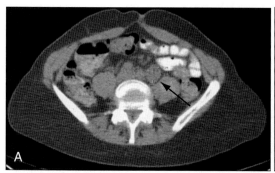
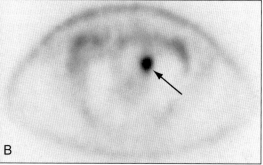

Figure 17-2. A 65-year-old woman underwent a laparoscopic sigmoidectomy for T3N0 colon cancer in 2003. Only two lymph nodes were found in the specimen. After referral to a tertiary care center, adjuvant therapy was recommended (capecitabine [Xeloda]). Nine months after her original operation, the patient was noted to have an elevated carcinoembryonic antigen (CEA) level on routine follow-up visit. The CEA elevation prompted the medical oncologist to request a positron emission tomography/computed tomography (PET-CT) scanning, which revealed a left iliac enlarged lymph node (*black arrows*) on CT (**A**); this was highly [18]fluorodeoxyglucose (FDG)-avid on PET (**B**), confirming a locoregional recurrence. Both the identification and confirmation of this locoregional recurrence on CT clearly were significantly aided by the correlative PET scan. The patient was started on FOLFOX and bevacizumab, and no other evidence of disease was seen on subsequent follow-up visits. The local recurrence responded to therapy with a decrease in size but remained.

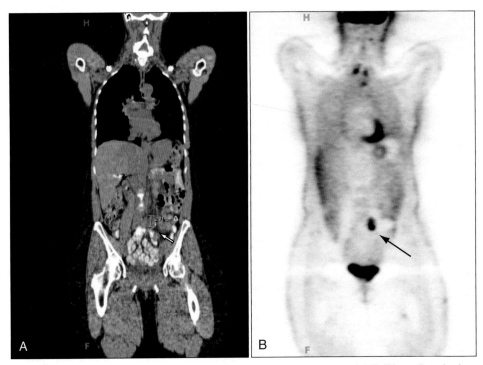

Figure 17-3. These coronal views on CT (**A**) and positron emission tomography (PET) (**B**) confirm the locoregional recurrence (*arrows*) in the same 65-year-old woman described in Figure 17-2. Note that no other site of metastatic disease can be seen; the remainder of FDG uptake seen on the PET scan (**B**) is physiologic. After 7 months of no other evidence of disease (while on chemotherapy), the patient underwent a low anterior resection of the 2.4 × 2.7 cm left iliac lymph node, and she remains disease-free.

Of the three other meta-analyses described in this chapter, one does not include comments on individual methods; the remaining two support the use of CEA as significantly improving aspects of postoperative surveillance, but the method, number, and combination of studies by which they came to this conclusion differed. In Figueredo and colleagues,[15] the analysts concluded that only trials using serial measurement of CEA in combination with liver imaging were able to demonstrate significant improvement in overall survival (relative risk [RR] 0.71 [95% CI, 0.60–0.85], P = .0002). Renehan and associates[19] concluded that the greatest reduction in mortality produced by post–curative intent therapy surveillance was seen in trials in which serial CT scan and CEA measurements were performed as an overall surveillance strategy (P = .002).

In a multicenter prospective randomized trial studying the optimal delivery of adjuvant chemotherapy for resected stage II and III colorectal cancer, the presence of symptoms uncovered as many patients with recurrence as did CEA among those who were able to undergo curative intent surgery for recurrence.[35] The trial included a 5-year surveillance strategy incorporating serial clinical examinations with CEA measurement and CT scans performed at 12 and 24 months of follow-up. Although symptoms and CEA might have appeared to be relatively equal contributors to the detection of recurrence in this report, the majority of resectable hepatic and pulmonary metastases were uncovered by CEA, CT, or a combination of these tests (91%) and not by symptoms[35] (Fig. 17-4; see Fig. 17-1). CEA testing is certainly helpful in identifying patients with asymptomatic recurrences, but this study revealed that a significant plurality of patients with resectable recurrences have normal CEA levels and require surveillance CT to uncover this disease[35] (Fig. 17-5; see Fig. 17-4). Among patients who had recurrences only 3% of symptomatic compared with 23% of asymptomatic patients detected by surveillance were able to undergo curative intent hepatic or pulmonary resection.[35] The authors concluded that surveillance CT and CEA, in combination, are important elements in the postoperative follow-up of resected stage II and III colorectal cancer.

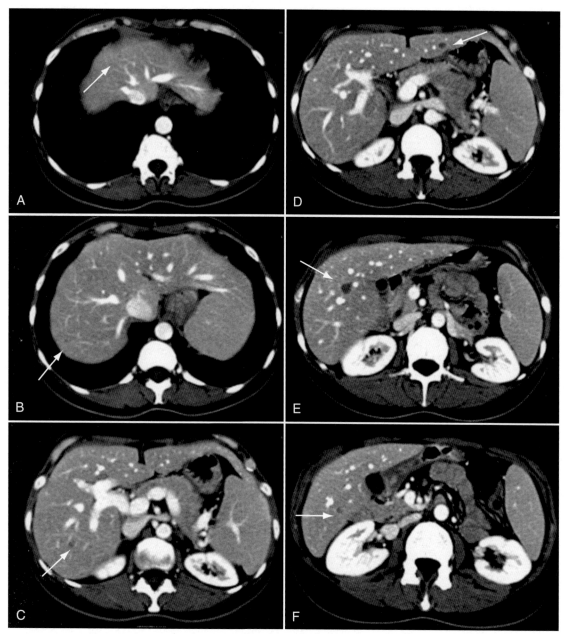

Figure 17-4. A 41-year-old woman presented in 2007 with T3N1 sigmoid colon cancer and underwent primary margin-negative resection. Her serum carcinoembryonic antigen (CEA) level remained normal, but surveillance CT scan revealed bilobar hepatic metastases (*white arrows*) 1 year later, as seen in **A** through **F**. Though bilobar, the metastases were technically resectable. The woman underwent right hepatectomy and wedge resection of three left liver lesions in segments 3 (**D**) and 4a (**A**) (*white arrow*).

The detection of recurrence of colon cancer by the serial measurement of CEA is optimal when CEA is elevated preoperatively and declines postoperatively. In general, a rising or persistently elevated CEA indicates disease progression[40] but should not be solely considered in this determination.[41,42] The initiation of adjuvant chemotherapy, especially oxaliplatin,

can transiently increase serum CEA levels,[42] presumably being at least partially related to chemotherapy-induced changes in hepatic function[41] and other non–cancer-related conditions, such as gastritis, diverticulitis, and diabetes, and can also result in or be associated with elevations in CEA.[43] Although discussion is outside the scope of this chapter, a persistently elevated

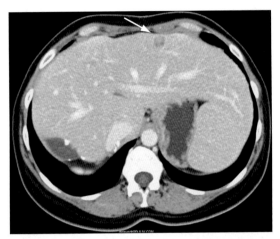

Figure 17-5. The same patient described in Figure 17-4 remained without evidence of disease for 16 months, at which time a surveillance CT revealed a solitary liver metastasis (*white arrow*) in segment 2 of her remnant hypertrophied left liver. Carcinoembryonic antigen (CEA) serum level remained within normal limits and was uninformative. She underwent a curative resection and remains disease free.

and/or rising CEA level should prompt a comprehensive investigation for evidence of distant and/or local recurrence. This examination should be initiated by a history and physical examination and concluded with a thoracoabdominopelvic CT scan and colonoscopy.

In the face of a rising or persistently elevated CEA, a positron emission tomography (PET) scan can be performed to identify a recurrence not identified by these modalities[44]—in particular when the CT is unrevealing (see Figs. 17-2 and 17-3). In addition, a PET scan should be considered before curative surgery for local and/or distant (liver, lung) recurrences to evaluate for evidence of incurable disease (see Fig. 17-3). A general consensus exists, supported by a panel of experts from the NCCN, that CEA-directed or "blind" laparotomy or laparoscopy should not be performed,[45] despite a rising or persistently elevated CEA level in the face of a negative comprehensive workup.[46]

The primary intent of including serial CEA measurement in the ASCO surveillance guidelines is to detect and treat isolated asymptomatic hepatic metastases,[40] an intent that may be developing increasing importance given the almost universal acceptance of the significantly expanded criteria for resecting hepatic metastases. An additional intent of measuring serum CEA in postoperative surveillance strategies is

to identify recurrent incurable metastatic disease as early as possible, given the growing evidence that systemic therapy of asymptomatic disease provides a significant survival advantage over the best supportive care,[19,22,47-49] even while preserving quality of life.[50] Although the use of CEA measurements with these intentions cannot be definitively shown to improve outcomes, the rationale of performing serial measurement of CEA in the postoperative surveillance of colon cancer is clearly based on evidence-based conclusions. CEA is a valuable component, in conjunction with clinical examination and CT scan, in the follow-up of resected colon cancer patients.

Computed Tomography

In this age of high-quality CT imaging and aggressive curative resection of hepatic metastases, the CT scan may have particular value in the postoperative surveillance. Unfortunately, most of the prospective randomized studies were performed before these advances; no evidence from any one of these studies definitively supports the use of surveillance CT in improving survival. With this lack of definitive evidence, all five meta-analyses cited in this chapter support a survival benefit of intensifying surveillance,[15,19,20,23,24] which includes several individual studies that investigated the use of surveillance CT or other form of liver imaging to improve survival. Four meta-analyses specifically addressed the contributions of individual components to surveillance, and all four comprehensive examinations support the use of CT or other form of liver imaging in improving overall survival.[15,19,20,23]

Excluding the most recent meta-analysis published by Tjandra and Chan,[20] the major reason why the most recent ASCO Guidelines[51] now include surveillance CT is based on the analysis of the remaining three meta-analyses.[15,19,23] All three of these meta-analyses showed an approximately 25% lower mortality rate in patients undergoing liver imaging compared with those who had no surveillance imaging. In contrast to the previous 1999 ASCO Guidelines[52] and 2000 Update,[53] which actually recommended against surveillance CT, the ASCO 2005 Guidelines now recommend annual surveillance chest and abdominal CT for the first 3 years for all higher-risk patients (who are also candidates for curative intent surgery),[51] a position the NCCN has also adopted.[45]

Evaluation of the most recent and arguably the most up-to-date meta-analysis by Tjandra and Chan[20] is illustrative of the difficulties involved in making conclusions based on these meta-analyses. The investigators in these meta-analyses concluded that although no survival benefit could be definitively attributed to abdominal or pelvic CT ($P = .06$), detection of asymptomatic tumor recurrences ($P = .007$) and curative re-operation rate ($P = .01$) was increased with the use of CT[20] (see Figs. 17-4 and 17-5). The investigators surmised that the lack of survival benefit for CT in the meta-analysis[20] may be attributable in part to the apparent disappointingly low rate of detection of curable pelvic or local recurrence found in four of the individual studies.[21,26-28] This low rate may be due to the inclusion of rectal cancer patients, in whom the investigators surmised that local recurrence was more likely to be incurable. The inclusion of the benefit of other tests for liver imaging, such as liver ultrasound, as an overall promotion of the argument for a survival benefit to surveillance CT can be easily criticized but is nonetheless a reasonable argument to make, given the limitation of available data. As such, in the same meta-analysis, the analysts also concluded that the use of surveillance liver ultrasound did significantly reduce mortality ($P = .008$), although intensifying the frequency of this liver imaging technique did not significantly improve this beneficial effect ($P = .73$).[20]

As previously described, surveillance chest CT is also included in the most recent ASCO recommendations. No evidence exists to support its use in routine surveillance for providing a survival benefit. Chest radiography is not as easily extrapolated to overall chest imaging techniques as a surrogate for chest CT, as is liver ultrasound to liver imaging and abdominal CT. Nonetheless, proceeding with a suspension of this disbelief, the most recent meta-analysis demonstrated that chest radiography reduced overall mortality ($P = .0005$); however, like liver ultrasound, increasing the frequency of this test did not provide any additional benefit ($P = .79$).[20] The finding that performing any type of surveillance chest imaging, compared with none at all, might have a survival benefit is in itself compelling. Yet, in comparison to the rate of metachronous liver metastases (1 of 5) in patients who

have completed potentially curative intent therapy, only about 1 of 12 such patients are estimated to develop pulmonary metastases.[54] Despite being less common, long-term survival rates after resection of pulmonary colorectal cancer metastases rival those rates after hepatic metastases resection (30%–60%),[55-59] and long-term survivors have been reported after sequential resection of both pulmonary and hepatic metastases.[55] Pulmonary colon cancer metastases tend to be peripheral and more amenable to resection than hepatic metastases. The rationale that supports chest CT thus centers not just on its potential to make meaningful, though numerically small, contributions to improving survival but also on its presumed ability to detect the greatest proportion, if not absolute number, of resectable recurrences.

In a relatively recent randomized, adjuvant chemotherapy trial, the authors separately reported on the use of a surveillance strategy of serial clinical examination with CEA measurement as well as the performance of chest, abdominal, and pelvic CT at 12 and 24 months of follow-up.[35] From a total of 530 patients, 154 subjects had recurrences, of which only 33 were eligible for curative intent surgical therapy. Of these 33 patients, almost one third ($n = 9$) underwent pulmonary resection. Most patients who underwent pulmonary resection (7 of 9) were asymptomatic and did not have an elevated CEA, and their recurrences were able to be found only on chest CT. Of the original 154 patients who had recurrence, almost one third ($n = 49$) were detected first by chest, abdomen, or pelvic CT; 39 of these 49 patients had solitary recurrences, 11 of which were found on chest CT and 22 on abdominal CT. It is interesting that more than 70% of the recurrences found on chest CT were treatable by curative resection for solitary recurrence compared with only 36% of the recurrences found on abdominal CT. Thus, chest CT identified the largest relative proportion of solitary recurrence among patients who could undergo curative intent surgical therapy.[35]

Colonoscopy

The primary role of endoscopic surveillance in colon cancer is to detect the low rate of both intramural local recurrence and metachronous new primary tumors in the hope of promoting long-term survival. In one of the meta-analyses, rates of intramural recurrence and metachronous cancer have been reported to be as low as 3.2% and 1.3%, respectively,[19] in contrast to the rates detailed in the introduction of this chapter. These low rates have caused the authors in another meta-analysis to conclude, despite a statistically significant reduction in mortality rates attributed to colonoscopy ($P = .0006$), that intensive efforts focused on intramural detection would be of little additional benefit.[20] In a meta-analysis, Figueredo and associates[15] stated clearly that effective surveillance requires an emphasis on CEA monitoring and liver imaging—not colonoscopy—since the trials that include these modalities show a survival benefit compared with the trials that did not include them and showed no gain. Despite the previous promise of colonoscopy, the intensification of frequency of this test, even in the first 2 to 3 years of follow-up, does not improve survival. Surveillance colonoscopy should be done but should not be the focus of a surveillance strategy.

The ASCO recommends a preoperative or perioperative colonoscopy to document that the colon is free of other metachronous cancers or polyps. Once this colonoscopy has been performed, additional surveillance colonoscopies are recommended at 3 years and then every 5 years if normal.[51] The NCCN differs in their guidelines, recommending a surveillance colonoscopy at 1 year and every 3 (advanced adenoma) to 5 (normal) years thereafter; if the colonoscopy at 1 year is abnormal, it should be repeated in 1 year.[45] The ASCO recommendation is more in line with the most recent American Gastroenterology Association's guideline, which is to perform a perioperative colonoscopy and, if findings are low risk or no polyps, to repeat the colonoscopy in 3 to 5 years. With high-risk polyp findings—defined as villous adenoma or tubular adenomas larger than 1 cm or high-grade dysplasia—excision and yearly colonoscopies are recommended until the absence of such polyps is documented.[60]

The cost and morbidity of endoscopy have been scarcely mentioned in the literature, but a general consensus exists that the cost is very high and morbidity is generally low. Yet no prospective colon cancer surveillance trial has examined and reported the inevitable harmful consequences of these tests to help assess the cost-benefit ratio of such a strategy. One study reports two perforations and two bleeding episodes in a total of 731 colonoscopies, which calculates to about a 0.55% morbidity rate.[21] This rate compared favorably with those of other series,[61,62] but nonetheless highlights the limitations of our understanding of true costs and benefits to intensive surveillance, given the small number of patients who might potentially benefit.

Despite this more pessimistic viewpoint of the contribution of surveillance colonoscopy, at least one recent prospective randomized trial comparing surveillance regimens for stage II and III resected colorectal cancer patients advocates an annual colonoscopy through 5 years of follow-up.[17] In this study, patients were randomized to either the intensive strategy or the simple strategy. In both arms, patients underwent clinical examination and serial CEA measurement every 3 months for the first 2 years and then every 6 months for the next 3 years. Patients randomized to the intensive arm also underwent serial abdominal CT or ultrasound, annual chest radiography, and annual colonoscopy through 5 years of follow-up. Although no overall survival benefit could be demonstrated, subset analysis suggested that stage II and rectal cancer patients did experience a survival benefit for this intensification of surveillance. Colonoscopy uncovered almost as many recurrences (26%) as abdominal CT or ultrasonography (31%) and more than serum CEA measurements (23%). In closer analysis, in the intensive strategy, colonoscopy uncovered more resectable recurrences than any other method (44%).[17] This outcome was surprising, given the relatively low percentage (about 25%) of rectal cancer patients in this study, in whom the risk of local recurrence is much higher. Similar to chest CT, the yield, or relative proportion, of resectable to discovered recurrences with colonoscopy was the highest of any method.[17] Yet the local recurrence rate of more than 30% is much higher than expected, especially in a trial in which colon cancer (more than 70%) predominated over rectal cancer (about 25%), as the authors themselves point out.[17]

The use of colonoscopy in the surveillance of colon cancer remains relatively controversial. It seems clear that the addition of colonoscopy is an important adjunct, but it is not clear whether the addition of more frequent endoscopic surveillance would significantly contribute to a survival benefit. Although the morbidity of surveillance colonoscopy is probably low, the cost-benefit ratio of more frequent colonoscopies remains blurred by the lack of quality data.

Positron Emission Tomography

Use of [18]fluorodeoxyglucose (FDG)-positron emission tomography (FDG-PET) is largely limited as an adjunct in the surveillance of colon cancer. There is no role for surveillance PET and no prospective randomized evidence to support its use. As an adjunct, however, PET combined with CT can be useful to help guide or change management. CEA and PET-CT can be helpful in managing the patient with a rising or persistently elevated CEA but with no other clinical, radiographic, or endoscopic evidence of recurrence (see Figs. 17-2 and 17-3).

In addition to the study by Libutti and associates[44] already described in the section on CEA, several reports have attempted to study the usefulness of PET in the management of patients with recurrent colorectal cancer, although the number of patients has been small (17 to 50). Like the Libutti study, Flanagan and associates[63] investigated PET in the management of patients with an abnormal CEA level but with negative comprehensive radiographic and endoscopic workup. Although this analysis included only 22 patients, of whom 17 had an abnormal PET, the authors reported 89% positive predictive value and 100% negative predictive value, identifying 7 resected for cure and 8 not amenable to curative intent therapy.[63] An additional retrospective analysis investigating PET in the same setting revealed a sensitivity of almost 80% and a positive predictive value of 89%.[64]

For patients with evidence of a local or distant recurrence that appears amenable to curative intent, PET can often change management (in about 30%) by detecting additional spread of disease that renders the patient incurable.[65] In particular, FDG-PET can help prevent nontherapeutic liver resection in patients with apparently curable hepatic metastases by identifying extrahepatic disease. In this setting, a recent meta-analysis of several nonrandomized studies suggests that FDG-PET changes clinical management 25% to 30% of the time.[66] In doing so, FDG-PET can facilitate better patient selection and thereby improve outcomes from liver resec-

tion and increase 5-year survival rates from about 30% to nearly 60%.[67]

Despite the significant increase in effectiveness of FDG-PET when used concurrently with CT,[68] the use of PET-CT has several limitations, including the normal physiologic accumulation of FDG in several organs, the inability to identify lesions smaller than 1 cm (including peritoneal carcinomatosis), the poor uptake of mucinous adenocarcinoma, and reliance on a dedicated CT interpreter.[68] Availability of PET imaging is limited largely to tertiary referral centers and remains a costly procedure.[69] Despite these limitations, the usefulness of PET as an adjunct to the management of recurrent colon cancer is growing,[70] but it is doubtful that it will become a part of the routine surveillance of colon cancer.

Summary

Despite the approximately 500,000 patients in the United States who undergo postoperative surveillance of apparently cured colon cancer every year,[71] the surveillance guidelines of several major organizations differ significantly. These differences underscore a lingering concern that seems to remain in the general medical community that either more or less should be done postoperatively to salvage the 30% to 50% of patients whose cancer recurs. For now, the minimalist versus unapologetic intensivist argument seems to be here to stay. This concern is highlighted by a recent survey of colorectal surgeons, about 30% of whom perform surveillance CT in the first year with more than 50% of these not performing routine surveillance CT at all.[72] The limitations of the literature have been extensively outlined in this chapter. The eight prospective randomized studies display significant heterogeneity in surveillance strategies; lack significant power; are hampered by small sample size and are single institutional; and were performed in the era before high-quality CT, more effective and tolerable chemotherapy, and aggressive and safe hepatic resection. In addition, the outcomes can be coalesced in different well-intentioned analyses and result in different conclusions. Yet, despite these limitations, the general consensus of physicians and patients alike, bolstered by carefully designed meta-analyses, support that more intensive surveillance saves lives.

The question of the optimal frequency and combination of tests that should make up this surveillance remains. It is likely that a definitive schedule and frequency will never be fully agreed upon. Given the timing of recurrences, clearly more frequent examinations in the first 2 or 3 years and follow-up for at least 5 years make sense. Clinical examination and serial measurement of CEA clearly form the backbone of this surveillance. Colonoscopy should be a part of the strategy but probably at less frequent intervals than many of the earlier enthusiasts argued for. CT has an increasingly prominent role in detecting both hepatic and pulmonary metastases; in the age of improving quality imaging and of more effective systemic therapy, more aggressive resection of such metastatic disease is likely to yield significant dividends. PET scan is likely to have an increasing role in patient selection, but given its high cost, limited availability, low resolution, and low specificity even when combined with CT, PET is unlikely to become a part of routine surveillance. Given these unanswered questions, we eagerly await the results of at least three multicenter, prospective, randomized trials. Considering the recent pace of advancement and the inherent challenge in comparing even more intensive surveillance with intensive surveillance strategies, it is likely that the oncology community will continue to have significant unanswered questions after these trials have been reported. The ability to salvage patients with recurrent colon cancer will predictably improve even more. Despite the unanswered questions and our own limitations in answering these questions, the role of surveillance will only strengthen during this time.

References

1. Jemal A, Siegel R, Ward E, et al: Cancer statistics, 2009. CA Cancer J Clin 59(4):225–249, 2009.
2. Abulafi AM, Williams NS: Local recurrence of colorectal cancer: the problem, mechanisms, management and adjuvant therapy. Br J Surg 81(1):7–19, 1994.
3. Devesa JM, Morales V, Enriquez JM, et al: Colorectal cancer. The bases for a comprehensive follow-up. Dis Colon Rectum 31(8):636–652, 1988.
4. Obrand DI, Gordon PH: Incidence and patterns of recurrence following curative resection for colorectal carcinoma. Dis Colon Rectum 40(1):15–24, 1997.
5. Safi F, Beyer HG: The value of follow-up after curative surgery of colorectal carcinoma. Cancer Detect Prev 17(3):417–424, 1993.
6. Sargent DJ, Wieand HS, Haller DG, et al: Disease-free survival versus overall survival as a primary end point for adjuvant colon cancer studies: individual patient data from 20,898 patients in 18 randomized trials. J Clin Oncol 23(34):8664–8670, 2005.
7. Steele G Jr, Ravikumar TS: Resection of hepatic metastases from colorectal cancer. Biologic perspective. Ann Surg 210(2):127–138, 1989.
8. Scheele J, Stangl R, Altendorf-Hofmann A, Gall FP: Indicators of prognosis after hepatic resection for colorectal secondaries. Surgery 110(1):13–29, 1991.
9. Russell AH, Tong D, Dawson LE, Wisbeck W: Adenocarcinoma of the proximal colon. Sites of initial dissemination and patterns of recurrence following surgery alone. Cancer 53(2):360–367, 1984.
10. Willett CG, Tepper JE, Cohen AM, et al: Failure patterns following curative resection of colonic carcinoma. Ann Surg 200(6):685–690, 1984.
11. Abdalla EK, Vauthey JN, Ellis LM, et al: Recurrence and outcomes following hepatic resection, radiofrequency ablation, and combined resection/ablation for colorectal liver metastases. Ann Surg 239(6):818–825; discussion 825–817, 2004.
12. Choti MA, Sitzmann JV, Tiburi MF, et al: Trends in long-term survival following liver resection for hepatic colorectal metastases. Ann Surg 235(6):759–766, 2002.
13. Fong Y, Fortner J, Sun RL, et al: Clinical score for predicting recurrence after hepatic resection for metastatic colorectal cancer: analysis of 1001 consecutive cases. Ann Surg 230(3):309–318; discussion 318–321, 1999.
14. Kjeldsen BJ, Kronborg O, Fenger C, Jorgensen OD: The pattern of recurrent colorectal cancer in a prospective randomised study and the characteristics of diagnostic tests. Int J Colorectal Dis 12(6):329–334, 1997.
15. Figueredo A, Rumble RB, Maroun J, et al: Follow-up of patients with curatively resected colorectal cancer: a practice guideline. BMC Cancer 3:26, 2003.
16. Galandiuk S, Wieand HS, Moertel CG, et al: Patterns of recurrence after curative resection of carcinoma of the colon and rectum. Surg Gynecol Obstet 174(1):27–32, 1992.
17. Rodriguez-Moranta F, Salo J, Arcusa A, et al: Postoperative surveillance in patients with colorectal cancer who have undergone curative resection: a prospective, multicenter, randomized, controlled trial. J Clin Oncol 24(3):386–393, 2006.
18. Cunliffe WJ, Hasleton PS, Tweedle DE, Schofield PF: Incidence of synchronous and metachronous colorectal carcinoma. Br J Surg 71(12):941–943, 1984.
19. Renehan AG, Egger M, Saunders MP, O'Dwyer ST: Impact on survival of intensive follow up after curative resection for colorectal cancer: systematic review and meta-analysis of randomised trials. BMJ 324(7341):813, 2002.
20. Tjandra JJ, Chan MK: Follow-up after curative resection of colorectal cancer: a meta-analysis. Dis Colon Rectum 50(11):1783–1799, 2007.
21. Schoemaker D, Black R, Giles L, Toouli J: Yearly colonoscopy, liver CT, and chest radiography do not influence 5-year survival of colorectal cancer patients. Gastroenterology 114(1):7–14, 1998.
22. Group NGTAT: Expectancy or primary chemotherapy in patients with advanced asymptomatic colorectal cancer: a randomized trial. J Clin Oncol 10(6):904–911, 1992.
23. Jeffery M, Hickey BE, Hider PN: Follow-up strategies for patients treated for non-metastatic colorectal cancer. Cochrane Database Syst Rev (1):CD002200, 2007.
24. Renehan AG, Egger M, Saunders MP, O'Dwyer ST: Mechanisms of improved survival from intensive followup in colorectal cancer: a hypothesis. Br J Cancer 92(3):430–433, 2005.
25. Kjeldsen BJ, Kronborg O, Fenger C, Jorgensen OD: A prospective randomized study of follow-up after radical surgery for colorectal cancer. Br J Surg 84(5):666–669, 1997.
26. Makela JT, Laitinen SO, Kairaluoma MI: Five-year follow-up after radical surgery for colorectal cancer. Results of a prospective randomized trial. Arch Surg 130(10):1062–1067, 1995.
27. Ohlsson B, Breland U, Ekberg H, et al: Follow-up after curative surgery for colorectal carcinoma. Randomized comparison with no follow-up. Dis Colon Rectum 38(6):619–626, 1995.
28. Pietra N, Sarli L, Costi R, et al: Role of follow-up in management of local recurrences of colorectal cancer: a prospective, randomized study. Dis Colon Rectum 41(9):1127–1133, 1998.
29. Secco GB, Fardelli R, Gianquinto D, et al: Efficacy and cost of risk-adapted follow-up in patients after colorectal cancer surgery: a prospective, randomized and controlled trial. Eur J Surg Oncol 28(4):418–423, 2002.
30. Wattchow DA, Weller DP, Esterman A, et al: General practice vs surgical-based follow-up for patients with colon cancer: randomised controlled trial. Br J Cancer 94(8):1116–1121, 2006.

31. Grossmann EM, Johnson FE, Virgo KS, et al: Follow-up of colorectal cancer patients after resection with curative intent—the GILDA trial. Surg Oncol 13(2–3):119–124, 2004.
32. Group FS: The Follow-up After Colorectal Surgery (FACS) Study 2004. http://www.facs.soton.ac.uk. Accessed 23 February 2010.
33. Wille-Jorgensen P, Laurberg S, Pahlman S, et al: An interim analysis of recruitment to the COLOFOL trial. Colorectal Dis 11(7):756–758, 2009.
34. Bohm B, Schwenk W, Hucke HP, Stock W: Does methodic long-term follow-up affect survival after curative resection of colorectal carcinoma? Dis Colon Rectum 36(3):280–286, 1993.
35. Chau I, Allen MJ, Cunningham D, et al: The value of routine serum carcino-embryonic antigen measurement and computed tomography in the surveillance of patients after adjuvant chemotherapy for colorectal cancer. J Clin Oncol 22(8):1420–1429, 2004.
36. Goldberg RM, Fleming TR, Tangen CM, et al: Surgery for recurrent colon cancer: strategies for identifying resectable recurrence and success rates after resection. Eastern Cooperative Oncology Group, the North Central Cancer Treatment Group, and the Southwest Oncology Group. Ann Intern Med 129(1):27–35, 1998.
37. Stiggelbout AM, de Haes JC, Vree R, et al: Follow-up of colorectal cancer patients: quality of life and attitudes towards follow-up. Br J Cancer 75(6):914–920, 1997.
38. Renehan AG, O'Dwyer ST, Whynes DK: Cost effectiveness analysis of intensive versus conventional follow up after curative resection for colorectal cancer. BMJ 328(7431):81, 2004.
39. Arnaud JP, Koehl C, Adloff M: Carcinoembryonic antigen (CEA) in diagnosis and prognosis of colorectal carcinoma. Dis Colon Rectum 23(3):141–144, 1980.
40. Locker GY, Hamilton S, Harris J, et al: ASCO 2006 update of recommendations for the use of tumor markers in gastrointestinal cancer. J Clin Oncol 24(33):5313–5327, 2006.
41. Moertel CG, Fleming TR, Macdonald JS, et al: An evaluation of the carcinoembryonic antigen (CEA) test for monitoring patients with resected colon cancer. JAMA 270(8):943–947, 1993.
42. Sorbye H, Dahl O: Carcinoembryonic antigen surge in metastatic colorectal cancer patients responding to oxaliplatin combination chemotherapy: implications for tumor marker monitoring and guidelines. J Clin Oncol 21(23):4466–4467, 2003.
43. Clinical Practice Guidelines for the Use of Tumor Markers in Breast and Colorectal Cancer. Adopted on May 17, 1996 by the American Society of Clinical Oncology. J Clin Oncol 14(10):2843–2877, 1996.
44. Libutti SK, Alexander HR Jr, Choyke P, et al: A prospective study of 2-[18F] fluoro-2-deoxy-D-glucose/positron emission tomography scan, 99mTc-labeled arcitumomab (CEA-scan), and blind second-look laparotomy for detecting colon cancer recurrence in patients with increasing carcinoembryonic antigen levels. Ann Surg Oncol 8(10):779–786, 2001.
45. Guidelines NCCN. www.nccn.org. Accessed 5 January 2009.
46. Martin EW Jr, Minton JP, Carey LC: CEA-directed second-look surgery in the asymptomatic patient after primary resection of colorectal carcinoma. Ann Surg 202(3):310–317, 1985.
47. Cunningham D, Pyrhonen S, James RD, et al: Randomised trial of irinotecan plus supportive care versus supportive care alone after fluorouracil failure for patients with metastatic colorectal cancer. Lancet 352(9138):1413–1418, 1998.
48. Glimelius B, Hoffman K, Graf W, et al: Cost-effectiveness of palliative chemotherapy in advanced gastrointestinal cancer. Ann Oncol 6(3):267–274, 1995.
49. Scheithauer W, Rosen H, Kornek GV, et al: Randomised comparison of combination chemotherapy plus supportive care with supportive care alone in patients with metastatic colorectal cancer. BMJ 306(6880):752–755, 1993.
50. Simmonds PC: Palliative chemotherapy for advanced colorectal cancer: systematic review and meta-analysis. Colorectal Cancer Collaborative Group. BMJ 321(7260):531–535, 2000.
51. Desch CE, Benson AB III, Somerfield MR, et al: Colorectal cancer surveillance: 2005 update of an American Society of Clinical Oncology practice guideline. J Clin Oncol 23(33):8512–8519, 2005.
52. Desch CE, Benson AB III, Smith TJ, et al: Recommended colorectal cancer surveillance guidelines by the American Society of Clinical Oncology. J Clin Oncol 17(4):1312, 1999.
53. Benson AB III, Desch CE, Flynn PJ, et al: 2000 Update of American Society of Clinical Oncology Colorectal Cancer Surveillance Guidelines. J Clin Oncol 18(20):3586–3588, 2000.
54. Kievit J: Follow-up of patients with colorectal cancer: numbers needed to test and treat. Eur J Cancer 38(7):986–999, 2000.
55. Ike H, Shimada H, Togo S, et al: Sequential resection of lung metastasis following partial hepatectomy for colorectal cancer. Br J Surg 89(9):1164–1168, 2002.
56. Regnard JF, Grunenwald D, Spaggiari L, et al: Surgical treatment of hepatic and pulmonary metastases from colorectal cancers. Ann Thorac Surg 66(1):214–218; discussion 218–219, 1998.
57. Rena O, Casadio C, Viano F, et al: Pulmonary resection for metastases from colorectal cancer: factors influencing prognosis. Twenty-year experience. Eur J Cardiothorac Surg 21(5):906–912, 2002.
58. Sakamoto T, Tsubota N, Iwanaga K, et al: Pulmonary resection for metastases from colorectal cancer. Chest 119(4):1069–1072, 2001.
59. Zink S, Kayser G, Gabius HJ, Kayser K: Survival, disease-free interval, and associated tumor features in patients with colon/rectal carcinomas and their resected intra-pulmonary metastases. Eur J Cardiothorac Surg 19(6):908–913, 2001.
60. Winawer S, Fletcher R, Rex D, et al: Colorectal cancer screening and surveillance: clinical guidelines and rationale—update based on new evidence. Gastroenterology 124(2):544–560, 2003.
61. Araghizadeh FY, Timmcke AE, Opelka FG, et al: Colonoscopic perforations. Dis Colon Rectum 44(5):713–716, 2001.
62. Bowles CJ, Leicester R, Romaya C, et al: A prospective study of colonoscopy practice in the UK today: are we adequately prepared for national colorectal cancer screening tomorrow? Gut 53(2):277–283, 2004.
63. Flanagan FL, Dehdashti F, Ogunbiyi OA, et al: Utility of FDG-PET for investigating unexplained plasma CEA elevation in patients with colorectal cancer. Ann Surg 227(3):319–323, 1998.
64. Flamen P, Hoekstra OS, Homans F, et al: Unexplained rising carcinoembryonic antigen (CEA) in the postoperative surveillance of colorectal cancer: the utility of positron emission tomography (PET). Eur J Cancer 37(7):862–869, 2001.
65. Huebner RH, Park KC, Shepherd JE, et al: A meta-analysis of the literature for whole-body FDG PET detection of recurrent colorectal cancer. J Nucl Med 41(7):1177–1189, 2000.
66. Wiering B, Krabbe PF, Jager GJ, et al: The impact of fluor-18-deoxyglucose-positron emission tomography in the management of colorectal liver metastases. Cancer 104(12):2658–2670, 1995.
67. Fernandez FG, Drebin JA, Linehan DC, et al: Five-year survival after resection of hepatic metastases from colorectal cancer in patients screened by positron emission tomography with F-18 fluorodeoxyglucose (FDG-PET). Ann Surg 240(3):438–447; discussion 447–450, 2004.
68. Kamel IR, Cohade C, Neyman E, et al: Incremental value of CT in PET/CT of patients with colorectal carcinoma. Abdom Imaging 29(6):663–668, 2004.
69. Abir F, Alva S, Longo WE, et al: The postoperative surveillance of patients with colon cancer and rectal cancer. Am J Surg 192(1):100–108, 2006.
70. Meyerhardt JA, Mayer RJ: Follow-up strategies after curative resection of colorectal cancer. Semin Oncol 30(3):349–360, 2003.
71. Pfister DG, Benson AB III, Somerfield MR: Clinical practice. Surveillance strategies after curative treatment of colorectal cancer. N Engl J Med 350(23):2375–2382, 2004.
72. Johnson FE, Virgo KS, Fossati R: Follow-up for patients with colorectal cancer after curative-intent primary treatment. J Clin Oncol 22(8):1363–1365, 2004.

Clinical Trials: Why Participate?

18

Jamila Mwidau and David Chang

KEY POINTS

- A clinical trial is any investigation in human subjects intended to discover or verify the effects of a product, device, or procedure.
- Clinical trials fall into five basic types: prevention, screening, diagnostic, treatment, and quality-of-life trials.
- An intervention is evaluated through preclinical studies and four phases of clinical trials to ensure its safety and efficacy for human subjects.
- Conducting clinical trials at multiple sites improves participant enrollment, ensures a more representative sample, and promotes collegiality.

Introduction

Many of the advances that have been made in medicine can be attributed to the participation of individuals in clinical trials. In 1747, James Lind performed one of the most famous clinical trials. By comparing the effects of various fruits on afflicted sailors, he was able to demonstrate that citrus fruits cured scurvy.

Strictly defined, a clinical trial or study is

> any investigation in human subjects intended to discover or verify the clinical, pharmacological, and/or other pharmacodynamic effects of an investigational product(s), and/or to identify any adverse reactions to an investigational product(s), and/or to study absorption, distribution, metabolism, and excretion of an investigational product(s) with the object of ascertaining its safety and/or efficacy.[1]

Although this definition specifically addresses pharmacologic agents, clinical trials may also include surgical procedures, diagnostic tests, and medical devices, with the intent to discover or verify safety and/or efficacy.

The strength of the conclusions from any study is dependent on the quality of the scientific approach and the principles used during the trial. For instance, surgical trials are particularly prone to operator bias because of the implications for patient referrals and the surgeon's reputation. Furthermore, elderly patients are often excluded from clinical trials, and this could affect the outcome of a trial. Although the elderly make up only 14% of the population, they consume more than one third of all drugs. There are other types of clinical research (e.g., case studies), but the clinical trial is viewed as the strongest source of evidence to support safety and efficacy statements. The clinical trial is an experiment in which the conditions are specified in a detailed document called the *protocol*. This detailed document allows the use of scientific methods to analyze the effects of the treatment.

Types of Clinical Trials

Several types of clinical trials can be conducted, depending on the goal of the study. These types are outlined below.

Prevention trials find better ways to prevent disease in people who have never had the disease or to prevent a disease from returning. The approaches tested in these trials may include medicines, vitamins, vaccines, minerals, and lifestyle changes.

Screening trials test the best way to detect certain diseases or health conditions.

Diagnostic trials are conducted to find better tests or procedures for diagnosing a particular disease or condition. Diagnostic trials usually include people who have signs or symptoms of the disease or condition being studied.

Treatment trials test new treatments, new combinations of drugs, or new approaches to surgery or radiation therapy.

Quality-of-life trials (or supportive care trials) explore ways to improve comfort and quality of life for individuals with a chronic illness.

Phases of a Clinical Trial

Clinical trials are traditionally classified into preclinical trials and four phases, although it is important to note that precise distinctions between the phases are not always possible in practice. Each phase of development leads to a greater understanding of the attributes and uses or indications of the compound or treatment.

The phases of a clinical trial are described in detail in Table 18-1. Briefly, phase 0 trials follow preclinical trials to look at dosing in humans and to speed up the development of a new intervention. Phase I trials are the first step in evaluating whether a new therapy is safe as administered. Phase II trials focus on how a given therapy may affect a specific group of participants for whom

the therapy is recommended. Phases I and II usually occur with the help of healthy volunteers. Phase III trials are randomized trials that compare a new therapy with the present standard therapy or placebo therapy (a pill or procedure that does not include active ingredients). However, most cancer trials do not use placebos. Most drugs are not released to the public for general use by the Federal Drug Agency (FDA) until at last two phase III trials have been completed. Finally, phase IV trials are conducted to study the long-term effectiveness of a therapy and may take several years to complete.

Clinical Trial Designs

The prospective randomized controlled trial (RCT) is considered the highest level of scientific evidence because it avoids bias in patient selection. RCTs typically also have the most regulatory oversight and study process. Therefore, RCTs are labor intensive and time consuming and can be expensive. In the 1990s, Europe, Japan, and the United States formed a joint regulatory industry initiative on international harmonization entitled the International Con-

Table 18-1. Clinical Research Phases

Phase	Description
Phase 0: Human microdosing (preclinical trials)	These studies and are designed to speed up the development of promising drugs or imaging agents by establishing very early on whether the drug or agent behaves in human subjects.
Phase I: Human pharmacology	Determines the metabolic and pharmacologic actions and the maximally tolerated dose. The experimental drug is administered to small numbers of normal human volunteers or to a carefully defined subject population under controlled conditions to obtain preliminary data on drug toleration, pharmacokinetics, and pharmacodynamics. Sample size: 20–80
Phase II: Therapeutic exploratory	The experimental drug is administered to limited numbers of subjects for whom it appears to be indicated in order to define a therapeutic dose range and to establish efficacy, side effects, and clinical toxicity of the drug. Often the phase is separated into phase II (a), which focuses on dosage, and phase II (b), which studies efficacy. Sample size: 100–300
Phase III: Therapeutic confirmatory	The experimental drug is administered in large-scale trials to establish safety and efficacy. These studies are required for submission to the regulatory authorities in support of a product license application for the new drug. Sometimes phase III studies are divided into phase III (a), before the drug is submitted for regulatory approval, and phase III (b), when the application has been submitted but approval is still pending. Sample size: 1000–3000
Phase IV: Therapeutic use	This phase is conducted after regulatory approval has been obtained; trials are limited to the drug's approved indications, dosage forms, dosage ranges, routes of administration, and subject population. The objective of this phase is to monitor ongoing safety in large populations and identify additional uses of the agent that may be approved by the regulatory authority.

Box 18-1. Key Principles of RCT

1. Underpowered trials or trials without enough participants are prone to error (false positives or false negatives).
2. Any reporting of data that may be significant but is underpowered can lead to false assumptions and the performance of even more costly RCTs.
3. Multicenter trials establish greater credence and generalizability than single-center trials.
4. Blind studies are preferred to eliminate bias.
5. Declaring a treatment superior is a much more desirable outcome than demonstrating that a treatment is not inferior.
6. Consider carefully the bias that may occur in a RCT as a result of accepting industry support over investigator-initiated support

Data from Stone G, Pocock S: Randomized trials, statistics, and clinical inference. J Am Coll Cardiol 55:428–430, 2010.

ference on Harmonization of Technical Requirements for Registration of Pharmaceuticals for Human Use (ICH) The goal of the ICH is to ensure that the interest of public health remains of foremost importance. ICH guidelines are aimed at ensuring that high-quality, safe, and effective medicines are developed and registered in the most efficient and cost-effective manner. Currently, most clinical trials follow ICH guidelines.

The RCT is not without flaws, however. In their recent article, Stone and Pocock[2] discuss some of the weaknesses of the RCT (Box 18-1). Many of the problems that arise in a RCT result from poorly defined primary and secondary objectives and an insufficient number of study participants. Any RCT requires prespecified primary objectives. In addition, secondary objectives can be specified. These objectives are used to determine the number of participants necessary to adequately answer the scientific question. The process of determining this number is called the *power analysis*. In analyzing the data of a RCT, regardless of whether the results are significant, the study must include the number of participants needed to prove that the results are truly significant. If the study is underpowered, the probability of the presence of false positives or false negative results is higher. Furthermore, the analysis of the data should reflect the objectives in which sufficient power was achieved. Stone and Pocock discuss this error in a study in which an observation of improved survival following percutaneous coro-

nary intervention for an acute myocardial infarction with the administration of a drug called pexelixumab was reported. However, the effect of this drug was not the primary objective of this study, and thus the study was underpowered to report this result as positive. This reporting resulted in a costly 8500-patient RCT to evaluate the use of this drug and its effect on mortality. This study was stopped early for futility.

In designing a clinical trial, the most desired outcome is demonstrating that one treatment is superior to another. However, this type of study requires many more participants than studies designed to demonstrate noninferiority of a treatment. Often, this type of design is used to demonstrate that a less expensive or less invasive treatment is just as good as the more expensive or more invasive treatment. To perform a noninferiority study, a study margin is set, and this margin may be inaccurate, allowing one to declare noninferiority when actually the study is inferior. Other common difficulties discussed by Stone and Pocock[2] that are encountered include unblinded studies and studies supported by industry, both of which are prone to bias.

Participation in a Clinical Trial

A clinical trial is the best method to identify new therapies that directly benefit patient care. Without clinical trials, scientific advancement in health care is nearly impossible. Because medical care has improved dramatically in the past few decades, we seldom see dramatic risk reduction from a single intervention. Therefore, a large number of participants is required to demonstrate that a therapy results in significant improvement. The graph in Figure 18-1 shows the results of a power analysis determining how many participants are necessary to demonstrate a significant (50%) risk reduction for each percentage difference expected to be seen. Most clinical studies today demonstrate only a 10% to 20% advantage over the existing treatment. Therefore, in order to complete must studies today, a large number of participants will be required.

Participants in a clinical study can experience a number of benefits. In addition to aiding the advance of medical care, patients may gain access to promising new approaches that may not be available otherwise. They will also receive careful attention from a research team that typically includes a variety of health care profession-

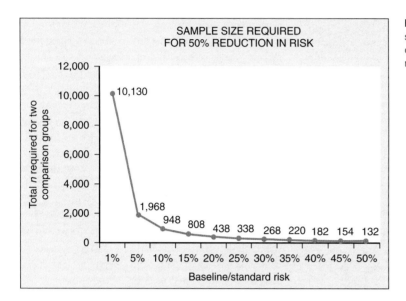

Figure 18-1. Estimated sample size of participants required for demonstration of a percentage of risk reduction in a clinical trial.

als. It should be noted, however, that a clinical trial may not always directly benefit the individual participant. There may be unexpected side effects from the trial treatment, and insurance coverage may be limited. For more information on participation in clinical trials see the *National Cancer Institute Fact Sheet*.[3,4]

Multicenter Clinical Trial

Clinical trials can be run at a single institution or at multiple institutions within the United States and abroad. Multi-institutional clinical trials have the advantage of increased patient participation and may provide more meaningful results, depending on the clinical question being studied. A multicenter clinical trial is a collaborative effort that involves more than one independent center in the implementation of a protocol, which includes enrolling and following the study patients. The main rationale for conducting multicenter trials is to recruit an adequate number of participants within a reasonable amount of time.

Another advantage of multicenter trials is that they ensure a more representative sample of the study or target population. Geography, race, socioeconomic status, and lifestyle of participants may be more representative of the general population when participants are enrolled by many centers. A large multicenter trial allows the treating physician to be de-identified and therefore offers more accurate reporting of complications. These factors may be important

in the researchers' ability to generalize the findings of the trial. Furthermore, a multicenter trial enables investigators with similar interests and skills to work together on a common problem. Science and medicine, like many other disciplines, are competitive. Nevertheless, investigators in clinical trials often find that collaboration serves their own interests as well as medical science in general.

Multicenter trials are not without flaws. The flaws among RCTs, whether single institution studies or multicenter trials, are similar. Zwitter outlined what he believes to be the major weaknesses of current multicenter studies.[5] First, the scientific question is formulated on the basis of what is available and feasible. Often a scientific question or hypothesis is rejected regardless of how good it may be secondary to feasibility. Second, the design of the trial is a reflection of the statistical analysis. Because of the inability to obtain the number of participants required (large sample size), the primary objective may not be the initial desired outcome variable and a different objective may be chosen. Finally, because of the increasing cost of a multicenter trial, there has been an increase in industry support of such trials.

Finally, a multicenter trial gives capable, clinically oriented persons who might otherwise not be involved in research activities the opportunity to contribute to science. For all of these reasons, we encourage health care professionals to collaborate in clinical trials whenever the protocols are appropriate for the patients concerned.

Several government agencies support the work on collaborative groups. The National Institute of Diabetes, Digestive and Kidney Disease (NIDDK) supports groups like the Urinary Incontinence Treatment Network (UITN). With regard to cancer research, the National Cancer Institute sponsors the Clinical Trials Cooperative Group Program, which is designed to promote and support clinical research on new cancer therapies. Several of these oncology groups, including the National Surgical Adjuvant Breast and Bowel Project (NSABP), the American College of Surgeons Oncology Group (ACOSOG), the Eastern Cooperative Oncology Group (ECOG), and the Radiation Therapy Oncology Group (RTOG), run colorectal cancer trials. For more information on the National Cancer Institute and Cooperative Group program, visit the NCI website.[3,4]

References

1. Guideline for Industry: E6 Good Clinical Practice: Consolidated Guidance. Washington, DC: U.S. Department of Health and Human Services, 1996, p 3.
2. Stone G, Pocock S: Randomized trials, statistics, and clinical inference. J Am Coll Cardiol 55:428–430, 2010.
3. National Cancer Institute Fact Sheet: Clinical Trials. Available at http://www.cancer.gov/cancertopics/factsheet/Information/clinical-trials.
4. National Cancer Institute Fact Sheet: NCI's Clinical Trials Cooperative Group Program. Available at http://www.cancer.gov/cancertopics/factsheet/NCI/clinical-trials-cooperative-group.
5. Zwitter M: A personal critique: evidence-based medicine, methodology, and ethics of randomised clinical trials. Crit Rev Oncol Hematol 40:125–130, 2001.

Vaccines and Immunotherapy

19 *Ajay Jain and Richard Schulick*

KEY POINTS

- Immunotherapy is a therapeutic strategy in which a patient's immune responses are modulated to eradicate malignant cancer cells.
- Immunotherapy includes both passive and active approaches.
- Passive immunotherapy involves administration of immunoactive agents such as antibodies that exert direct antitumor effects. No sustained, reproducible antitumor immune responses are generated.
- Active immunotherapy induces the host's own immune system to generate effector populations capable of mounting a long-term antitumor response. Active immunotherapy includes both nonspecific and specific immunotherapy strategies. A nonspecific active immunotherapy approach that has been tested in colorectal cancer with negative results is the use of Bacillus Calmette-Guérin (BCG), an inactivated form of tuberculosis that induces generalized inflammatory immune responses. An example of specific immunotherapy strategy is the use of tumor vaccines that generate antigen-specific antitumor immune responses in the host. Vaccine strategies that have been used in colorectal cancer include autologous whole cell vaccines, anti-idiotype antibodies, and dendritic cell vaccines.
- Methods such as vaccines that will generate a long-term, tumor-specific immune response are considered the most promising.
- Many small trials have addressed the various immune modalities. To date, the data, although promising, have been equivocal, and no clear advantage over traditional modalities such as surgery, chemotherapy, and radiation has been seen. Future strategies may target patients with micrometastatic disease who may derive the most benefit.

Introduction

Colorectal cancer is the second leading cause of cancer death in the United States. The standard treatment options for colorectal cancer, as with many other gastrointestinal malignancies, include surgery, chemotherapy, and radiation, depending on the location and stage of disease at clinical presentation. Although early-stage colon cancer (stages I and II) has an excellent prognosis when treated with surgical therapy alone, recurrence-free and overall survival rates drop significantly with regional nodal metastases or distant metastases (stages III and IV disease, respectively). Even with standard adjuvant treatments such as chemotherapy and radiation, for patients with stage III disease, the overall 5-year survival rate is anywhere from 44% to 83%. Patients with the more advanced stage IV disease have a 5-year survival rate of about 10%. Given the fact that advanced colorectal cancer has a poor prognosis, it is even more unfortunate that in the United States only 39% of patients are diagnosed with early-stage disease. It is therefore critical to develop better adjuvant therapies for advanced colorectal cancer in addition to the standard modalities such as chemotherapy and radiation.[1]

Immunotherapy—An Overview

One of the most intriguing strategies that has been considered for adjuvant treatment of colorectal cancer is immunotherapy. Immunotherapy and the numerous strategies by which it can be used are broad topics of discussion. Immunotherapy has been investigated in the treatment of a number of cancers with varying degrees of success. To adequately discuss the subject, we must first define what immunotherapy is. Stated simply, immunotherapy is a therapeutic strategy that uses a person's own immune system to eradicate malignant cancer cells. There are a number of ways in which the immune system can be primed to eradicate tumor cells, and it is important to understand the distinctions among the major classes of immunotherapy.[2]

The broadest division of immunotherapy strategies is into passive and active approaches. In the passive immunotherapy approach, immunoactive agents such as tumor antigen-specific antibodies are administered to patients to exert antitumor effects. The antitumor immune responses induced in these patients are therefore "passive," since no native, long-term antitumor immune responses are generated in the host. In contrast, the active immunotherapy approach uses the host's own immune system to elicit long-term antitumor responses. The active immunotherapy approach can be further subdivided into nonspecific and specific immunotherapy strategies. In the nonspecific approach, the immune system is activated in a non–tumor antigen-specific fashion, which results in the eradication of cancer cells.

Among the most famous historical examples of the active, nonspecific approach are the experiments of Dr. William B. Coley, a surgeon at the Memorial Hospital for Cancer and Allied Diseases in New York City during the 1890s. Coley noted that patients with incurable soft tissue sarcomas who developed wound infections had higher disease-free survival and overall survival rates than patients who did not develop infectious wound complications. Coley actually conducted experiments in which he administered live streptococcal culture to patients with sarcomas to generate systemic infections. Then, he observed regression of the primary tumors in a significant number of patients. Coley postulated that the immune responses against the bacterial infection somehow cross-reacted with the tumor tissue, resulting in eradication of the malignant disease. For his early experiments, Coley has often been referred to as the "Father of Cancer Immunotherapy."[3] In contemporary times, the active nonspecific approach to immunotherapy continues to be used. An example is the systemic administration of interferon-α (IFN-α) or high-dose interleukin-2 (IL-2) to patients with advanced melanoma. In contrast to the active nonspecific approach, the active specific approach focuses on selective activation of the immune system only against primary tumor antigens. These responses are most typically mediated by T cells and B cells. In addition to short-term antitumor responses, the active specific approach ideally generates tumor antigen-specific memory T cells that can respond to a future tumor challenge. Currently, the most promising method being investigated to generate long-term active specific immunity is the use of tumor vaccines.[2,4]

In considering immunotherapy to treat colorectal cancer, a number of unique challenges must be addressed. Not all cancers are equal, and some cancers are better than others at evading host immune responses. There are multiple reasons for this. Some cancers lack major antigens that can be the target of a host-derived immune response. Historically, many researchers have considered colon tumors as being relatively deficient in immunodominant antigens when compared with other cancers such as melanoma, in which more than 10 major antigens have been identified.[5]

Many research efforts have focused on identifying antigens that could be the targets of vaccine-induced immune responses. It is highly likely that most of the aberrant antigens that arise on colorectal cancer cells do so as normal colonic cells undergoing malignant transformation. The transformation from normal colonic tissue into cancer is a complex, multistep process in which multiple genes can undergo a variety of point mutations. Indeed, most colon cancers have several mutations rather than one discrete genetic anomaly. This results in a heterogeneous group of colon tumors with wide genotypic and histologic variation. Therefore, it is unlikely that an individual antigen will be isolated that can be the target of a single colon cancer vaccine.[2,6,7]

To date, a number of potential target antigens have been identified. These include, but are not limited to, the proto-oncogene K-ras, the tumor suppressor gene p53, carcinoembryonic antigen (CEA), transforming growth factor-β receptor type II (TGFβRII), squamous cell antigen recognized by T cells 3 (SART-3), and cyclophylin.[4] In addition, even when a vaccine is active against a particular patient's tumor antigen profile, the antigen profile can change as tumors continue to transform. This may result in some tumor cell clones "escaping" the vaccine. Therefore, it may become necessary to administer polyvalent vaccines that are active against an entire spectrum of cancer antigens or to administer vaccines for early-stage disease before tumors have a chance to grow and change their molecular profiles.[8]

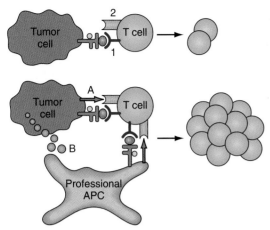

Figure 19-1. Mechanisms of T-cell tolerance. T-cell tolerance occurs when tumor cells present tumor antigens on major histocompatibility complex molecules (1) to T cells without a second costimulatory signal (2). Genetically engineered tumor cells express either costimulatory molecules on their cell surface (A) to activate T cells directly or to release cytokines (B) to attract professional antigen-presenting cells (APCs), which subsequently activate antigen-specific T cells. (From Greten TM, Jaffee EF: Cancer vaccines. Clin Oncol 17[3]:1047–1060, 1999, Fig 2.)

Table 19-1. Summary of Major Immunotherapy Modalities

Approach	Examples
Passive Immunotherapy	
Antitumor antibodies[27]	Edrecolomab (mAB 17-1A); antibody to Ep-CAM, an epithelial cell adhesion molecule
Passive and Possible Active	
Adoptive immunotherapy[25,26]	Tumor-infiltrating lymphocyte (TIL) therapy involving transfer of activated CD8 and CD4 TILs
Active Immunotherapy	
Nonspecific[79]	Bacillus Calmette-Guérin (BCG) Systemic interleukin 2 Interferon-α Interferon-γ Bacterial toxins (mainly in animal models)
Specific	Whole cell tumor vaccines Anti-idiotype antibodies Dendritic cell tumor vaccines Peptide vaccines Ganglioside vaccines DNA vaccines Viral vector vaccines

An additional problem is that even though vaccination may induce tumor antigen-specific responses in a host, this does not always result in sustained antitumor activity. These activated, tumor antigen-specific immune effectors often become attenuated over time. This may be due to secondary host immune responses that downregulate the activity of these cells, or it may be due to the lack of sufficient costimulatory signals that maintain host immune cell activation. This downregulation in activity of tumor antigen-specific immune effector cells is referred to as *tolerance*. One proposed mechanism for tolerance induction is illustrated in Figure 19-1.[8] For vaccine strategies to become effective, these issues of tumor antigen identification, antigen escape, and tolerance are a few of many challenges that need to be resolved.

Passive Immunotherapy

First, we address some of the passive immunotherapy approaches that have been used against colorectal cancer. A classic passive immunotherapy approach involves the administration of antitumor antibodies. Table 19-1 shows a synopsis of some of these modalities. Antibodies that are specific for tumor antigens can elicit antitumor activity in a number of ways. First, the Fc (nonbinding, free terminus) regions of tumor-specific antibodies might be able to bind complement and facilitate lysis of tumor cells, or they may result in opsonization and tumor cell destruction. Some antibodies are designed to cross-link tumor cells and native T cells in circulation to result in more efficient antigen encounter and possible activation by native T cells.

A final class of antibodies, referred to as *T bodies*, have variable regions that are specific for tumor antigens and Fc regions that act as cytosolic T-cell activation domains. These T bodies can bind tumor antigens and then intercalate into the membranes of T cells, triggering a cascade that results in T-cell activation. Figure 19-2 depicts some of the different antibody-mediated, passive immunity strategies.[4] In clinical practice, a few of these strategies have been used in human trials. Some of these human trials have involved the use of mAB 17-1A (edrecolomab), an antibody that targets Ep-CAM, an epithelial cell adhesion molecule. Edrecolomab causes cell death by complement-dependent cytotoxicity (CDC) and antibody-dependent

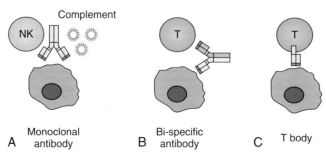

Figure 19-2. Antibody-mediated immunotherapeutic strategies of passive immunity. Mechanisms of antitumor activity exploited by immunotherapy approaches based on monoclonal antibodies (mAbs) and their structural derivatives. mABs directed against tumor antigens (**A**) can opsonize tumor cells and promote their elimination either by activation of cellular immune effectors such as natural killer (NK) cells (antibody-dependent cell-mediated cytoxicity [ADCC]) or by activation of the complement cascade (complement-dependent cytotoxicity [CDC]). Bi-specific antibodies (**B**) are chimeric antibodies whose two binding domains recognize two different antigens: bi-specific antibodies directed against the CD3 molecule and a surface tumor antigen that can cross-link T cells with tumor cells, triggering T-cell activation and tumor cell killing. T bodies (**C**) are chimeric receptors composed of antibody-derived variable regions joined to signaling subunits of antigen receptors (i.e., T-cell receptors); T bodies can be used to redirect T-cell cytotoxicity against antibody-defined tumor antigens and are currently developed for adoptive immunotherapy approaches. (From Dalerba P, Maccalli C, Casati C, et al: Immunology and immunotherapy of colorectal cancer. Crit Rev Oncol Hematol 36[1]:33–57, 2003, Figure 4.)

cellular cytotoxicity (ADCC).[9] Riethmüller and colleagues[10] published the 7-year results of a prospective, randomized trial in which 189 patients with resected Dukes C colorectal cancer were assigned to receive either vaccination with mAB 17-1A or no additional therapy. At 7 years, administration of the antibody therapy reduced overall mortality and recurrence rates by 32% and 23%, respectively.

Not all studies with mAB 17-1A have been so promising, however. In contrast, in another large study reported by Punt and colleagues,[11] 2761 patients with stage III colon cancer were assigned to receive either adjuvant 5-fluorouracil (5-FU) and folinic acid alone or in combination with edrecolomab. The authors reported no difference in 3-year overall survival, but surprisingly they found that the patients who received the antibody therapy had a higher incidence of cancer recurrence. There have also been a number of other smaller studies investigating the use of edrecolomab alone or in combination with chemotherapy and/or cytokines such as granulocyte macrophage colony-stimulating factor (GM-CSF) or IL-2. Some of these studies showed no therapeutic benefit, whereas others showed partial regression of tumors in patients with advanced metastatic cancers. The data in these smaller studies are by no means definitive, and they have to be weighed against the potential toxicities of the drug including allergic infusion reactions to the antibody.[12-16]

An even more complex passive immunotherapy technique that has been tested in humans is adoptive immunotherapy. In adoptive immunotherapy, active immune cells are administered to host with cancer. Initial attempts at the treatment of cancer focused on the adoptive transfer of non–tumor antigen-specific T cells stimulated in vitro. Several human trials have been conducted using various immune effector cell lines and stimulatory agents. In some of the early experiments carried out by Rosenberg and colleagues,[17,18] lymphocytes were stimulated in vitro with IL-2 and then transferred to patients with various gastrointestinal cancers. Initially, the data suggested that the transfer of these "lymphokine-activated killer cells" (LAKs) might confer a survival benefit to patients with malignancy when administered along with systemic doses of IL-2. Later experiments revealed that the benefit of administering non–tumor antigen-specific lymphokine-activated killer cells was no greater than that of administering IL-2 alone.[17,18]

In one small phase I/II French series, monocytes from 15 patients with colorectal cancer were isolated, cultured, and stimulated in vitro with interferon-γ (IFN-γ). These activated monocytes were then readministered. In the 14 patients who were followed up, no significant clinical responses were noted.[19] A similar treatment regimen was administered to nine patients with advanced colorectal cancer in a phase I German trial. These patients were treated with an infusion of autologous monocytes that had been cultured with IFN-γ and lipopolysaccharide in vitro. One of these nine patients had stabilization of previously progressive disease for 12 weeks.[20] Given these rather disappointing results with adoptive transfer of nonspecific immune effectors, emphasis shifted toward the adoptive transfer of effector cells, which might be more specific for the tumors they were targeted against. One such strategy focuses on the adoptive transfer of activated tumor-infiltrating lymphocytes (TILs) isolated ex vivo from resected cancer specimens. Rosenberg and Dudley[21] have demonstrated dramatic clinical responses in some patients with advanced metastatic melanoma who have been treated with adoptive transfer of TILs expanded in vitro with IL-2 and administered after myeloablative chemotherapy.

The adoptive transfer of TILs is well described for melanoma[22] (Fig. 19-3) The data regarding its efficacy in the treatment of colorectal cancer are more limited. In a nonrandomized, prospective study published by Gardini and colleagues,[23] 47 patients with colorectal cancer hepatic metastases underwent surgical hepatic resection. Fourteen patients received adjuvant infusion of IL-2-activated TILs isolated from their surgical specimens, and 14 received adjuvant chemotherapy. The remaining 19 patients received no additional therapy. No difference in disease-free or overall survival was seen at 1, 3, and 5 years. In another Italian study, nine patients with advanced colorectal cancer were treated with adoptive immunotherapy of IL-2-stimulated TILs along an infusional course of systemic IL-2. An additional 19 patients were treated with the same treatment regimen after surgical resection of their metastases to increase the ratio of TILs to solid tumor cells. No major treatment effects were seen in patients who did not undergo surgical resection of their disease. In 8 of the 19 patients who underwent surgical resection, 8 remained disease-free at a median follow-up time of 21 months.[24]

Although adoptive transfer of TILs has traditionally been thought of as a passive immunotherapy approach, it is possible that adoptive transfer may also result in active immunity. Rosenberg and colleagues[25] have shown that tumor-specific TILs can ultimately reconstitute the host recipient's native immune system (immediately following nonmyeloablative che-

motherapy regimen) so that up to 75% of the circulating CD8 T cells are antigen specific. It is possible that these cells could produce a "recall" response if additional tumor cells were encountered at a later date (an active response). Most recently, it has been shown that CD4 cells can also be adoptively transferred, resulting in regression of established tumor burden (melanoma) in at least one human subject.[26] Since CD4 T-cells are critical mediators of active immunity, adoptive transfer techniques may someday be capable of generating sustained, adaptable, long-term immune responses.

Active Immunotherapy

Nonspecific Strategies

In addition to passive immunotherapy strategies and adoptive immunotherapy strategies, another area of intensive research is active immunotherapy techniques. Some of the earliest efforts to treat colorectal cancer involved active nonspecific techniques. The results of the National Surgical Adjuvant Breast and Bowel Project (NSABP) Protocol C-01 were presented in 1988. In this study, 166 patients with Dukes B and C carcinoma of the colon who were entered into NSABP C-01 between November 1977 and February 1983 were randomized to one of three therapeutic categories: (1) no further treatment after curative resection ($n = 394$); (2) postoperative chemotherapy consisting of 5-FU, semustine, and vincristine ($n = 379$); or (3) postoperative Bacillus Calmette-Guérin [BCG], an inactivated form of tuberculosis ($n = 393$). BCG is a potent, nonspecific immune adjuvant that has been studied as a possible therapeutic agent in the treatment of various cancers for many years. It has even been found to be effective in treating transitional carcinoma of the bladder.[27] The initial results of the NSABP C-01 study were published in 1988. At 5 years of follow-up, patients treated with surgery alone had a 1.29 times greater risk of developing a treatment failure and a 1.31 times greater likelihood of dying, as did similar patients treated with combination adjuvant chemotherapy. Comparison of the BCG-treated group with the group treated with surgery alone indicated no statistically significant difference in disease-free survival ($P = .09$). It is interesting that adjuvant treatment with BCG alone did result in an overall survival

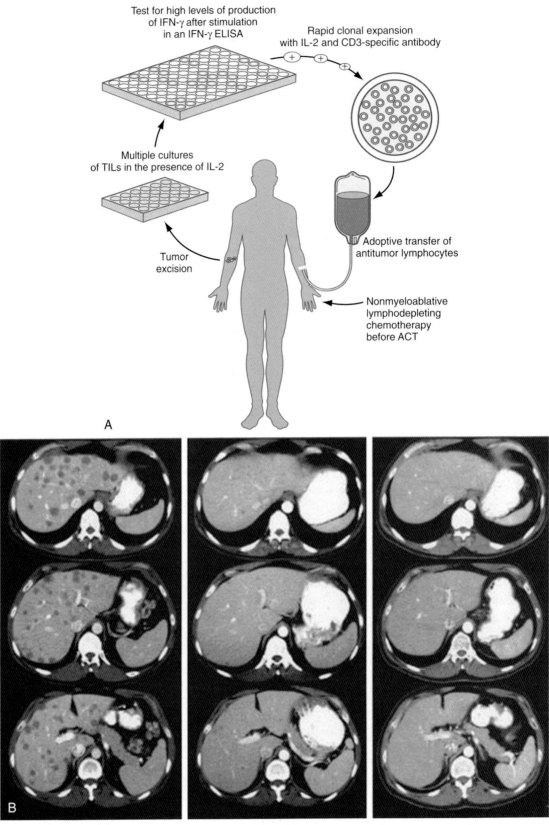

Test for high levels of production
of IFN-γ after stimulation
in an IFN-γ ELISA

Rapid clonal expansion
with IL-2 and CD3-specific antibody

Multiple cultures
of TILs in the presence of IL-2

Tumor
excision

Adoptive transfer of
antitumor lymphocytes

Nonmyeloablative
lymphodepleting
chemotherapy
before ACT

A

B

Pretreatment   1 month   18 months

Figure 19-3. Adoptive immunotherapy (described in melanoma). **A,** Adoptive cell therapy (ACT) requires the generation of highly avid tumor antigen-reactive T cells. Tumor-specific T cells, derived from tumor-infiltrating lymphocytes (TILs), can be efficiently isolated ex vivo from melanoma lesions using high levels of interleukin-2 (IL-2). TILs are successively selected for their ability to secrete high levels of interferon-γ (IFN-γ) when cultured with autologous or allogeneic major histocompatibility complex–matched tumor cell lines. Alternatively, cell-mediated lysis has been used to identify tumor-reactive T cells for transfer. Highly avid, tumor antigen-reactive T-cell populations selected for ACT are rapidly expanded (up to 10^{11} cells) using CD3-specific antibody, exogenously supplied IL-2, and irradiated allogeneic peripheral blood mononuclear "feeder" cells; these are validated for activity before transfer. Patients now receive systemic immunosuppression before the adoptive transfer of antitumor lymphocytes. Published lymphodepleting regimens consist of a nonmyeloablative, but lymphodepleting, conditioning chemotherapy comprising cyclophosphamide and fludarabine before administration of T cells. Newer, as yet unpublished, regimens also include total body irradiation. **B,** Computed tomography scans of the liver in a patient with metastatic melanoma show dramatic tumor regression of liver metastases after the administration of tumor-reactive TILs after lymphodepletion. The patient is still disease-free after 27 months. (**A** and **B** from Gattinoni L, Powell DJ Jr, Rosenberg SA, Restifo NP: Adoptive immunotherapy for cancer: building on success. [Review]. Nat Rev Immunol 6(5):383–393, 2006, Figures 1 and 2. Copyright © 2006 Nature Publishing Group.)

advantage when compared with that for surgery alone. This survival advantage was attributed to a decrease in the number of non–cancer-related deaths. When only cancer-specific survival was evaluated, then adjuvant BCG therapy offered no advantage over surgery alone.[28] The 10-year follow-up of this study was also recently published—with more intriguing results. At 10 years, the patients randomized to surgery and chemotherapy had no significant increase in overall survival. When the surgery-alone cohort was compared with the group who received surgery and BCG, it was found that BCG significantly increased overall 10-year survival rates. This improvement in overall survival appeared to be due to a smaller number of cardiac-related deaths rather than to a decrease in deaths after recurrent colon cancer.[29] A number of other large, prospective randomized trials have cast doubt on the efficacy of BCG as adjuvant therapy for colorectal cancer after resection. These trials included the Veterans Administration Surgical Oncology Group study ($n = 204$), the Gastrointestinal Tumor Study Group trial ($n = 621$), the Southwest Oncology Group trial ($n = 626$), and a Canadian study done at the Cross Cancer Institute ($n = 253$), which all failed to demonstrate any benefit to adding adjuvant BCG, either as a single agent or in combination with chemotherapy.[30-33]

In addition to BCG, other nonspecific immune adjuvants that have been investigated include systemic IL-2, IFN-α, and IFN-γ. All these nonspecific, cytokine-based adjuvant treatment strategies have proved to be ineffective in the treatment of colorectal cancer. Also, many of these cytokine regimens carry significant toxicities, especially when administered in high doses.[34-42]

Specific Immunotherapy

Unlike active nonspecific immunotherapy strategies such as treatment with BCG, active specific immunotherapy generates selective immune responses against specific tumor antigens. In addition to generating a short-term response against cancer cells, successful active specific immunotherapy strategies should generate sustained, long-term "immunity" in the future against tumors with the same antigenic makeup. During the 1990s, a number of vaccination strategies to generate active specific immune responses against colon cancer were investigated. One of these strategies was the use of whole cell tumor vaccines.[4] In this technique, autologous or cultured tumor cells are irradiated so that they are no longer viable and capable of proliferating, and they are administered to patients as a vaccine (most often as a subcutaneous injection). As the irradiated tumor cells die, they shed antigens and prime the immune system. This may result in an antigen-specific, antitumor immune response. Most often, these whole cell tumor vaccines are administered with some form of nonspecific, immunostimulatory agent, such as cytokines or BCG. This nonspecific immunostimulatory adjuvant is added to ensure that the tumor antigens shed by the vaccines are encountered in an inflammatory context that facilitates immune activation against these antigens. Otherwise, the antigens might be ignored by the immune system.[2] This is a fundamentally different strategy than that of administering active nonspecific adjuvants, such as BCG alone, without the vaccine and its associated antigens. Following some of the initial interest in using BCG alone in treatment of colon cancer, it was then tested as costimulatory adjuvant along with autologous, irradiated, whole cell colonic tumor cells administered as a subcutaneous vaccine.

In one early study, 24 patients whose colon cancers were resected received intradermal vaccinations of irradiated cells derived from their surgical resection specimens along with intradermal BCG. Sixteen of the 24 (67%) vaccinated patients demonstrated delayed cutaneous hypersensitivity (DCH) reactions when rechallenged with a subcutaneous injection of their own irradiated tumor cells. These patients did not exhibit DCH responses when challenged with subcutaneous experimental control injections of autologous cells derived from normal mucosal tissues. Furthermore, no significant DCH responses against autologous tumor or mucosa cells were detected in a group of nonimmunized control patients.[43]

Another small, randomized trial published by the same group suggested that there might be a clinical benefit to therapy with autologous colon cancer vaccines along with BCG. In this study, patients with colorectal cancer who had transmural extension of their primary tumor or nodal metastases were randomized to treatment by resection alone (control) or resection plus vaccine and BCG therapy. With a mean follow-up of 28 months at the time the results were reported (range 14–24), only 3 of 20 treatment patients had recurrences and none had died, whereas 9 of 20 control patients had recurrences and 4 died.[44] These results led to bigger clinical trials.

To date, three major phase III trials have tested the efficacy of autologous whole tumor cell vaccines administered with intradermal BCG. In the first trial, published in 1993, 98 patients with Dukes B2-C3 colon and rectal adenocarcinoma were randomized to receive either resection alone or resection and immunotherapy. All rectal cancer patients also received pelvic radiation. Eight patients ultimately met eligibility criteria for the study, and the final data analysis revealed no clinical benefit with the addition of immunotherapy to surgical resection. When a cohort analysis was done that excluded the rectal cancer patients (who all received radiation), however, a significant improvement in overall survival ($P = .02$) and disease-free survival ($P = .039$) was noted in all eligible colon cancer patients who received adjuvant immunotherapy.[45]

A larger, prospective study published in 1999 showed that adjuvant autologous, whole cell vaccination along with BCG conferred a significant recurrence-free survival advantage to patients with stage II colon cancer compared with those with surgery alone (42% risk reduction for recurrence or death, $P = .032$). A trend toward improved overall survival was also noted, but this was not statistically significant ($P = .14$). No benefit was noted for patients with stage III disease.[46] The results of a separate phase III trial were reported in 2000. In this series, 297 patients with stage II colon cancer and 115 patients with stage III colon cancer were assigned to receive either surgery alone or surgery followed by autologous tumor vaccine and BCG. After a median follow-up of 7.6 years, no significant difference was noted in recurrence-free or overall survival between the control and treatment groups. The authors conducted a subset analysis of the patients and evaluated clinical outcomes in patients who were compliant with all of their postoperative vaccinations and who also demonstrated significant DCH responses (indicative of induced cell-mediated immunity). In these vaccine- and BCG-treated patients, there was a trend toward increased disease-free survival ($P = .078$) and overall survival ($P = .12$), which did not reach statistical significance.[47]

In addition to BCG, a number of other immunostimulatory adjuvants have been tested along with whole tumor vaccines in small phase I studies, including IL-2, *Mycobacterium phlei* cell wall and *Salmonella minnesota* lipid A, IFN-1a, IL-7, and GM-CSF.[48–51] Although some of these studies have been promising, none has convincingly demonstrated a clinical benefit. In summation, although clinical trials with autologous whole cell tumor vaccines have provided some tantalizing data that suggest that these vaccines may confer a clinical benefit to certain subsets of patients (e.g., those with minimal residual disease who complete immunotherapy and have good DCH responses), the data have not been convincing enough to justify their use in preference to the standard treatments available today.

Anti-idiotype Antibodies

In addition to autologous whole cell vaccines, other vaccination strategies are being investigated for the treatment of colorectal cancer. Autologous whole cell vaccines are difficult and expensive to generate because every patient must have his or her tumor individually manufactured into a vaccine. The expense and effort for such an endeavor are prohibitive. Cultured whole cell vaccines generated from a human cell line might be considered as an alternative to the expensive autologous vaccines strategy, but cultured cells might not have the same antigen profile as the patient's own tumor. One novel method of active immunotherapy is the use of anti-idiotype antibodies. Although mABs have previously been discussed in this chapter as a form of *passive* immunotherapy, mABs should not be confused with anti-idiotype antibodies, which generate *active, specific* antitumor responses in the host. The anti-idiotype antibody strategy is a clever one that can be used when the immunodominant antigen of a tumor is not known. To make an anti-idiotype antibody, a mouse (mouse A) is injected with a human colorectal cancer. The animal can then generate many antibodies against this foreign human cancer's multiple unidentified antigens. In simple terms, mouse A forms antibodies directed against multiple tumor antigen epitopes. The variable domains of the antitumor antibodies contain "mirror images" of these tumor antigen epitopes. If the antibodies from mouse A are isolated and then injected into a second mouse with a different genotype (mouse B), then new antibodies (anti-idiotype antibodies) are formed in mouse B that are directed against epitopes in the variable region of mouse A's antibodies, thus forming a "mirror image of a mirror image" and resembling the original tumor antigen epitope. If the anti-idiotype antibodies are humanized and injected into the original patient with the tumor, then the human should mount a T-cell– and B-cell–mediated immune response against the mouse epitopes in the humanized antibody. Because these epitopes are morphologically identical to the epitopes of the tumor antigens in the patient, immune responses will also be directed against tumor

epitopes in the host. This process is better summarized in Figure 19-4 (keep in mind that this figure is a simplified graphic illustration of a complex process and that the anti-idiotype antibodies that form are specific for small epitopes and not entire, large surface proteins).

Foon and colleagues[52] generated anti-idiotype antibodies against the well-known colorectal cancer antigen CEA (CeaVac). Thirty-two patients with resected Dukes B, C, and D, and incompletely resected Dukes D disease were treated with 2 mg of CeaVac every other week for four injections and then monthly until tumor recurrence or progression. Fourteen of these 32 patients also received concurrent 5-FU-based chemotherapy. All 32 patients developed high titers of immunoglobulin G and T-cell responses against CEA. No definitive clinical benefit was achieved this study, although several patients with advanced, completely resected Dukes D disease remained in the study from 12 to 33 months postoperatively.

In another recently published phase III trial, 630 patients with previously untreated metastatic colorectal cancer were randomized in a 2:1 fashion to receive bolus 5-FU and leucovorin (LV) plus either a novel anti-CEA idiotype antibody 3H1 ($n = 422$) or placebo ($n = 208$). Seventy percent of the patients who received the vaccine generated immune responses against CEA. There was no statistically significant improvement in overall survival in patients who received vaccine compared with placebo, but when the subset of patients who had an induced immune response against CEA was analyzed, there was a suggestion that a survival advantage might exist.[53]

Anti-idiotype antibody vaccine trials against other colorectal cancer antigens such as Ep-CAM and CD55 have also been conducted. In one interesting study done in the United Kingdom, 35 patients with colorectal cancer were vaccinated before surgical resection with an anti-idiotype antibody vaccine that was almost identical to an anti-CD55 vaccine. The study showed that vaccination resulted in increased tumor infiltration by CD4 cells and natural killer cells.[54] Although many studies have documented that patients generate immune response after receiving anti-idiotype antibodies, it is unclear whether these agents truly confer a survival benefit. More prospective trials are needed to definitively answer this question.[55-59]

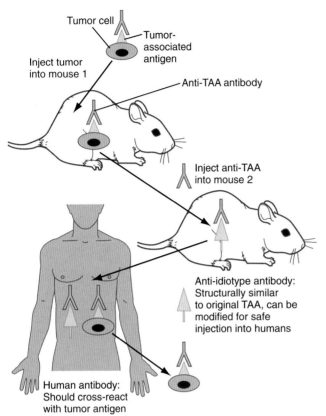

Tumor cell

Tumor-associated antigen

Inject tumor into mouse 1

Anti-TAA antibody

Inject anti-TAA into mouse 2

Anti-idiotype antibody: Structurally similar to original TAA, can be modified for safe injection into humans

Human antibody: Should cross-react with tumor antigen

Figure 19-4. Anti-idiotype antibodies for treatment of cancer.   Tumors express tumor-associated antigens (TAA) not recognized by the host immune system. Tumor cells can be injected into mice to generate anti-TAA antibodies. These anti-TAA antibodies can be injected into a second line of mice to generate anti-idiotype antibodies that contain similar epitopes as the tumor antigen. They can be modified (humanized) for safe injection into the tumor-bearing host. The immune response elicited by injecting this foreign antibody may generate cross-reactivity with the host's own cancer cells.

In addition to anti-idiotype antibodies, a number of other active, specific vaccination strategies are in development. As we have discussed, simply generating a pool of tumor-specific effector cells in a host with cancer does not ensure that antitumor activity and cancer regression will result. These cells must remain activated rather than becoming tolerized for antitumor effects to be maintained. This is the basis for adding immunostimulatory adjuvants to autologous whole tumor cell vaccines.

Other investigators have taken a different approach to overcoming this obstacle. Vaccines constructed from engineered, nonreplicating canarypox viruses have been tested in humans in phase I trials. These engineered vaccines express the colorectal cancer antigen CEA along with a costimulatory molecule B7-1. When T cells encounter tumor antigens with B7-1 costimulation, the resulting signal cascade that occurs should favor activation of the T cell rather than tolerance. In this small trial, three cohorts of six patients, each with advanced colorectal cancers, were treated with escalating doses of vaccine. Three of these patients devel-

oped clinically stable disease, and their T cells showed elevated secretion of IFN-γ in-vitro (indicative of increased activation) when stimulated by CEA peptide. This suggests that the modified viral vaccines were able to generate CEA-specific, T-cell–mediated antitumor responses in subject patients.[60]

Dendritic Cells

One of the exciting new frontiers in the development of tumor vaccines is the use of dendritic cells. The term *dendritic cell* refers to a complex group of immune effector cells that are capable of maturation, differentiation, migration, and antigen presentation. In addition to presenting antigens, dendritic cells can mediate antigen-specific immune responses via T-cell, B-cell, and natural killer cell pathways. We have only begun to understand the complex immune cascades mediated by dendritic cells, some of which result in immune system activation and others that result in tolerance, depending on the context in which the dendritic cells present antigens to immune effectors. Nevertheless, a significant body of evidence suggests that dendritic cells may be a powerful tool for inducing antitumor responses in cancer patients.[61] Dendritic cell vaccines have been studied extensively in melanoma patients. We have earlier stated that many melanoma antigens have already been identified, and tumor antigen peptides have been synthesized in vitro. Tumor antigen peptides or even whole tumor lysates are loaded onto empty MHC-I and MHC-II receptors on dendritic cells in vitro, and these cells are then administered as vaccines to melanoma patients along with a stimulatory adjuvant.[62]

In one benchmark study reported by Nestle and colleagues,[63] dendritic cells pulsed with tumor lysates were administered to 16 patients with advanced melanoma. DCH responses were seen in all patients in response to re-challenge with a tracer peptide that had been added to the vaccine. In addition, 11 of 16 patients exhibited continued DCH responses to booster vaccines with the dendritic cells, suggesting successfully established T-cell–mediated immunity. Peptide-specific cytotoxic lymphocytes were found to migrate into the sites of vaccination, and clinical responses were seen in 5 of the 16 patients (two complete responses, three partial responses) with regression of metastases in various organs (skin, soft tissue, lung, pancreas). Since this report, numerous other studies have suggested that peptide-pulsed dendritic cell vaccines may be effective in treating melanoma.[64–66] Most of these trials have been small phase I or phase II trials, and larger studies are needed. Work with dendritic cell vaccine in the treatment of colorectal cancer is still largely in the preclinical phase. In murine models, dendritic cell vaccines have been shown to induce antitumor responses.[67–69] The experimental evidence in humans to date has mainly been limited to studies of antitumor activity of dendritic cell vaccines against cultured human tumor cell lines in vitro.[70]

Immunotherapy and Metastases

Finally, immunotherapy has also been investigated as a means of addressing one of the most challenging clinical problems associated with colon cancer, which is the high incidence of hepatic metastases. Colorectal cancer often first presents at an advanced stage, and the most common site of metastasis is to the liver. Treatment options for colorectal cancer hepatic

metastases include surgical resection, ablation, and chemotherapy, but even with these techniques, 5-year survival rates range only from 30% to 40%. Recurrence of disease after surgical resection is typically attributed to incomplete removal of residual microscopic disease.[71,72] This residual microscopic disease makes an ideal target for immunotherapy strategies. Several varieties of immunotherapy have been attempted in the treatment of colorectal cancer hepatic metastases. Some interesting attempts in the 1990s used CEA-specific, radiolabeled mABs to localize small, occult colorectal cancer metastases. The occult metastases that were imaged by the radiolabeled CEA-specific antibodies were then treated with focused external radiation or direct hyperthermia with limited success.[73,74]

Nonspecific immunotherapy techniques have also been used to treat unresectable liver metastases. In one report, 75 patients with advanced cancer (including 48 patients with colorectal cancer) were treated with nonspecific therapies: either the cytokine IFN-γ or the cytokine tumor necrosis factor (TNF) followed by a course of OK-432, a biological adjuvant derived from *Streptococcus pyogenes*. OK-432 does not have the toxic properties of *Streptococcus* but it still has immunostimulatory properties as a foreign antigen. Partial responses were seen in 17% of the colorectal cancer patients, and patients with liver lesions who received more than five courses of this nonspecific therapy were found to have increased survival compared with that of control patients.[75]

Other nonspecific therapies that have been tested with limited success in the treatment of colorectal cancer hepatic metastases include administration of IL-2, IFN-β, and TNF.[35,76,77] Specific forms of immunotherapy have also been tested in the treatment of colorectal cancer hepatic metastases, but most have focused on treatment of large-volume unresectable disease. Although data on the treatment of hepatic micrometastases in animal models are extensive, data on the efficacy of immunotherapy in the treatment of hepatic micrometastases in humans are very limited. As previously mentioned, micrometastases might be the ideal target for adjuvant vaccine strategies, since low tumor burden might be easier to treat and induce less tolerization of vaccine-activated immune effectors. Some phase I and II dendritic cell vaccine trials have been conducted in humans with resected colorectal cancer hepatic metastases. Data from one trial conducted at Duke University have shown that dendritic cell vaccines can induce delayed type hypersensitivity–type immune responses at injection sites and in the peripheral blood. They are also safe to administer.[78]

Conclusion

"Immunotherapy" is actually a broad-based field that uses a number of different strategies to use the immune system to eradicate cancer. Some of these strategies use passive immunity; others nonspecifically activate immune effector cells. The methods that offer the greatest promise in the treatment of colon cancer are those that focus on generating tumor-specific, sustained, and reproducible activation of the immune system against host cancer cells. To date, none of these experimental treatments has proved more effective than conventional surgery, chemotherapy, or radiation. The preliminary data from a number of clinical trials are encouraging, however, and it may be that immunotherapy strategies need to be tested in a context in which they offer the greatest clinical advantage. This may involve focusing on treatment of micrometastatic rather than gross disease, and it may also involve targeting of immune responses in the liver, the most common organ of colorectal cancer metastasis.

References

1. American Cancer Society: Cancer Facts & Figures. Atlanta: American Cancer Society, 2006.
2. Laheru DA, Jaffee EM: Potential role of tumor vaccines in GI malignancies. Oncology (Williston Park, NY) 14(2):245–256; discussion 259–260, 265, 2000.
3. Zacharski LR, Sukhatme VP: Coley's toxin revisited: immunotherapy or plasminogen activator therapy of cancer? J Thromb Haemost 3(3):424–427, 2005.
4. Dalerba P, Maccalli C, Casati C, et al: Immunology and immunotherapy of colorectal cancer. Crit Rev Oncol Hematol 46(1):33–57, 2003.
5. Vandeneynde BJ, Vanderbruggen P: T cell defined tumor antigens. Curr Opin Immunol 9:684–693, 1997.
6. Hinoi T, Loda M, Fearon ER: Silencing of CDX2 expression in colon cancer via a dominant repression pathway. J Biol Chem 278(45):44608–44616, 2003.
7. Fearon ER, Jones PA: Progressing toward a molecular description of colorectal cancer development. FASEB J 6(10):2783–2790, 1992.
8. Greten TM, Jaffee EF. Cancer vaccines. Clin Oncol 17(3):1047–1060, 1999.
9. Harris M: Monoclonal antibodies as therapeutic agents for cancer. Lancet Oncol 5(5):292–302, 2004.
10. Riethmüller G, Holz E, Schlimok G, et al: Monoclonal antibody therapy for resected Dukes' C colorectal cancer: seven-year outcome of a multicenter randomized trial. J Clin Oncol 16(5):1788–1794, 1998.
11. Punt C, Nagy A, Douillard J, et al: Edrecolomab alone or in combination with fluorouracil and folinic acid in the adjuvant treatment of stage III colon cancer: a randomised study. Lancet 360:671–677, 2002.
12. Hartung G, Hofheinz RD, Dencausse Y, et al: Adjuvant therapy with edrecolomab versus observation in stage II colon cancer: a multicenter randomized phase III study. Onkologie 28(6–7):347–350, 2005.
13. Fiedler W, Kruger W, Laack E, et al: A clinical trial of edrecolomab, interleukin-2 and GM-CSF in patients with advanced colorectal cancer. Oncol Rep 8(2):225–231, 2001.
14. Liljefors M, Ragnhammar P, Nilsson B, et al: Anti-EpCAM monoclonal antibody (MAb17-1A) based treatment combined with alpha-interferon, 5-fluorouracil and granulocyte-macrophage colony-stimulating factor in patients with metastatic colorectal carcinoma. Int J Oncol 25(3):703–711, 2004.
15. Makower D, Sparano JA, Wadler S, et al: A pilot study of edrecolomab (Panorex, 17-1A antibody) and capecitabine in patients with advanced or metastatic adenocarcinoma. Cancer Invest 21(2):177–184, 2003.
16. Hjelm Skog A, Ragnhammar P, Fagerberg J, et al: Clinical effects of monoclonal antibody 17-1A combined with granulocyte/macrophage-colony-stimulating factor and interleukin-2 for treatment of patients with advanced colorectal carcinoma. Cancer Immunol Immunother 48(8):463–470, 1999.
17. Rosenberg SA, Lotze MT, Muul LM, et al: A progress report on the treatment of 157 patients with advanced cancer using lymphokine-activated killer cells and interleukin-2 or high-dose interleukin-2 alone. N Engl J Med 316(15):889–897, 1987.
18. Rosenberg SA, Lotze MT, Yang JC, et al: Prospective randomized trial of high-dose interleukin-2 alone or in conjunction with lymphokine-activated killer cells for the treatment of patients with advanced cancer. J Natl Cancer Inst 85(8):622–632, 1993.
19. Eymard JC, Lopez M, Cattan A, et al: Phase I/II trial of autologous activated macrophages in advanced colorectal cancer. Eur J Cancer 32A(11):1905–1911, 1996.
20. Hennemann B, Beckmann G, Eichelmann A, et al: Phase I trial of adoptive immunotherapy of cancer patients using monocyte-derived macrophages activated with interferon gamma and lipopolysaccharide. Cancer Immunol Immunother 45(5):250–256, 1998.
21. Rosenberg SA, Dudley ME: Cancer regression in patients with metastatic melanoma after the transfer of autologous antitumor lymphocytes. Proc Natl Acad Sci U S A 101(Suppl 2):14639–14645, 2004.
22. Gattinoni L, Powell DJ Jr, Rosenberg SA, Restifo NP: Adoptive immunotherapy for cancer: building on success. Nat Rev Immunol 6(5):383–393, 2006.
23. Gardini A, Ercolani G, Riccobon A, et al: Adjuvant, adoptive immunotherapy with tumor infiltrating lymphocytes plus interleukin-2 after radical hepatic resection for colorectal liver metastases: 5-year analysis. J Surg Oncol 87(1):46–52, 2004.
24. Fabbri M, Ridolfi R, Maltoni R, et al: Tumor infiltrating lymphocytes and continuous infusion interleukin-2 after metastasectomy in 61 patients with melanoma, colorectal and renal carcinoma. Tumori 86(1):46–52, 2000.
25. Rosenberg SA, Restifo NP, Yang JC, et al: Adoptive cell transfer: a clinical path to effective cancer immunotherapy. Nat Rev Cancer 8(4):299–308, 2008.
26. Hunder NN, Wallen H, Cao J, et al: Treatment of metastatic melanoma with autologous CD4+ T cells against NY-ESO-1. N Engl J Med 358(25):2698–2703, 2008.
27. Shelley MD, Court JB, Kynaston H, et al: Intravesical Bacillus Calmette-Guerin in Ta and T1 bladder cancer. Cochrane Database Syst Rev (4):[CD001986], 2000.
28. Wolmark N, Fisher B, Rockette H, et al: Postoperative adjuvant chemotherapy or BCG for colon cancer: results from NSABP protocol C-01. J Natl Cancer Inst 80(1):30–36, 1988.
29. Smith RE, Colangelo L, Wieand HS, et al: Randomized trial of adjuvant therapy in colon carcinoma: 10-year results of NSABP protocol C-01. J Natl Cancer Inst 96(15):1128–1132, 2004.
30. Higgins GA, Donaldson RC, Rogers LS, et al: Efficacy of MER immunotherapy when added to a regimen of 5-fluorouracil and methyl-CCNU following resection for carcinoma of the large bowel. A Veterans Administration Surgical Oncology Group report. Cancer 54(2):193–198, 1984.
31. Adjuvant therapy of colon cancer—results of a prospectively randomized trial. Gastrointestinal Tumor Study Group. N Engl J Med 310(12):737–743, 1984.

32. Panettiere FJ, Goodman PJ, Costanzi JJ, et al: Adjuvant therapy in large bowel adenocarcinoma: long-term results of a Southwest Oncology Group Study. J Clin Oncol 6(6):947–954, 1988.

33. Abdi EA, Hanson J, Harbora DE, et al: Adjuvant chemoimmuno- and immunotherapy in Dukes' stage B2 and C colorectal carcinoma: a 7-year follow-up analysis. J Surg Oncol 40(3):205–213, 1989.

34. Rosenberg SA: Karnofky Memorial Lecture. The immunotherapy and gene therapy of cancer. J Clin Oncol 10:180–199, 1992.

35. Barni S, Lissoni P, Ardizzola A, et al: Immunotherapy with low-dose subcutaneous interleukin-2 plus beta-interferon as a second-line therapy for metastatic colorectal carcinoma. Tumori 79(5):343–346, 1993.

36. Douillard JY, Bennouna J, Vavasseur F, et al: Phase I trial of interleukin-2 and high-dose arginine butyrate in metastatic colorectal cancer. Cancer Immunol Immunother 49(1):56–61, 2000.

37. Palmeri S, Meli M, Danova M, et al: 5-Fluorouracil plus interferon alpha-2a compared to 5-fluorouracil alone in the treatment of advanced colon carcinoma: a multicentric randomized study. J Cancer Res Clin Oncol 124(3–4):191–198, 1998.

38. Thirion P, Piedbois P, Buyse M, et al: Alpha-interferon does not increase the efficacy of 5-fluorouracil in advanced colorectal cancer. Br J Cancer 84(5):611–620, 2001.

39. Chang AE, Cameron MJ, Sondak VK, et al: A phase II trial of interleukin-2 and interferon-alpha in the treatment of metastatic colorectal carcinoma. J Immunother Emphasis Tumor Immunol 18(4):253–262, 1995.

40. Piga A, Cascinu S, Latini L, et al: A phase II randomised trial of 5-fluorouracil with or without interferon alpha-2a in advanced colorectal cancer. Br J Cancer 74(6):971–974, 1996.

41. Wiesenfeld M, O'Connell MJ, Wieand HS, et al: Controlled clinical trial of interferon-gamma as postoperative surgical adjuvant therapy for colon cancer. J Clin Oncol 13(9):2324–2329, 1995.

42. O'Connell MJ, Ritts RA Jr, Moertel CG, et al: Recombinant interferon-gamma lacks activity against metastatic colorectal cancer but increases serum levels of CA 19-9. Cancer 63(10):1998–2004, 1989.

43. Hoover HC Jr, Surdyke M, Dangel RB, et al: Delayed cutaneous hypersensitivity to autologous tumor cells in colorectal cancer patients immunized with an autologous tumor cell: Bacillus Calmette-Guerin vaccine. Cancer Res 44(4):1671–1676, 1984.

44. Hoover HC Jr, Surdyke MG, Dangel RB, et al: Prospectively randomized trial of adjuvant active-specific immunotherapy for human colorectal cancer. Cancer 55(6):1236–1243, 1985.

45. Hoover HC Jr, Brandhorst JS, Peters LC, et al: Adjuvant active specific immunotherapy for human colorectal cancer: 6.5-year median follow-up of a phase III prospectively randomized trial. J Clin Oncol 11(3):390–399, 1993.

46. Vermorken JB, Claessen AM, van Tinteren H, et al: Active specific immunotherapy for stage II and stage III human colon cancer: a randomised trial. Lancet 353(9150):345–350, 1999.

47. Harris JE, Ryan L, Hoover HC Jr, et al: Adjuvant active specific immunotherapy for stage II and III colon cancer with an autologous tumor cell vaccine: Eastern Cooperative Oncology Group Study E5283. J Clin Oncol 18(1):148–157, 2000.

48. Tarasov VA, Filatov MV, Kisliakova TV, et al: Combined surgical and immunotherapeutic treatment of patients with fourth stage colon cancer. Hybridoma 18(1):99–102, 1999.

49. Woodlock TJ, Sahasrabudhe DM, Marquis DM, et al: Active specific immunotherapy for metastatic colorectal carcinoma: phase I study of an allogeneic cell vaccine plus low-dose interleukin-1 alpha. J Immunother 22(3):251–259, 1999.

50. Sobol RE, Shawler DL, Carson C, et al: Interleukin 2 gene therapy of colorectal carcinoma with autologous irradiated tumor cells and genetically engineered fibroblasts: a Phase I study. Clin Cancer Res 5(9):2359–2365, 1999.

51. Wittig B, Marten A, Dorbic T, et al: Therapeutic vaccination against metastatic carcinoma by expression-modulated and immunomodified autologous tumor cells: a first clinical phase I/II trial. Hum Gene Ther 12(3):267–278, 2001.

52. Foon KA, John WJ, Chakraborty M, et al: Clinical and immune responses in resected colon cancer patients treated with anti-idiotype monoclonal antibody vaccine that mimics the carcinoembryonic antigen. J Clin Oncol 17(9):2889–2895, 1999.

53. Chong G, Bhatnagar A, Cunningham D, et al: Phase III trial of 5-fluorouracil and leucovorin plus either 3H1 anti-idiotype monoclonal antibody or placebo in patients with advanced colorectal cancer. Ann Oncol 17(3):437–442, 2006.

54. Durrant LG, Maxwell-Armstrong C, Buckley D, et al: A neoadjuvant clinical trial in colorectal cancer patients of the human anti-idiotypic antibody 105AD7, which mimics CD55. Clin Cancer Res 6(2):422–430, 2000.

55. Herlyn D, Wettendorff M, Schmoll E, et al: Anti-idiotype immunization of cancer patients: modulation of the immune response. Proc Natl Acad Sci U S A 84:8055–8059, 1987.

56. Mittelman A, Chen ZJ, Yang H, et al: Human high molecular weight melanoma-associated antigen (HMW-MAA) mimicry by mouse anti-idiotypic monoclonal antibody MK2-23: induction of humoral anti-HMW-MAA immunity and prolongation of survival of patients with stage IV melanoma. Proc Natl Acad Sci U S A 89:466–470, 1992.

57. Magliani W, Polonelli L, Conti S, et al: Neonatal mouse immunity against group B streptococcal infection by maternal vaccination with recombinant anti-idiotypes. Nat Med 4:705–709, 1998.

58. Chatterjee SK, Tripathi PK, Chakraborty M, et al: Molecular mimicry of carcinoembryonic antigen by peptides derived from the structure of an anti-idiotype antibody. Cancer Res 58:1217–1224, 1998.

59. Ruiz P, Wolkowicz R, Waisman A, et al: Idiotypic immunisation induces immunity to mutant p53 and tumor rejection. Nat Med 4:710–712, 1998.

60. Horig H, Lee DS, Conkright W, et al: Phase I clinical trial of a recombinant canarypoxvirus (ALVAC) vaccine expressing human carcinoembryonic antigen and the B7.1 co-stimulatory molecule. Cancer Immunol Immunother 49(9):504–514, 2000.

61. Nestle FO, Farkas A, Conrad C: Dendritic-cell-based therapeutic vaccination against cancer. Curr Opin Immunol 17(2):163–169, 2005.

62. Kim CJ, Dessureault S, Gabrilovich D, et al: Immunotherapy for melanoma. Cancer Control 9(1):22–30, 2002.

63. Nestle FO, Alijagic S, Gilliet M, et al: Vaccination of melanoma patients with peptide- or tumor lysate-pulsed dendritic cells. Nat Med 4(3):328–332, 1998.

64. Thurner B, Haendle I, Roder C, et al: Vaccination with mage-3A1 peptide-pulsed mature, monocyte-derived dendritic cells expands specific cytotoxic T cells and induces regression of some metastases in advanced stage IV melanoma. J Exp Med 190(11):1669–1678, 1999.

65. Bancherau J, Palucka AK, Dhodapkar M, et al: Immune and clinical responses in patients with metastatic melanoma to CD34(+) progenitor-derived dendritic cell vaccine. Cancer Res 61(17):6451–6458, 2001.

66. Hersey P, Menzies SW, Halliday GM, et al: Phase I/II study of treatment with dendritic cell vaccines in patients with disseminated melanoma. Cancer Immunol Immunother 53(2):125–134, 2004.

67. DeMatos P, Abdel-Wahab Z, Vervaert C, Seigler HF: Vaccination with dendritic cells inhibits the growth of hepatic metastases in B6 mice. Cell Immunol 185(1):65–74, 1998.

68. Heckelsmiller K, Beck S, Rall K, et al: Combined dendritic cell- and CpG oligonucleotide-based immune therapy cures large murine tumors that resist chemotherapy. Eur J Immunol 32(11):3235–3245, 2002.

69. Wu Y, Wan T, Zhou X, et al: Hsp70-like protein 1 fusion protein enhances induction of carcinoembryonic antigen-specific CD8+ CTL response by dendritic cell vaccine. Cancer Res 65(11):4947–4954, 2005.

70. Nair SK, Morse M, Boczkowski D, et al: Induction of tumor-specific cytotoxic T lymphocytes in cancer patients by autologous tumor RNA-transfected dendritic cells. Ann Surg 235(4):540–549, 2002.

71. Knol J: Colorectal cancer metastasis to the liver: hepatic arterial infusion chemotherapy. In Cameron JL (ed): Current Surgical Therapy, 6th ed. Philadelphia: Mosby, 1998, pp 355–361.

72. Jain A, Slansky JE, Matey LC, et al: Synergistic effect of a granulocyte-macrophage colony-stimulating factor-transduced tumor vaccine and systemic interleukin-2 in the treatment of murine colorectal cancer hepatic metastases. Ann Surg Oncol 10(7):810–820, 2003.

73. Mittal BB, Zimmer MA, Sathiaseelan V, et al: Phase I/II trial of combined 131I anti-CEA monoclonal antibody and hyperthermia in patients with advanced colorectal adenocarcinoma. Cancer 78(9):1861–1870, 1996.

74. Meredith RF, Khazaeli MB, Plott WE, et al: Phase II study of dual 131I-labeled monoclonal antibody therapy with interferon in patients with metastatic colorectal cancer. Clin Cancer Res 2(11):1811–1818, 1996.

75. Kato M, Shinohara H, Goto S, et al: Clinical experience of EET therapy for 75 advanced cancer patients. Anticancer Res 18(5D):3941–3949, 1998.

76. Lillis PK, Brown TD, Beougher K, et al: Phase II trial of recombinant beta interferon in advanced colorectal cancer. Cancer Treat Rep 71(10):965–967, 1987.

77. IJzermans JN, Scheringa M, van der Schelling GP, et al: Injection of recombinant tumor necrosis factor directly into liver metastases: an experimental and clinical approach. Clin Exp Metastasis 10(2):91–97, 1992.

78. Morse MA, Nair SK, Mosca PJ, et al: Immunotherapy with autologous, human dendritic cells transfected with carcinoembryonic antigen mRNA. Cancer Invest 21(3):341–349, 2003.

79. Veronese ML, O'Dwyer PJ: Monoclonal antibodies in the treatment of colorectal cancer. Eur J Cancer 40(9):1292–1301, 2004.

20

Genetic Profiling in Colorectal Cancer

Debashish Bose and Nita Ahuja

KEY POINTS

- Genetic profiling is the attempt to classify disease states by the molecular characteristics of tumor tissue or non-tumor tissue. Molecular characteristics include features of the tissue at the chromosomal level (karyotypic features) as well as features of the tissue at the nucleotide level (point mutations or variation of sequences) and nucleotide-modification level (epigenetic features).

- A genetic profile is a mathematical construct by which a particular set of features is linked with a clinical pattern in a statistically meaningful way. This includes linking profiles to diagnosis, prognosis, response to therapies, and identification of novel pathogenetic mechanisms.

- Genetic techniques have identified polyposis syndromes in families and kindred groups who are predisposed to colorectal cancer. This has allowed screening of patients and their family members for early or aggressive disease that can be treated before the development of advanced disease.

- Microsatellite instability, a characteristic of DNA at the chromosomal level, is the basis for the classification of some colorectal cancers into categories such as microsatellite instability "high" (MSI-H), microsatellite instability "low" (MSI-L), and microsatellite stable (MSS). This information is relevant to the screening implica-

tions for the patient and family, as well as for the clinical pattern of a patient's disease.

- Molecular lesions in individual genes have been associated with patterns of disease progression, response to therapy, and prognosis. Molecular characterization of patients' cancers may allow us to tailor therapy based on the genetic profile.

- Microarray technology reveals expression data for potentially many thousands of genes at once in a given tissue. Although data on individual genes can be obtained from the data, it is more important that patterns of expression can be recognized.

- Information and computing technology have made possible the development of molecular profiles using microarrays. Millions of operations are required to identify an expression pattern and link the pattern to a statistically definable clinical group. A critical appreciation of microarray data requires an understanding of statistical and computational methods.

- The TailoRx trial using the Oncotype Dx chip seeks to determine whether specific profiles can be used to effectively manage early-stage breast disease. Similar work has been done in Europe with the Mammaprint technology. These studies can serve as templates for further trials in other areas such as colorectal cancer to answer important clinical questions.

Introduction

Genetic profiling represents one way in which molecular methods are brought to the bedside in human disease. Loosely defined, "genetic profiling" has been applied to a variety of ways in which investigators have attempted to characterize tissues, disease, or individuals in a genetically meaningful way. The term itself implies that a particular disease state is characterized by a set of genetic lesions that is consistent across individuals with similar clinical disease and with similar tumor behavior. As a consequence,

genetic profiling has the potential to distinguish subsets of individuals with disease that is otherwise broadly categorized according to "gross" clinical features, thereby offering a basis for the clinical differences observed among patients thought otherwise to have the same disease.

The project of creating genetic profiles involves the molecular characterization of large groups of individuals and/or tissue samples and then discerning patterns in the information gathered. Analysis of the data has been enormously advanced by recruiting statistics, computing, and bioinformatics methods to the enterprise of pattern recognition and validation of the profiles created. In this chapter, we discuss the genetic profiling of colorectal cancer with a specific focus on high-throughput technologies, their potential and current applications, and the future of genetic profiling in our understanding and management of colorectal cancer. This chapter presupposes some familiarity on the reader's part with the basic models of the development of colorectal cancer, but some of the classic methods of genetic analysis are discussed as they relate to the basic assumptions upon which newer methods of analysis rely.

Types of Genetic Profiling

Genetic Analysis

Although most colorectal cancer is understood as sporadic, up to 5% is thought to result from inherited genetic lesions (see Chapter 3), and another 10% to 15% of colorectal cancers may have a familial predisposition.[1] The identification of such familial syndromes of colorectal cancer as Lynch syndrome, Gardner syndrome, Peutz-Jeghers syndrome, and juvenile polyposis syndrome has contributed to our understanding of disease. Familial adenomatous polyposis (FAP) and hereditary nonpolyposis colorectal carcinoma (HNPCC) were identified initially from pedigree analysis, as are many heritable diseases[2,3] (see Chapter 3 for further details). Conventional techniques such as linkage analysis were ultimately combined with molecular techniques to identify specific genes involved in the transmission of these diseases, but a thorough understanding of family history remains the mainstay

of screening patients for familial cancer syndromes. Thus, the Amsterdam criteria remain an important means of identifying HNPCC patients and their families (Table 20-1), who have an underlying genetic defect in the mismatch repair genes and also display microsatellite instability. The Amsterdam criteria, as revised, include non-colorectal tumors as well, reflecting a broader understanding of HNPCC, whereas the Bethesda criteria identify patients with HNPCC who should undergo further molecular characterization to look for microsatellite instability.[4,5]

Cytogenetic Analysis

Cytogenetics refers to "gross" chromosomal analysis, in which lesions such as large deletions are detected and initial genetic mapping is carried out. Techniques in chromosomal analysis include G-band analysis, fluorescence in situ hybridization (FISH), and comparative genomic hybridization (CGH) among others. Indeed, the initial involvement of the *p53* and *DCC* genes was discovered on the basis of chromosomal studies on the 17p and 18q loci, respectively. These investigations subsequently led to the recognition of microsatellite instability as a marker of chromosomal aberrations that incur loss of tumor suppressor gene activity.[6-8] Table 20-2 lists some chromosomal alterations associated with the development and progression of colorectal cancer that were identified in early studies of the progression of colorectal tumorigenesis. The initial adenoma-carcinoma progression model of colorectal cancer has now evolved further into models that recognize differences in

Table 20-1. Amsterdam and Bethesda Criteria for Hereditary Nonpolyposis Colorectal Cancer

Amsterdam I	Three relatives with colorectal cancer *and* all of the following: One first-degree relative of the other two Two or more generations At least one individual diagnosed before age 50 Not FAP
Amsterdam II	Expanded inclusion criteria to tumors of endometrium, stomach, ovary, ureter/renal pelvis, brain, small bowel, hepatobiliary, and skin (sebaceous)
Bethesda	Test for microsatellite instability (MSI) when: 1. Diagnosis of CRC in age <50 2. Presence of synchronous or metachronous HNPCC lesions 3. CRC in patient < age 60 with MSI-specific pathology 4. CRC in one or more first-degree relatives with HNPCC lesions and < age 50 5. CRC in two or more first- or second-degree relatives with HNPCC lesions, regardless of age

CRC, colorectal cancer, FAP, familial adenomatous polyposis; HNPCC, hereditary nonpolyposis colon cancer.

Table 20-2. Classic Chromosome Alterations Associated with Colorectal Cancer

Chromosome	Alteration	Role in Carcinogenesis
5q21	*APC* gene mutation/loss	Early event in adenoma-carcinoma sequence; induces degradation of β-catenin
12p	KRAS mutation	Middle event in adenoma-carcinoma sequence; growth promotion through MAP kinases
17p	*p53* gene deletion	Late event in adenoma-carcinoma sequence; G1 cell cycle arrest, induction of apoptosis
18q	*DCC* gene deletion	Late event in adenoma-carcinoma sequence; transmembrane protein that interacts with netrin
31q	β-catenin mutation/loss	Possible alternate germline mutation in familial adenomatous polyposis, target of APC activity, growth promoter when active form accumulates

the sequence and character of genetic lesions apparent in different subsets of colorectal cancer. Most important, cytogenetic analysis has clearly identified two pathways in which genetic instability occurs: (1) the microsatellite instability (MIN) pathway and (2) the chromosomal instability (CIN) pathway. Each pathway has a specific and different complexion of genetic lesions with chromosomal instability pathway tumors carrying multiple gross chromosomal lesions versus an accumulation of more subtle mutations in microsatellite instability pathway cancers.[9]

Classical Molecular Analysis

Concurrent with genetic and cytogenetic analysis, numerous investigations into the molecular biology of colorectal cancer have enriched our understanding of the disease process, but initially at the individual gene level in what can now be described as the "classical" molecular biology era. Newtonian in approach, the project of identifying genes that play a role in disease revolved mainly around the identification of mutations in individual genes that then had to (1) be associated with a disease state with some degree of specificity, (2) satisfy the rules of causality (e.g., Koch's postulates), and (3) be reliably attributed with some pathogenetic feature in terms of diagnosis, prognosis, or response to treatment, and so on. The result in the field of colorectal cancer is the now classic description of the stepwise progression to cancer of Vogelstein and colleagues[10] (Fig. 20-1). Such studies were critical to the development of the technical capacity to study mutations and gene expression in a "quantum" fashion. The estab-

lishment of cDNA libraries, the cataloging of expressed sequence tags (ESTs) and the use of serial analysis of gene expression (SAGE), subtractive hybridization, and polymerase chain reaction (PCR) techniques remain ways in which molecular biology allows the investigation of a multitude of genes. Aside from the genes listed in Table 20-2, other genes discovered to have pathogenetic roles in colorectal cancer include members of the matrix metalloprotease family of proteins, *p16*, *SMAD4*, *c-src*, phosphatidylinositol-3-kinase, and epidermal growth factor receptor family members, to name but a few.[11-17] Individually, some of these genes have been identified as prognostic in terms of survival, response to therapy, presence of metastatic disease, and other clinical characteristics in small retrospective studies. Identification of robust biomarkers for determining cancer prognosis and recurrence remains one of the core goals of genetic profiling.

Microarray Analysis

Microarray analysis of gene expression has developed into a powerful tool for the characterization of many pathophysiologic processes. The basic idea is that RNA isolated from tissue is hybridized to probes for specific genes that are fixed in a grid in small microscopic spots. Figure 20-2 provides a schematic that shows a typical arrangement of a microarray. Depending on the design of the experiment, the signal intensity of the hybridization is normalized to internal controls and other tissues to yield a result for each gene that tells the investigator whether a particular gene has an increased, decreased, or normal expression. The result for the sample, then, is an

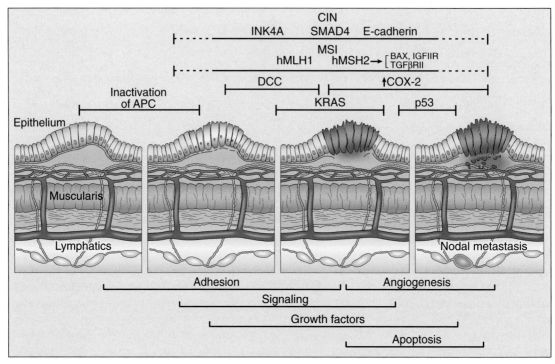

Figure 20-1. Adenoma-to-carcinoma sequence and the associated molecular alterations involved in colon cancer development. CIN, chromosomal instability; MSI, microsatellite instability. (From Abeloff MD, Armitage JO, Niederhuber JE, et al: Abeloff's Clinical Oncology, 4th ed. Philadelphia: Churchill Livingstone, 2008, Fig. 81-2.)

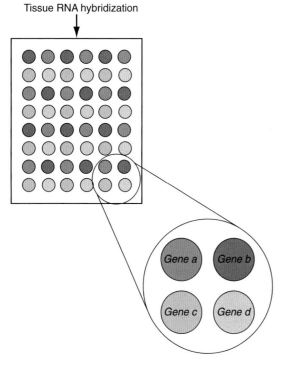

Tissue RNA hybridization

Figure 20-2. Schematic depiction of a microarray chip. Nucleotide oligomer probes specific to genes being interrogated are adhered to the chip in a grid. Sample mRNA converted to cDNA by reverse transcription-polymerase chain reaction is hybridized to the chip and the attached probes. The amount of hybridization is then analyzed by comparison to reference hybridization, with the relative amount of hybridization indicated colorimetrically on the chip.

answer for each gene included in the microarray as to whether the gene is up- or downregulated; the composite data represent a gene expression profile for the sample. When a large number of samples are thus tested, depending on the experimental design, the use of microarrays makes possible the establishment of gene expression profiles for any given disease state, the comparison of subsets to determine molecular predictors of clinical behavior, and so on (Fig. 20-3). As the technology has advanced, the sophistication of microarray analysis has likewise provided increasingly powerful ways of discriminating the molecular characteristics of disease states, including the identification of methylation status of genes (an epigenetic modification of expression) and alternative splicing.[18-20]

In colorectal cancer studies, microarray studies have provided a great deal of data in terms of genetic profiles. Table 20-3 provides a partial list of studies that identified expression profiles that correlate with features of disease that the studies were designed to query.[18-34] Some studies are listed to highlight molecular subsets that may be clinically significant. The table illustrates the use of microarray analysis to ask critical questions, including primary site of origin, prognosis, response to therapy, methylation status, and even diagnosis. Microarray analysis also exhibits particular robustness in that a properly designed and validated array can be derived from the analysis of a relatively small number of probes. This is hoped to make microarray analysis a potentially low-cost and easily reproducible assay that could be readily put into clinical practice.

The cost of development of microarray assays is relatively high in the case of colorectal cancer and requires a large investment before the establishment of clinical significance. First,

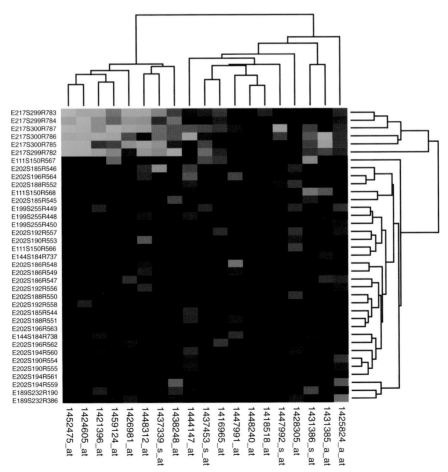

Figure 20-3. Heat map generated by relative up- or downregulation of genes. (Available at http://en.wikipedia.org/wiki/Image:Heatmap.png; originally created by Miguel Andrade.)

as a surgical and oncologic disease, the development of clinically meaningful assays requires the collection of tissue from surgical specimens and subsequent long-term follow-up on a large number of patients. Some of this cost may be mitigated by developing assays using existing tissue banks and patient databases, but *expression* analysis may be problematic if significant mRNA degradation has occurred in banked specimens. Second, after validation and testing (see text that follows), the assay must be supported by a clinical trial that demonstrates its value to the management of patients. Until a specific microarray assay emerges as particularly significant in the potential management of colorectal carcinoma, we will not be able to specifically perform cost-benefit analysis, but, under the assumption that improved patient care and selection for treatment will result, an overall savings would be expected. Such analysis

has been performed for the use of microarray analysis in breast cancer.[35]

Practical Issues in Genetic Profiling

Applications of Genetic Profiling

As Table 20-3 illustrates, numerous applications are possible for genetic profiling. Identification of individuals at risk, diagnosis, prognosis, tumor aggressiveness, and prediction of response to therapy can be achieved through genetic profiling. Expression profiles are also a powerful basic science tool in the investigation of disease at the cellular level. Cardoso and colleagues[36] have nicely summarized the results of a comprehensive review of profiling studies in colorectal cancer in terms of adenoma-carcinoma progression, markers of poor prognosis, differences between tumors with chromosomal instability

Table 20-3. Studies in Gene Profiling of Colorectal Cancer

Author (Year)	Query	Result
Croner et al (2005)[21]	Normal mucosa versus carcinoma	Differentiation based on 23 genes
Gardina et al (2006)[19]	Validation of alternative splicing assay and expression	Identification of cancer-specific alternative splicing and differential expression of genes involved in cell motility
Friederichs et al (2005)[22]	Expression profiles and progression	Identification of profiles associated with progression and systemic vs. lymphatic metastasis
Mori et al (2004)[23]	Expression and methylation profile of MSI-H tumors	Identification of specific hypermethylation of RAB32, hMLH1
Banerjea et al (2004)[24]	MSI-H vs MSS tumors	Higher expression of proinflammatory genes in MSI-H tumors
Barrier et al (2006)[25]	Prognosis in stage II patients	30-gene profile predictive of disease free survival
Zou et al (2002)[28]	Cancer vs normal mucosa	250 differentially expressed genes
Barrier et al (2007)[27]	Prognosis in stage II patients using non-neoplastic sample	70 differentially expressed genes correlate with disease free survival
Mori et al (2003)[30]	MSS vs MSI-H vs MSI-L tumors	Microarray data distinguish MSI-L as a distinct subset of MSI tumors
Matsuyama et al (2006)[29]	Response to 5-FU	Three-gene profile predictive of response
Eschrich et al (2005)[31]	Prognosis	43-gene set predictive of 36 month survival, better than Dukes' staging
Sui et al (2006)[32]	Profiling preneoplastic mitochondrial DNA	Array analysis of mtDNA feasible and may provide screen for preneoplastic lesions of GI tract
Glebov et al (2003)[33]	Right vs left colon	Expression differences between right and left colon confirmed by expression profile
Suzuki et al (2002)[34]	Array analysis of methylated genes	Methylation-dependent expression distinctly assayed
Schuebel et al (2007)[20]	Array analysis of methylated genes	Genome wide analysis of genes that are methylated and compares this to range of mutational events

5-FU, 5-fluorouracil; MSI-H, microsatellite instability-high; MSI-L, microsatellite instability-low; MSS, microsatellite stable.

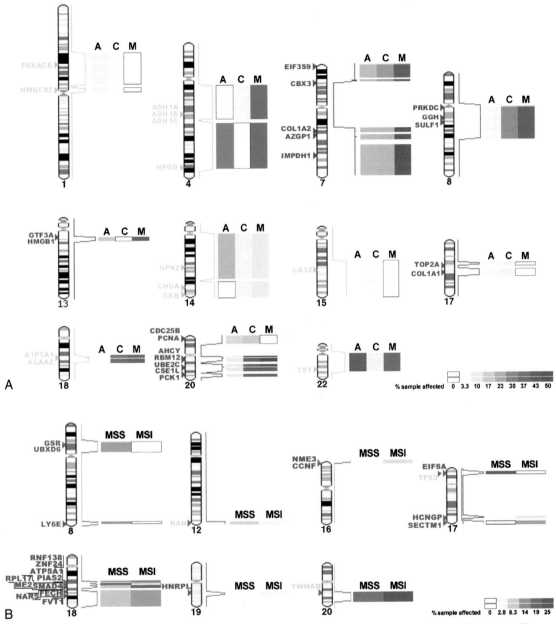

Figure 20-4. Molecular events associated with the adenoma-carcinoma sequence on colorectal cancer. (From Cardoso J, Boer J, Morreau H, Fodde R: Expression and genomic profiling of colorectal cancer. Biochim Biophys Acta 1775:103–137, 2007, Fig 1.)

versus microsatellite instability, response to therapy, and progression to metastasis (Fig. 20-4). Genetic profiles identified thus far have yet to penetrate common clinical practice because of the need for further validation and variation among studies in terms of technology and analytical methods (see further discussion in following text). As the data derived from these studies become more uniform in their results and interpretation, it is reasonable to expect that genetic profiling of individuals will identify patients at risk and who may benefit from closer surveillance. Subsequent use of expression arrays to analyze biopsy specimens may aid in the detection of field defects in colonic mucosa or polyps that place patients at risk for the development of cancer. Once colorectal cancer has been identified, genetic profiling should aid in management, perhaps even identifying patients that may benefit from neoadjuvant therapy before resection, adjuvant therapy, or increased vigilance after resection.

Information Technology and Genetic Analysis

A primary issue in the use of array data to create genetic profiles arises from variation in the analytical methods and specific technologies used. First, microarrays are not currently standardized across studies. The availability of commercial chips (e.g., Affymetrix, Agilent) opens the possibility of uniform methods in the actual sample analysis. The next step revolves around the ways in which the resulting data are analyzed. To discern patterns in a large amount of information, investigators have recruited techniques from computing and statistics to develop ways of fitting the data from large numbers of samples into meaningful patterns. Typically, this involves using one set of samples as a training set to initially identify profiles that are then tested against a validation set of samples to determine whether the profiles can correctly sort new samples. The validation-testing process may also occur by creating multiple training and validation sets from a limited group of samples by rotation of individual samples in different combinations between training and validation sets and by repeating the process for each permutation thus generated. Insofar as the actual pattern recognition process goes, computing methods typically involve hierarchical clustering, neural networks, and other procedures, which are beyond the scope of this chapter. Puzstai and Hess[37] have recently discussed the basics of the design of microarray trials that aim to identify multigene signatures that have clinical value.

In general, the validation process in large clinical trials remains the most effective means of confirming that a specific profile has value; on the other hand, these supervised studies in which a preconceived pattern is tested against data can lead to an "overfitting" bias in which random data are made to comply with the profile, a pitfall that tends to occur with smaller sample sizes. Unsupervised methods of analysis are available that allow queries of data sets to identify novel patterns, however, and these types of studies have value as an initial step toward the identification of profiles. Ideally, such studies would be additionally validated against new sample sets in the hands of independent investigators.

The recent FDA approval of the Mammaprint (Agendia, Amsterdam, Netherlands) gene expression chip for breast cancer helps to illustrate the practical issues involved in microarray technology.[35,38–40] The Mammaprint assay is a microarray assay developed at the Netherlands Cancer Institute that assigns patients to a low- or high-risk category based on a 70-gene expression profile. The profile was initially developed in a group of node-negative young (under 55) patients with tumors smaller than 5 cm, who either developed distant metastasis within 5 years or stayed disease-free for at least 5 years.[38] The 70-gene profile was developed with a goal of identifying patients at risk for the early development of distant metastases, thereby defining them as high-risk patients who might benefit from systemic therapy. In 295 patients who were young with stage I or II tumors, overall survival and disease-free survival were significantly different for high- and low-risk patients (55% versus 95% 10-year overall survival; 51% versus 85% disease-free survival, respectively), regardless of nodal status.[39] In a European multicenter study of 307 patients with node-negative tumors less than 5 cm and who were younger than 61 years of age, the 70-gene signature outperformed the use of clinicopathologic criteria for risk assessment.[40] The developers of this assay ultimately hope to show that the Mammaprint assay will help eligible patients avoid adjuvant therapy, and a large consortium trial is in the planning stages in Europe—the MINDACT (Microarray In Node negative Disease may Avoid ChemoTherapy) trial.[41]

A similar 21-gene profile has been developed by the National Surgical Adjuvant Breast and Bowel Project (NSABP) and is marketed as Oncotype DX (Genomic Health, Redwood City, California) and is due to undergo a phase III prospective trial known as TailoRx.[42,43] The Recurrence Score, as it is called, not only provides prognostic classification but also specifically predicts that low-risk patients will not benefit from adjuvant chemotherapy.[44] The use of both assays is predicted to be cost-effective in avoiding chemotherapy in low-risk patients.[35,45] As Mammaprint and Oncotype DX stand poised for clinical trial, it will be important to consider whether these assays are (1) better than clinico-pathologic risk assessment in direct prospective comparison for prognosis, (2) able to improve overall and disease-free survival when used to manage patients, and (3) cost-effective in the management of patients with early breast cancer.

The development of these assays represents potential pathways for the development of similar assays in colorectal cancer. Microarray data may identify genetic profiles that help us clarify areas of uncertainty in the management of colorectal cancer. In particular, in stage II colon cancer (i.e., node-negative disease) the groups of patients who may benefit from adjuvant chemotherapy remain to be clearly identified. The project of creating a prognostically valuable gene expression profile has begun in Europe (see Barrier and colleagues[25–27]), and one can anticipate that such a profile could be applied to identify stage II patients who might benefit from adjuvant therapy. Also, some rectal cancers treated with neoadjuvant chemotherapy and radiation that display complete pathologic response may not require resection; a gene profile may be developed to identify this subset as well. Likewise, extension of gene profiling to anticipate chemotherapy responses may also aid in the rational tailoring of specific regimens to individual patients.

A recent study by Arango and colleagues[46] demonstrates the potential benefits and some limitations to future expression profiling studies. These authors used expression profiling to predict recurrence for Dukes' C colorectal cancer patients. The authors used a cohort of Dukes' C patients from the mid 90s before the universal adoption of adjuvant chemotherapy for such patients in order to identify an expression signature that will predict recurrence. The authors had 281 Dukes' C patients among their tissue bank of 1042 patients who had frozen tissue available. Among these 281 patients, only 25 samples had an optimal amount of RNA to perform the expression array. The expression profiling using unsupervised hierarchical clustering showed that tumors with bad prognoses (i.e., recurrence within 5 years) clustered separately from tumors with good prognosis (i.e., no recurrence within 5 years) (Fig. 20-5). Expression profiling was superior to single-gene biomarkers such as K-ras mutation or 18q allelic loss in

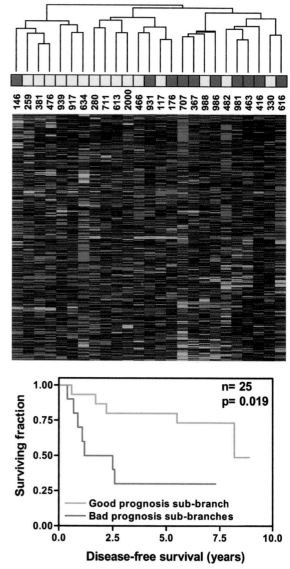

Figure 20-5. Hierarchical clustering. The *top panel* shows how 25 patients with Dukes' C colorectal cancer could be separated according to expression profile, which correlated with recurrence-free survival (*bottom panel*). Such clustering is achieved by creating a statistically generated hierarchy based on the expression profile of each tumor. It is "unsupervised" in that the analysis looks for similarity of the expression profiles to determine the closeness of samples in the hierarchy without bias, that is, the samples are arranged in the hierarchy prior to relating the clusters to clinical behavior. (From Arango D, Laiho P, Kokko A, et al: Gene expression profiling predicts recurrence in Dukes' C colorectal cancer. Gastroenterology 29:874–884, 2005, Fig 1.)

predicting recurrence and survival. One of the genes that was significantly downregulated in the poor prognosis patients was *RHOA*. The authors then validate that downregulation of this one gene was also associated with shorter

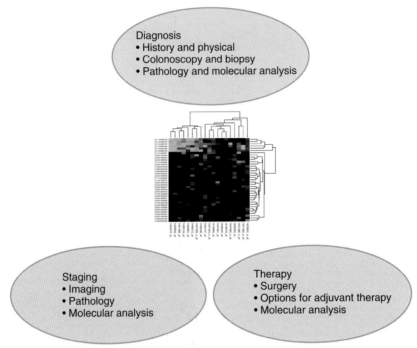

Figure 20-6. Schematic depicting clinical arenas in which genetic profiling of tumors may play an important role.

survival. The study points to the limitations of expression profiling including the need for fresh-frozen cancer sample tissue banks and the inability to perform such a study with current samples on Dukes' C patients in which most patients would have received adjuvant therapy and it would be harder to identify a signature profile.

Future Directions

As surgeons, we anticipate the movement of genetic profiling into the clinical arena in several ways (Fig. 20-6; see Fig. 20-5). Preoperative workup by colonoscopy would be enhanced by the microarray analysis of biopsy specimens in that correlation of specific profiles with specific outcomes would influence decisions regarding the timing and nature of surgery. For example, a patient with synchronous colon and liver lesions may benefit from treatment with chemotherapy before surgery in order to undergo less extensive hepatic resection. Conversely, if such a patient had a tumor genetic profile that was particularly unfavorable, and a poor outcome was inevitable despite surgery, the morbidity and risk of mortality attending surgery might be avoided. Resected specimens could be analyzed in real time during surgery to guide management

as well as postoperatively. Ultimately, genetic profiles may lead to such well-tailored, specific therapies that, with or without resection, patients could be provided with increasingly successful outcomes and disease-free survival.

References

1. Lynch HT, de la Chapelle A: Hereditary colorectal cancer. N Engl J Med 348:919–932, 2003.
2. Lynch HT, Lynch JF: Hereditary non-polyposis colorectal cancer. Semin Surg Oncol 18:305–313, 2000.
3. Leppert M, Burt R, Hughes JP, et al: Genetic analysis of an inherited predisposition to colon cancer in a family with a variable number of adenomatous polyps. N Engl J Med 322: 904–908, 1990.
4. Lackner C, Hoefler G: Critical issues in the identification and management of patients with hereditary non-polyposis colorectal cancer. Eur J Gastroenterol Hepatol 17:317–322, 2005.
5. Ahuja N, Baylin SB: Subclassification of microsatellite-unstable tumors in colorectal cancer. Curr Colorectal Cancer Rep 3(4): 212–219, 2007.
6. Jen J, Kim H, Piantadosi S, et al: Allelic loss of chromosome 18q and prognosis in colorectal cancer. N Engl J Med 331:213–221, 1994.
7. Baker SJ, Fearon ER, Nigro JM, et al: Chromosome 17 deletions and p53 mutations in colorectal carcinomas. Science 244: 217–221, 1989.
8. Fearon ER, Cho KR, Nigro JM, et al: Identification of a chromosome 18q gene that is altered in colorectal cancers. Science 247:49–56, 1990.
9. Lindblom A: Different mechanisms in the tumorigenesis of proximal and distal colon cancers. Curr Opin Oncol 13(1): 63–69, 2001.
10. Vogelstein B, Fearon ER, Hamilton SR, et al: Genetic alterations during colorectal tumor development. N Engl J Med 319: 525–532, 1988.

11. Toyota M, Ohe-Toyota M, Ahuja N, et al: Distinct genetic profiles in colorectal tumors with or without the CpG island methylator phenotype. Proc Natl Acad Sci 97:710–715, 2000.

12. Gayet J, Shou X-P, Duval A, et al: Extensive characterization of genetic alterations in a series of human colorectal cancer cell lines. Oncogene 20:5025–5032, 2001.

13. Wagenaar-Miller RA, Gorden L, Matrisian LM: Matrix metalloproteinases in colorectal cancer: is it worth talking about? Cancer Metastasis Rev 23:119–135, 2004.

14. Takayama T, Miyanishi K, Hayashi T, et al: Colorectal cancer: genetics of development and metastasis. J Gastroenterol 41:185–192, 2006.

15. Weitz J, Koch M, Debus J, et al: Colorectal cancer. Lancet 365:153–165, 2005.

16. Zhou S, Kinzler K, Vogelstein B: Going mad with SMADs. N Engl J Med 341:1144–1146, 1999.

17. Woodford-Richens KL, Rowan AJ, Gorman P, et al: SMAD4 mutations in colorectal cancer probably occur before chromosomal instability, but after divergence of the microsatellite instability pathway. Proc Natl Acad Sci 98:9719–9723, 2001.

18. Kimura N, Nagasaka T, Murakami J, et al: Methylation profiles of genes using newly developed CpG island methylation microarray on colorectal cancer patients. Nucleic Acids Res 33:e46, 2005.

19. Gardina PJ, Clark TA, Shimada B, et al: Alternative splicing and differential gene expression in colon cancer detected by a whole genome exon array. BMC Genom 7:325, 2006.

20. Schuebel K, Chen W, Cope L, et al: Comparing the DNA hypermethylome with gene mutations in human colorectal cancer. PLoS Genet 3(9):1709–1723, 2007.

21. Croner RS, Foertsch R, Brueckl WM, et al: Common denominator genes that distinguish colorectal carcinoma from normal mucosa. Int J Colorectal Dis 20:353–362, 2005.

22. Friederichs J, Rosenberg R, Mages J, et al: Gene expression profiles of different clinical stages of colorectal carcinoma: toward a molecular genetic understanding of tumor progression. Int J Colorectal Dis 20:391–402, 2005.

23. Mori Y, Yin J, Sato F, et al: Identification of genes uniquely involved in frequent microsatellite instability colon carcinogenesis by expression profiling combined with epigenetic scanning. Cancer Res 64:2434–2438, 2004.

24. Banerjea A, Ahmend S, Hands RE, et al: Colorectal cancers with microsatellite instability display mRNA expression signatures characteristic of increased immunogenicity. Molecular Cancer 3:21, 2004.

25. Barrier A, Boëlle P-Y, Roser F, et al: Stage II colon cancer prognosis prediction by tumor gene expression profiling. J Clin Oncol 24:4685–4691, 2006.

26. Barrier A, Lemoine A, Boëlle P-Y, et al: Colon cancer prognosis by gene expression profiling. Oncogene 24:6155–6164, 2005.

27. Barrier A, Roser F, Boëlle P-Y, et al: Prognosis of stage II colon cancer by non-neoplastic mucosa gene expression profiling. Oncogene 26(18):2642–2648, 2007.

28. Zou T-T, Selaro FM, Xu Y, et al: Application of cDNA microarrays to generate a molecular taxonomy capable of distinguishing between colon cancer and normal colon. Oncogene 21:4855–4862, 2002.

29. Matsuyama R, Togo S, Shimizu D, et al: Predicting 5-fluorouracil chemosensitivity of liver metastases from colorectal cancer using

30. Mori Y, Selaru FM, Sato F, et al: The impact of microsatellite instability on the molecular phenotype of colorectal tumors. Cancer Res 63:4577–4582, 2003.

31. Eschrich S, Yang I, Bloom G, et al: Molecular staging for survival prediction of colorectal cancer patients. J Clin Oncol 23:3526–3535, 2005.

32. Sui G, Zhou S, Wang J, et al: Mitochondrial DNA mutations in preneoplastic lesions of the gastrointestinal tract: a biomarker for the early detection of cancer. Molecular Cancer 5:73, 2006.

33. Glebov OK, Rodriguez LM, Nakahara K, et al: Distinguishing right from left colon by the pattern of gene expression. Cancer Epidemiol Biomarkers Prev 12:755–762, 2003.

34. Suzuki H, Gabrielson E, Chen W, et al: A genomic screen for genes upregulated by demethylation and histone deacetylase inhibition in human colorectal cancer. Nat Genet 31:141–150, 2002.

35. Oestreicher N, Ramsey SD, Linden HM, et al: Gene expression profiling and breast cancer care: what are the potential benefits and policy implications. Genet Med 7:380–389, 2005.

36. Cardoso J, Boer J, Morreau H, Fodde R: Expression and genomic profiling of colorectal cancer. Biochim Biophys Acta 1775:103–137, 2007.

37. Pusztai L, Hess KR: Clinical trial design for microarray predictive marker discovery and assessment. Ann Oncol 15:1731–1737, 2004.

38. van't Veer LJ, Dai H, van de Vijver MJ, et al: Gene expression profiling predicts clinical outcome of breast cancer. Nature 415:530–536, 2002.

39. van de Vijver MJ, He Y, van't Veer LJ, et al: A gene-expression signature as a predictor of survival in breast cancer. N Engl J Med 347:1999–2009, 2002.

40. Buyse M, Loi S, van't Veer L, et al: Validation and clinical utility of a 70-gene prognostic signature for women with node-negative breast cancer. J Natl Cancer Inst 98:1183–1192, 2006.

41. Bogaerts J, Cardoso F, Buyse M, et al: Gene signatures evaluation as a prognostic tool: challenges in the design of the MINDACT trial. Nat Clin Pract Oncol 3:540–551, 2006.

42. Paik S, Shak S, Tang G, et al: A multigene assay to predict recurrence of tamoxifen-treated, node-negative breast cancer. N Engl J Med 351:2817–2826, 2004.

43. Paik S: Development and clinical utility of a 21-gene recurrence score prognostic assay in patients with early breast cancer treated with tamoxifen. Oncologist 12:631–635, 2007.

44. Paik S, Tang G, Shak S, et al: Gene expression and benefit of chemotherapy in women with node-negative, estrogen receptor-positive breast cancer. J Clin Oncol 24:3726–3734, 2006.

45. Hornberger J, Cosler LE, Lyman GH: Economic analysis of targeting chemotherapy using a 21-gene RT-PCR in lymph-node-negative, estrogen-receptor-positive, early stage breast cancer. Am J Manag Care 11:313–324, 2005.

46. Arango D, Laiho P, Kokko A, et al: Gene expression profiling predicts recurrence in Dukes' C colorectal cancer. Gastroenterology 29:874–884, 2005.

21

Coping with Colorectal Cancer

Eden R. Stotsky

KEY POINTS

- Colon and rectal cancers are among the most common adult cancers worldwide, and the number of survivors of colorectal cancer is likely to increase.
- Colorectal cancer is one of the most common invasive cancers, and it is responsible for considerable physical and psychosocial morbidity.
- After receiving a diagnosis of colorectal cancer, patients normally feel overwhelmed and stressed; however, there are things that the health care provider can suggest to help patients feel better.
- Many resources are available to provide support for cancer patients and their families.

Introduction

Hearing the words "you have cancer" can be devastating for anyone. The good news about colorectal cancer is that 80% to 90% of those diagnosed at stage I or stage II survive more than 5 years. However, when the cancer is diagnosed at stage III, only about 60% to 70% survive more than 5 years. Unfortunately, when cancer is diagnosed at stage IV, only 8.5% reach the 5-year survival milestone. Thanks to advances in the treatment of advanced colorectal cancer and better management of complications associated with disease and therapy, though, patients with this diagnosis are living longer and better, which creates a realistic sense of hope for the future among this patient population.[1]

It is important to realize that the key to survival is early detection and the key to prevention is screening.

Physical and Psychosocial Aspects of Colorectal Cancer

Colorectal cancer is one of the most common invasive cancers. It is responsible for considerable physical and psychosocial morbidity.[2] As part of the study entitled Dimensions of Quality of Life and Psychosocial Variables Most Salient to Colorectal Cancer Patients, a number of focus group participants spoke at length about how they had coped with the experience of colorectal cancer. Some participants said they had made themselves determined to recover and felt that having a positive attitude had been helpful.[2] Patients who had coped with previous traumatic events were able to draw on the strength and coping abilities learned earlier through their experience with cancer.[2] Participants also found that talking openly about their disease and the treatment they had undergone had been helpful. Learning to live with cancer seems to involve both accepting the situation and finding the inner resources to cope.

Another study, Reducing the Unmet Needs of Patients with Colorectal Cancer: A Feasibility Study of The Pathfinder Volunteer Program, discovered that the most common needs of patients concerned the fear of cancer's spreading or returning, the worries of others, changes in weight, changes in bowel habits or bowel movements, and bowel problems such as diarrhea, constipation, and pain.[3]

Patients who are facing life with a colostomy or ileostomy after surgery have serious concerns about how to deal with this situation—both physically and emotionally. It is important to remind such patients that their ostomy is allowing them to survive colorectal cancer and to be able to resume their lives.[4] Whether a patient needs an ostomy depends on the extent of the surgery. This discussion should occur with the patient before surgery, and the patient should meet with an ostomy nurse before surgery to familiarize him- or herself with the stoma and with living with an ostomy. Furthermore, the patient should become familiar with the appearance and location of the stoma, the various ostomy appliances and supplies, two-piece pouch versus one-piece pouch or pouch plate, how to care for the ostomy, how to clean the stoma as well as the skin, the different skin barriers and seals, how to empty the pouch, how to discard the waste, how to attach and reattach the pouch, how to handle the odor as well as the noises and other sensations, and finally how to resume activities.[4] This orientation, for the care of the stoma, may be better handled in the postoperative period once the patient has an ostomy and can really perform the daily care. Patients often find that living with a stoma is easier than they had imagined; reassurance and practical advice are key to a patient's comfort and acceptance of the situation.

It is normal for a patient who has just received a diagnosis of colorectal cancer to feel overwhelmed and stressed. Uncertainty about the future and financial concerns can trigger a number of reactions, including grief. Patients may have trouble sleeping at night, experience body aches and headaches, and just feel exhausted. All are common symptoms of stress. However, there are strategies you can suggest to your patients to help them feel better.

Supportive Strategies

There are many ways to cope with the stress and fear associated with cancer. With education and supportive care, patients should be able to deal with the diagnosis and treatment of their cancer. However, patients who are having intense trouble coping may need more extensive counseling.

The most important advice you can give to your patients is for them to seek help as soon as they feel less able to cope with their cancer. Taking action early enables them to understand and deal with the many effects of their illness. Learning to manage stress helps them maintain a positive physical, emotional, and spiritual outlook on life.

When a patient is facing cancer, stress can build up and affect how he or she feels about life. Prolonged stress can lead to frustration, anger, hopelessness, and, at times, depression. The person with cancer is not the only one affected. Family members also are influenced by the ongoing health changes of a loved one with cancer.

The following tips help patients reduce stress:

- Keep a positive attitude.
- Accept that there are events you cannot control.
- Be assertive rather than aggressive. "Assert" your feelings, opinions, or beliefs rather than becoming angry, combative, or passive.
- Learn to relax.
- Exercise regularly. Your body can fight stress better when you are physically fit.
- Eat well-balanced meals.
- Rest and sleep. Your body needs time to recover from stressful events.
- Don't rely on alcohol or drugs to reduce stress.

Furthermore, patients can perform a number of relaxation exercises. These exercises include specific types of breathing, muscle and mind relaxation, relaxation to music, and biofeedback. First, be sure your patient has a quiet, distraction-free location and that he or she can find a comfortable body position (i.e., sitting or reclining on a chair or sofa). Also, suggest that he or she maintain a positive state of mind and try to block out worries and troubling thoughts. The following are suggestions for stress-relieving exercises for patients.

- *Two-minute relaxation.* Concentrate your thoughts on yourself and your breathing. Take a few deep breaths, exhaling slowly. Mentally scan your body, noticing areas that feel tense or cramped. Loosen up these areas, letting go of as much tension as possible. Rotate your head in a smooth, circular motion once or twice. (If any movement causes pain, stop immediately.) Roll your shoulders forward and backward several times. Relax all your muscles. Recall a pleasant thought for a few seconds. Take another deep breath and exhale slowly. You should now feel relaxed.
- *Mind relaxation.* Close your eyes. Breathe normally through your nose. As you exhale, silently, say to yourself the word "one," a short word such as "peaceful," or a short phrase such as "I feel quiet." Continue for 10 minutes. If your mind wanders, gently remind yourself to think about your breathing and your chosen word or phrase. Let your breathing become slow and steady.
- *Deep-breathing relaxation.* Imagine a spot just below your navel. Breathe into that spot and fill your stomach with air. Let the air fill from the stomach up, then let it out, like deflating

a balloon. With every long, slow exhalation, you should feel more relaxed.

In addition to experiencing emotional distress, colorectal cancer patients experience physical side effects from treatment (surgery, radiation therapy, and chemotherapy). Therefore, it is important for health care providers to address both their emotional and physical concerns.

Perspective and Concerns of the Patient

Sexuality-related Issues

A study entitled Colorectal Cancer Patients' Informational Needs about Sexuality-Related Issues identified and described the importance of providing patients with information about sexuality-related issues during hospitalization.[5] Of the 87 patients who completed the structural questionnaire, 71% reported that their disease or its treatment had affected their sexuality. Effects on sexuality were reported by 77% of men and 64% of women with colorectal cancer. In addition, 75% of respondents younger than 40 and 67% of respondents older than 50 complained about the effect that colorectal cancer has had on their sexuality.[5] Of the total surveyed, 72% stated that it is necessary to discuss the effect of the disease and its treatment on sexuality during hospitalization,[5] and 87% of the patients felt that health care personnel should take the initiative in discussing sexuality-related issues. Only 12% said the initiative should come from the patient.

It is important for health care professionals to provide colorectal cancer patients with an opportunity to discuss issues related to sexuality. The clinician should develop, introduce, and evaluate action models to facilitate open discussion for these sensitive issues.[5]

Age-related Issues

The PAIS-SR (Psychosocial Adjustment to Illness Scale—Self-Report) measurement tool looked at the patient's vocational environment, domestic environment, sexual relationship, extended family environment, social environment, and psychological distress for two groups: seniors (older than 65 years) and non-seniors (younger than 65 years).[6] Psychosocial adjustment was found to differ by life stage only for "psychological distress." However, analysis of background factors related to psychosocial adjustment revealed distinct patterns in each life stage. This study suggests that life stage

should be considered when attempts are made to improve the psychosocial adjustment among cancer patients.[6]

Gender-related Issues

According to a study conducted in Israel— Gender and Psychological Distress among Middle- and Older-Aged Colorectal Cancer Patients and Their Spouses: An Unexpected Outcome—male patients reported higher distress scores than their healthy female partners, whereas healthy male spouses had higher distress scores than their sick wives.[7] Psychological distress is a common and shared symptom among cancer patients and their spouses, and it persists for years in up to 30% of cancer survivors.[7] Psychological interventions involve accurate clinical diagnoses and recognition of and communication of symptomatology by caregivers and patients according to the DSM-IV categorical diagnoses of depression and appropriate pharmacologic recommendations.[7]

For patients, an important part of coping with a diagnosis of colorectal cancer is understanding the medical information given to them. Patients should not be afraid to ask their doctor, nurse, or other health care provider to repeat any instructions or medical terms that they do not understand. By answering the patient's questions and addressing their concerns, the health care provider/clinician provides an important component of the patient's ability to cope with his or her cancer diagnosis.

The health care provider/clinician also should suggest that the patient make use of resources and support services offered by the local hospital as well as those available in the community. Encourage your patients to learn more about their disease, which will help them feel more comfortable with their illness and treatment. Furthermore, encourage them to ask their family and friends to help sort through the information they receive and also to bring a family member or friend to appointments. In addition, encourage your patients to talk with other patients and families about colorectal cancer and its treatment.

Fear of Cancer Recurrence

The fear of cancer recurrence is, to varying degrees, almost universal in cancer survivors.[8] The Fear of Cancer Recurrence Inventory (FCRI) is a multidimensional self-reporting scale for assessing the fear of cancer recurrence (Box 21-1).

Box 21-1. Fear of Cancer Recurrence Inventory (FCRI)

Factor 1: Triggers

Conversations about cancer or illness in general

Seeing or hearing someone who's ill

Television shows or newspaper articles about cancer or illness

Going to a funeral or reading the obituary section of the paper

An appointment with my physician or other health professional

Physical examination (annual check-up, blood tests, x-rays)

When I feel less well physically or when I am sick

Generally, I avoid situation or things that make me think about the possibility of cancer recurrence (PCR)

Factor 2: Severity

How long have you been thinking about the PCR?

How many times per day do you spend time thinking about the PCR?

How often do you think about the PCR?

In your opinion, what is your risk of having a cancer recurrence?

I am afraid of a cancer recurrence

I am worried or anxious about the PCR

I believe that I am cured and the cancer will not come back

I think it's normal to be anxious or worried about the PCR

When I think about PCR, other unpleasant thoughts or images come to mind (death, suffering, consequences for my family)

Factor 3: Psychological Distress

Frustration, anger, or outrage

Sadness, discouragement, or disappointment

Helplessness or resignation

Worry, fear or anxiety

Factor 4: Coping Strategies

I try to replace this thought with a more pleasant one

I try to convince myself that everything will be fine or I think positively

I try to get the idea out of my mind, to not think about it

I try to distract myself (e.g. do various activities, watch TV, read, work)

I try to understand what is happening and to deal with it

I tell myself "stop it"

I pray, meditate, or do relaxation

I try to find a solution

I talk to someone about it

Factor 5: Functioning Impairments

My social or leisure activities (e.g., outings, sports, travel)

My quality of life in general

My ability to make future plans or set life goals

My work or everyday activities

My relationship with my partner, my family, or those close to me

My state of mind or my mood

Factor 6: Insight

I feel that I worry excessively about the PCR

I think that I worry more about the PCR than other people who have diagnoses of cancer

Other people think that I worry excessively about the PCR

Factor 7: Reassurance

I go to the hospital or clinic for an examination

I call my doctor or another health professional

I examine myself to see if I have any physical signs of cancer

From Simard S, Savard J: Fear of Cancer Recurrence Inventory: development and initial validation of a multidimensional measure of fear of cancer recurrence. Support Care Cancer 17:241–251, 2009, Table 2.

The French-Canadian version of the FCRI contains 42 items coherent with the cognitive-behavioral conceptualization that underlined the development of the questionnaire. The FCRI should be used to gain a better understanding of a patient's fear of cancer recurrence.[8]

Types of Cancer Support Resources

Many resources are available to provide support for your cancer patients and their families. Among them are:

Social workers. Social workers are available to patients and their families to discuss concerns they may have about their diagnosis and treatment or about their personal situation. Social workers can provide education, counseling regarding lifestyle changes, and referrals to community or national agencies and support groups. They can also help families find temporary lodging, provide information about community resources, and help with other needs. Social workers are just one part of the caregiving team that can offer treatment in a compassionate setting.

Patient navigators. Patient navigators provide caring individual attention, compassion, and empathy to patients and their families. They are trained to identify clinical needs, issues, and care goals. They also work with all team members to assist with timely and resourceful problem solving for patients and families. Patient navigators also assist patients in overcoming barriers to the timely receipt of health care services.

Individual counseling. Sometimes patients have problems that are better addressed in a one-on-one environment (Fig. 21-1). By participating in individual counseling sessions, patients may more effectively express sensitive or private feelings they have about their illness and its impact on their lifestyle and relationships. Counseling services can help cancer patients and families to do the following:

- Discuss issues of concern
- Develop and enhance coping abilities
- Gain a sense of control
- Enjoy an improved quality of life

In addition, mental health care providers are available to create a treatment plan to meet the specific needs of each patient. Strategies can be designed to help patients regain a sense of control over their lives and improve their quality of life—something everyone deserves. If a patient is depressed, medication for this condition may be prescribed.

Support groups. Participating in support groups can be a very useful sharing experience. Such groups provide an environment in which patients can learn new ways of dealing with their illness. Others who have been through similar experiences may be able to explain things in a different manner from that of health care professionals and clinicians. Patients are also given the opportunity to share with others the approaches that they have

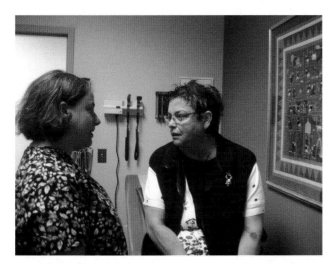

Figure 21-1. Therapeutic communication, the foundation of a healthcare provider-patient relationship, is an important part of helping patients cope with colorectal cancer.

discovered. Patients gain strength in knowing that they are not facing illness alone. Health care workers should remind patients that others may share information or experiences that do not pertain to them and should remind patients never to replace advice from a professional with that from another patient.

Other Considerations After a Diagnosis of Colorectal Cancer

Although no one likes to think about his or her own disability or mortality, it is something that everyone—not just those facing a serious illness such as cancer—should consider. Patients should be encouraged to think about advance directives. There are special documents that describe the patients' wishes regarding their medical care, including the following:

Living will. This document exercises a patient's right to accept or refuse medical treatment that artificially prolongs his or her life. The living will provides clear instructions regarding an individual's choice of extended medical care. It is prepared when a patient is fully competent in case he or she becomes unable to make such decisions at a later time. It is important for the patient to put some thought into developing a living will and think about what hospice and palliative care may offer. Hospice is a special concept of care designed to provide comfort and support to patients and their families when a life-limiting illness no longer responds to cure-oriented treatments. Hospice care neither prolongs life nor hastens death. Hospice staff and volunteers offer a specialized knowledge of medical care, including pain management.

Durable power of attorney for health care. This is a document in which a patient appoints a trusted friend or family member to speak on his or her behalf in the event that the patient becomes incapable of expressing medical treatment preferences. An attorney should create this document so that it conforms to state laws and other legal regulations.

An example of an advance directives information sheet is given in Box 21-2.

In addition, all patients should be encouraged to write a will to ensure that those who survive them will know how to carry out their wishes.

This document should be prepared with an attorney.

Late Effects versus Long-Term Side Effects of Cancer Treatment

Late effects of cancer treatment are side effects that become apparent after treatment has ended. Cancer survivors might experience late effects of cancer treatment a few months after treatment is completed or years later. An example of a late effect is "chemo brain," also known as chemotherapy-related cognitive impairment (CRCI).[9] CRCI is of significant concern to patients.[9] A variety of potential factors associated with CRCI have been identified, including age, education level, intelligence and social support; anxiety, depression, and fatigue; disease site, stage, and comorbidities; treatment regimen, timing, duration, and concomitant therapies; and hormonal levels, cytokine levels, damage to neural progenitor cells, and the presence of the apolipoprotein E 4 allele. Controversy exists as to the most suitable neurocognitive tests to evaluate this sequel of treatment. Neuroimaging techniques are beginning to reveal affected areas of the brain. A neuropsychologist is essential for the assessment, diagnosis, and recommendation of appropriate management strategies for this patient population.[9]

In contrast to late effects, side effects that start during cancer treatment and linger for months or years after treatment are called long-term side effects. Long-term side effects usually are different from late effects. For example, nerve damage (peripheral neuropathy) is common during some types of chemotherapy and may begin during treatment and linger for months or even years after cancer treatment is completed. Most long-term side effects decrease or completely resolve with time.

What Is It Like to Be a Cancer Survivor?

A cancer patient's fear and anxiety do not disappear over time, but they become more manageable. However, most patients do not express unmet needs for supportive care once treatment is finished.[10] Therefore, cancer survivors with unmet needs may benefit from the targeted application of psychosocial resources.

Colon and rectal cancers are among the most common adult cancers, and the number of sur-

Box 21-2. Advance Directives Information Sheet

What You Should Know About Advance Directives

Everyone has the right to make personal decisions about health care. Doctors ask whether you will accept a treatment by discussing the risks and benefits and working with you to decide. But what if you can no longer make your own decisions? Anyone can wind up hurt or sick and unable to make decisions about medical treatments. An advance directive speaks for you if you are unable to speak for yourself and helps make sure your religious and personal beliefs will be respected. It is a useful legal document for an adult of any age to plan for future health care needs. While no one is required to have an advance directive, it is smart to think ahead and make a plan now. If you don't have an advance directive and later you can't speak for yourself, then usually your next of kin will make health care decisions for you. But even if you want your next of kin to make decisions for you, an advance directive can make things easier for your loved ones by helping to prevent misunderstandings or arguments about your care.

What Can You Do in an Advance Directive?

An advance directive allows you to decide who you want to make health care decisions for you if you are unable to do so yourself. You can also use it to say what kinds of treatments you do or do not want, especially the treatments often used in a medical emergency or near the end of a person's life.

Health Care Agent. Someone you name to make decisions about your health care is called a *health care agent* (sometimes also called a *durable power of attorney for health care*, but, unlike other powers of attorney, this is not about money). You can name a family member or someone else. This person has the authority to see that doctors and other health care providers give you the type of care you want and that they do not give you treatment against your wishes. Pick someone you trust to make these kinds of serious decisions and talk to this person to make sure he or she understands and is willing to accept this responsibility.

Health Care Instructions. You can let providers know what treatments you want to have or not to have. (Sometimes this is called a "living will," but it has nothing to do with an ordinary will about property.) Examples of the types of treatment you might decide about are:

> Life support–such as breathing with a ventilator
> Efforts to revive a stopped heart or breathing (CPR)
> Feeding through tubes inserted into the body
> Medicine for pain relief

Ask your doctor for more information about these treatments. Think about how, if you become badly injured or seriously ill, treatments like these fit in with your goals, beliefs, and values.

How Do You Prepare an Advance Directive?

Begin by talking things over, if you want, with family members, close friends, your doctor, or a religious advisor. Many people go to a lawyer to have an advance directive prepared. You can also get sample forms yourself from many places. There is no one form that must be used. You can even make up your own advance directive document.

To make your advance directive valid, it must be signed by you in the presence of two witnesses, who will also sign. If you name a health care agent, make sure that person is not a witness.

Maryland law does not require the document to be notarized. You should give a copy of your advance directive to your doctor, who will keep it in your medical file, and to others you trust to have it available when needed. Copies are just as valid as the originals.

You can also make a valid advance directive by talking to your doctor in front of a witness.

Can You Change Your Advance Directive?

Yes, you can change or take back your advance directive at any time. The most recent one will count.

Where Can You Get Forms and More Information About Advance Directives?

There are many places to get forms, including medical, religious, aging assistance, and legal organizations. Your advance directive does not have to be on any particular form.

Adapted from Advance Directives Information Sheet. Maryland Department of Health and Mental Hygiene. Baltimore, Maryland.

vivors of these cancers is likely to increase. It is estimated that by the year 2030, the number of persons older than 65 years will have doubled and the number of persons older than 85 years will have quadrupled. Given this expanding and aging population, projections suggest that the number of colorectal cancer patients may increase by as much as 30%. With these significant demographic changes, it is imperative to comprehend more fully the late effects and health care needs of long-term colorectal cancer survivors.[7]

With advances in treatment, colorectal cancer is being transformed from a deadly disease into an illness that is increasingly curable.[11] With this transformation has come increased interest in the unique problems, risks, needs, and concerns of survivors who have completed treatment and are cancer-free. Research has shown that physical and mental qualities of life for colorectal cancer survivors are inferior compared with those of age-matched persons without cancer.[11] Although issues and symptoms are most prominent during the first 3 years after cancer treatment, long-term effects—including fatigue, sleep difficulty, fear of recurrence, anxiety, depression, negative body image, sensory neuropathy, gastrointestinal problems, urinary incontinence, and sexual dysfunction—can persist.[11] The unique challenges and issues of colorectal cancer survivors can and should be addressed by health care providers and the research community to ensure effective interventions and models of care to manage these problems.[11] Furthermore, it is vitally important to discuss a survivorship care plan with your patient, which includes a summary of treatment and a plan for follow-up/surveillance.

Coping with life after treatment for cancer can be a real challenge. Many cancer survivors feel that they have an abundance of support and information during their treatment. However, once treatment has stopped, they have entered a new world filled with new questions. Once again, it is important for the health care provider to discuss a survivorship care plan with the patient and to determine who is going to manage and coordinate follow-up care. Finally, it is important to provide patients with resources to use when these new questions arise.

The Caregiver's Perspective

When the health care professional/clinician is fortunate enough to meet the caregivers who take care of patients on a day-to-day basis, it is important to understand the role of those caregivers in the fight against cancer. Caregivers play an important role in ensuring that colon cancer patients receive the best possible care. When a person has cancer, the disease spreads throughout the lives of everyone who loves that person. It is important that the caregiver take care of him- or herself while also taking care of the person with cancer. One of the many important roles that a caregiver plays in treatment is facilitating communication with doctors and making sure the right questions are asked.

Tips for Family and Friends of Cancer Patients

Family members and friends of the person with cancer are also influenced by changes in a loved one's health. Following are some tips to help family and friends cope with a loved one's diagnosis:

- Feel free to ask the doctor questions when you accompany your loved one to appointments. Write down questions beforehand so you don't forget them.
- Be prepared for changes in your loved one's behavior and mood. Medications, discomforts, and stress can cause a person with cancer to become depressed or angry.
- Encourage your loved one to be active and independent as much as possible, to help him or her regain a sense of self-reliance and confidence.
- Be realistic about your own needs. Be sure you are sleeping enough, eating properly, and taking some time off for yourself. It is hard to offer much help when you are exhausted.
- Don't hesitate to ask other family members and friends for help. They will appreciate the opportunity.

Family members and friends of a person coping with cancer may also find themselves under a great deal of stress. To reduce their stress, they should:

- Keep a positive attitude.
- Accept that there are events they cannot control.
- Be assertive rather than aggressive. "Assert" their feelings, opinions, or beliefs rather than becoming angry, combative, or passive.
- Learn to relax.
- Exercise regularly. The body can fight stress better when physically fit.
- Eat well-balanced meals.
- Rest and sleep. The body needs time to recover from stressful events.
- Don't rely on alcohol or drugs to reduce stress.
- Consider joining a support group to share experiences and to learn from others. It may help to feel that they are not alone.

Conclusion

Despite advances in the treatment of colorectal cancer and improvements in the number of patients surviving this disease, a diagnosis of colorectal cancer can be devastating. Most patients and families experience significant stress and anxiety before, during, and after treatment. Ways to help patients and their families cope with this stress do exist, and health care professionals should reach out to patients and their families to offer help. It is especially important for providers to reach out to patients *after* treatment, when patients are less likely to seek help on their own. Survivors of colorectal cancer may have recurring fears of the return or later spread of the cancer and need help in coping with these fears just as they did when first diagnosed.

References

1. There Is No Place Like Hope: Chronicles of Colon Cancer Survivors. Spotlight on Symposia from the ONS 31st Annual Congress, Boston, Massachusetts, 2006.
2. Dunn J, Lynch B, Rinaldis M, et al: Dimensions of quality of life and psychosocial variables most salient to colorectal cancer patients. Psycho-Oncology 15:20–30, 2006.
3. Macvean ML, White VM, Pratt S, et al: Reducing the unmet needs of patients with colorectal cancer: a feasibility study of The Pathfinder Volunteer Program. Support Care Cancer 15:293–299, 2007.
4. Johnston L: Fact sheet about ostomy adapted from Colon and Rectal Cancer: A Comprehensive Guide for Patients and Families. Onconurse.com, retrieved November 22, 2009, Copyright 2000 by Patient-Centered Guides.
5. Karagiannis S, Heras P, Hatzopoulos A, et al: Colorectal cancer patients' informational needs about sexuality related issues. ASCO Annual Meeting Proceedings (Post-Meeting Edition) J Clin Oncol 24(18 Suppl):18569, 2006.
6. Nishigaki M, Kazuma K, Oya M, et al: The influence of life stage on psychosocial adjustment in colorectal cancer patients. J Psychosoc Oncol 25(4):71–87, 2007.
7. Goldzweig G, Hubert A, Walach N, et al: Gender and psychological distress among middle- and older-aged colorectal cancer patients and their spouses: an unexpected outcome. Crit Rev Oncol/Hematol 70:71–82, 2009.
8. Simard S, Savard J: Fear of cancer recurrence inventory: development and initial validation of a multidimensional measure of fear of cancer recurrence. Support Care Cancer 17:241–251, 2009.
9. Myers JS: Chemotherapy-related cognitive impairment: neuroimaging, neuropsychological testing, and the neuropsychologist. J Oncol Nurs 13(4):413–421, 2009.
10. Armes J, Crowe M, Colbourne L, et al: Patients' supportive care needs beyond the end of cancer treatment: a prospective, longitudinal survey. J Clin Oncol 27(36):6172–6179, 2009. Epub 2009 Nov. 2.
11. Denlinger CS, Barsevick AM: The challenges of colorectal cancer survivorship. J Natl Compr Cane Netw 7(8):889–893, 2009.

Websites

www.cancer.gov
www.cancer.org
www.ccalliance.org
www.fightcolorectalcancer.org
www.getyourrearingear.com
www.nccn.org
www.nccrt.org
www.preventcancer.org
www.preventingcolorectalcancer.org

Conclusion

22   *Susan L. Gearhart and Nita Ahuja*

Since 1984, death rates from colorectal cancer have decreased in both men and women, with an accelerated rate of decline after 1998. This reduction is attributed not only to the introduction of screening but also to newer systemic therapies and improvement in surgical techniques, such as the ones described in this volume.[1,2]

Over the past decade, considerable investigational work has resulted in the addition of new chemotherapeutic agents and more innovative combination strategies for the treatment of colorectal cancer. Furthermore, the ability to sequence the entire genome of individual patients allows for the translation of genomic knowledge into the clinical arena. For the first time, limited clinical data are being replaced by "personalized" target therapies. This information, coupled with newer surgical techniques such as total mesorectal excision (TME), transanal excision, sphincter-sparing surgery, and laparoscopic and robotic surgery, has resulted in significantly better quality of life for patients with colorectal cancer.

Although much has been accomplished in the prevention and treatment of colorectal cancer, the job is by no means complete. In the United States, despite the efforts of several organizations including the American Cancer Society, only about 50% of individuals 50 years or older have been screened for colorectal cancers. Identification of new hereditary forms of colorectal cancer and of better screening methods for hereditary colorectal cancer has been slow. Little improvement has been made in risk reduction for the general U.S. population. Medications to prevent polyp formation have shown minimal benefit. Finally, despite the advances detailed in this volume, the incidence of colorectal cancer is increasing worldwide.

Further improvements in outcomes from colorectal cancer will depend on increasing colorectal cancer screening, on the use of minimally invasive surgical techniques, and on translating the vast knowledge from the genomic revolution into the clinical arena. The emerging modalities described in this volume, such as expression profiling, vaccine therapies, and the use of DNA-based markers for early detection, will become increasingly important. Clearly, effective management of colorectal cancer requires a multidisciplinary approach.

We hope this volume will inspire health care practitioners to follow research advances closely and to adopt the most current practices for early diagnosis and multimodal treatment. With the techniques now at our disposal, we can aim not merely to raise survival rates but also to improve each patient's overall quality of life.

References

1. Jemal A, Siegel R, Ward E, et al: Cancer statistics, 2009. CA Cancer J Clin 59:225–249, 2009.
2. Edwards BK, Ward E, Kohler BA, et al: Annual report to the nation on the status of cancer, 1975–2006, featuring colorectal cancer trends and impact of interventions (risk factors, screening, and treatment) to reduce future rates. Cancer 116:544–573, 2010.

Index

Note: Page numbers followed by f indicate figures; those followed by t indicate tables; and those followed by b indicate boxed material.

Diabetes
  preoperative testing with, 119t
  as risk factor, 8, 52
Diagnostic trials, 219–220
Dialysis patient, preoperative testing of, 119t
Dietary modification, 7, 48–55, 56b, 71–72, 71f
  macronutrient(s) in, 48–53
    coffee and tea as, 52
    dairy food and probiotics as, 52–53
    fat as, 7, 49–50
    fiber as, 50–51, 50b, 71–72
    insulin and glycemic load as, 52
    red meat as, 48–49, 71
    USDA MyPyramid and, 58f
    vegetables and fruit as, 51–52, 71, 71f
  vitamin(s) and micronutrient(s) in, 53–55, 70–71
    antioxidants as, 55, 71, 71f
    calcium as, 53–54, 70
    folate as, 54–55, 70
    selenium as, 55, 70–71
    vitamin D as, 54
Distal margins, in rectal cancer, 155
Diuretics, on day of surgery, 120t
Diverting loop ileostomy, 161
DNA integrity assay (DIA), 101, 101f
DNA testing, for screening, 93–102
  advantages and disadvantages of, 97, 97b
  blood, 97–98
  rationale for, 94–97, 95t–96t
  stool, 98–102
    detection of methylation in, 98t, 99t, 100–101, 101f
    epigenetic inactivation of SFRP genes in, 100
    vs. fecal occult blood testing, 99–100
    multicolor digital protein truncation test in, 100, 100f
    rationale for, 98, 98t
    recommendations on, 93–94, 94b
    sensitivity and specificity of, 98–102, 99t
Double-contrast barium enema, for screening, 94b
DPC4 gene, in familial/juvenile polyposis coli, 26
Durable power of attorney for health care, 256, 257b
DVT (deep venous thrombosis), preoperative evaluation of risk of, 121–122, 121b, 122t

E

Eastern Cooperative Oncology Group (ECOG) E5202 trial, 179, 179t
EBRT. See External beam radiation therapy (EBRT).
E-cadherin gene, in classical molecular analysis, 242f
Economic burden, of colorectal cancer, 9, 10f
Edrecolomab, in immunotherapy, 227–228
EGF (epidermal growth factor), signaling pathway of, 171–172, 172f
EGFR (epidermal growth factor receptor) antibodies, for metastatic colorectal cancer, 167, 171–174, 174t
Electrocardiogram, in preoperative evaluation, 119b
EMLA (eutectic mixture of local anesthetic) cream, and methemoglobinemia, 124
EMR (endoscopic mucosal resection), 136–137, 137f, 138f
En bloc resection, of locally advanced, adherent colorectal tumors, 154
Endoluminal fly-through views, in virtual colonoscopy, 111, 113f
Endorectal ultrasound (ERUS), for local excision
  follow-up, 131
  preoperative, 129
Endoscopic mucosal resection (EMR), 136–137, 137f, 138f

Endoscopic resection, 135–139
  indications for, 136
  mucosal, 136–137, 137f, 138f
  outcomes of, 138–139
  technique(s) for, 136–138
    endoscopic mucosal resection as, 136–137, 137f, 138f
    endoscopic submucosal dissection as, 137–138
    polypectomy as, 136
Endoscopic submucosal dissection (ESD), 137–138
Endoscopic surveillance, 203t, 204t, 213–215
Endoscopic tattooing, 148
Endoscopy. See Colonoscopy; Flexible sigmoidoscopy.
End-stage renal disease, preoperative testing with, 119t
End-to-end anastomosis, 161–162, 161f
Enteral Wallflex Colonic Stent, 141t
Enteral Wallstent, 141t
Environmental risk factor(s), 7–8, 47–59
  alcohol as, 7–8, 56
  diet as, 7, 48–55, 56b, 71–72, 71f
    antioxidants in, 55, 71, 71f
    calcium in, 53–54
    coffee and tea in, 52
    dairy foods and probiotics in, 52–53
    fat in, 7, 49–50
    fiber in, 50–51, 50b, 71–72
    folate in, 54–55, 70
    glycemic index of, 52
    red meat in, 48–49, 71
    selenium in, 55, 70–71
    USDA MyPyramid and, 58fr
    vegetables and fruit in, 51–52, 71, 71f
    vitamin D in, 54
  immigration and, 47, 57–59, 57f
  insulin resistance and diabetes as, 7–8, 52
  obesity, 7–8, 57, 72
  physical activity as, 7, 56–57, 56b, 57f, 72
  smoking as, 7–8, 55–56
Ep-CAM, in immunotherapy, 227–228, 233
Epidemiology, of colorectal cancer, 1–5, 47, 48f, 93
  incidence in, 1, 2f–4f, 93
  lifetime risk in, 93
  location of primary tumor in, 4–5, 5f
  recurrent, 201–202
  stage at time of diagnosis in, 3–4, 4b, 4t
  types in, 1, 2f
  worldwide distribution in, 47, 47f
Epidermal growth factor (EGF), signaling pathway of, 171–172, 172f
Epidermal growth factor receptor (EGFR) antibodies, for metastatic colorectal cancer, 167, 171–174, 174t
Epidural anesthesia, for perioperative pain management, 123–124
Epigallocatechin gallate, in green tea, 52
Epigenetic alterations, stool screening for, 100–101, 101f
ER gene
  in colorectal cancer, 95t
  CpG island methylation of, 101
ERUS (endorectal ultrasound), for local excision
  follow-up, 131
  preoperative, 129
ESD (endoscopic submucosal dissection), 137–138
Esr1 gene, in colorectal cancer, 95t
Estrogen, for chemoprevention, 69–70, 69f
Eutectic mixture of local anesthetic (EMLA) cream, and methemoglobinemia, 124
EVEREST trial, 174
Exercise, in prevention, 7, 56–57, 56b, 57f, 72
Exercise tolerance, poor, preoperative testing with, 119t
EXO1 gene, in Lynch syndrome, 37
EXPLORE trial, 173